METALLIC BIOMATERIALS
Metals for Medical Devices

Takao Hanawa
Council Member, Science Council of Japan
Honorary Professor, Tokyo Medical and Dental University
Specially Appointed Professor, Osaka University
Visiting Professor, Kobe University
Japan

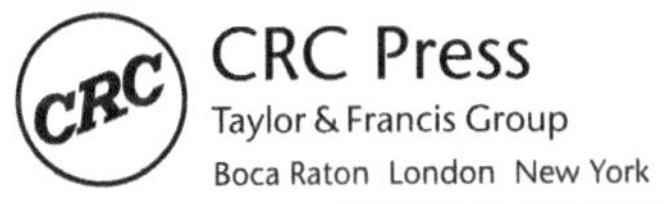
CRC Press
Taylor & Francis Group
Boca Raton London New York

CRC Press is an imprint of the
Taylor & Francis Group, an **informa** business
A SCIENCE PUBLISHERS BOOK

Cover credit: Images provided by:
Teijin Nakashima Medical Co., Ltd
LivaNova Japan K.K. with Courtesy of CORCYM Srl.
Striker Japan Co. Ltd.
Straumann Co., Ltd.

First edition published 2025
by CRC Press
2385 NW Executive Center Drive, Suite 320, Boca Raton FL 33431

and by CRC Press
4 Park Square, Milton Park, Abingdon, Oxon, OX14 4RN

CRC Press is an imprint of Taylor & Francis Group, LLC

Library of Congress Cataloging-in-Publication Data (applied for)

ISBN: 978-1-032-41377-8 (hbk)
ISBN: 978-1-032-41378-5 (pbk)
ISBN: 978-1-003-35782-7 (ebk)

DOI: 10.1201/9781003357827

Typeset in Times New Roman
by Prime Publishing Services

Preface

This book was written with the goal of helping students learn the essentials regarding metallic biomaterials and acquire knowledge that can be applied in a progressive manner. The target readers are students specializing in materials engineering who have learned the basics of metallurgical engineering, graduate students, engineers, and others who need knowledge about metallic biomaterials even without prior knowledge of medicine and dentistry. The book was also written for people who have not studied metallic materials in engineering or other fields of medicine and dentistry, with the goal of making it readable even without prior knowledge of metallic materials. Because I tried to fit the entire picture of metallic biomaterials into a limited amount of space and I tried not to obstruct the overall flow of understanding, some of the descriptions are vague from a materials engineering perspective. I recognize that there are many points in which medical explanations are insufficient. Furthermore, because the contents of each chapter are closely related to each other, terms may be explained in later chapters rather than the first time they appear. In order to understand the full picture of metallic biomaterials, a lot of knowledge about metallurgical engineering and materials science, life science, and clinical medicine is required, but it is difficult to explain these in the limited space available with my limited knowledge. If you would like to learn more about the contents of this book, please refer to the respective specialized books.

The overall writing policy for this book is as follows.

I. Make it clear who first invented or proposed materials, systems, methods, theories, etc., and how they have developed over time and how they are currently being used. We have made it clear what is expected of us going forward. Therefore, some of the cited documents are quite old. I believe that knowing the historical development of a field is essential for conducting research and development in that field. In recent years, an increasing number of papers ignore past research, do not properly cite it, and propagandize as if they were the first to do so, even though many similar studies have been conducted in the past. We cannot afford to ignore past epoch-making research, even if it was conducted decades ago.

II. I tried to focus on explaining the properties of metallic materials in an *in vitro* biological simulated environment and an *in vivo* human body environment. The explanation of mechanical properties and surface properties is not limited to general explanations, but instead tried to use examples of phenomena in the biological environment to clarify issues specific to metallic biomaterials.

III. In each chapter, I have tried to list textbooks and reviews that complement the content and help deepen understanding.

IV. To help you get an overall picture of metallic materials, I have shown the standards for materials that are standardized by ASTM or ISO whenever possible.

V. Biological evaluation methods depend on developments in life sciences, not just metallic biomaterials. In addition, skill in cell culture and animal experiments is essential for its implementation, and knowledge of cell biology, molecular biology, histology, etc. is required for interpretation of the results. These are outside the scope of this book, and we have only given an overview of them here.

VI. Weaknesses of metallic biomaterials and possible clinical problems were explained in detail using examples. Many explanations and textbooks on biomaterials only emphasize the advantages and expandability of the materials without clearly indicating their weaknesses and limitations. These explanations are what characterize this book.

Many materials are used to regenerate and reconstruct human body functions lost due to aging, disease, and accidents, and these materials have supported medical progress and contributed to lifesaving, treatment, and improved quality of life. The importance of materials in medical care is increasing, and the existence of materials is essential for implementing cutting-edge medical care. The performance required for medical purposes differs depending on the purpose of use, while the basics are replacements for human body functions, and it is necessary to create materials with diverse biological functions. To satisfy this demand, it is necessary to make materials biofunctional; however, dentists, and medical device development engineers in clinical settings do not necessarily pay attention to the importance of materials. This situation is common not only in medicine but also in engineering in general. Furthermore, attention is being turned to regenerative medicine as a means of rebuilding human body functions, and attention is being focused on gene therapy and drug delivery systems (DDS) as treatment technologies, which is also contributing to the neglect of materials. In particular, metals are typically artificial materials and are recognized to have no biological functions, and are often considered unattractive as medical materials. Nevertheless, metallic materials are still used in many medical devices due to their high mechanical reliability due to their excellent strength and toughness, and they account for more than 70% of internally implantable devices (implants). This discrepancy between the attention paid to research and its practical importance is particularly large in the field of biomaterials. I hope that this book will help you understand the necessity and problems of metallic materials used in medical applications.

Metals as materials have a long history, and the foundations of today's materials science and engineering were formed through research into metallic materials. It goes without saying that metallic materials are important among the materials used in our society, and it is a well-known fact that modern society cannot exist without them. However, when it comes to materials used in medical devices and biomaterials, there are people who think that metals are toxic and are "undesirable materials" as biomaterials because of the environmental destruction and damage caused to the human body by heavy metals. Furthermore, metals are typically artificial materials and are recognized to have no biofunction; they are often considered unattractive as biomaterials. This phenomenon is based on the idea that materials with excellent biocompatibility and biofunctionality are superior as biomaterials. However, this argument does not take into account the durability required over the period of use while implanted in the body. The most important property required of a material is that it continues to exhibit the required performance in the environment in which it is used for a long period of time. Rapid technological innovations in ceramics and polymers over the past 30 years have enabled a wide range of applications for these medical devices. In particular, the excellent tissue compatibility and biofunctionality of polymers and ceramics hold great promise as biomaterials, and in fact many metal medical devices have been replaced with ceramics and polymers. Nevertheless, metallic materials are still used in many medical devices due to their superior strength and toughness. At one time, it was thought that all devices would be made of ceramics or polymers, but the need for metallic materials for their mechanical reliability has not diminished at all. In addition, although it was thought that artificial materials would be eliminated due to advances in regenerative medicine, it has become clear that it will take a considerable amount of time to achieve this goal, especially for artificial joints, bone fixation, spinal fixation, etc. It is difficult for current treatments with metallic materials, such as artificial joints, bone fixators, spinal fixators, stents, and dental implants, to be replaced by treat with regenerative medicine in the future. Therefore, the importance of metallic materials is being recognized as a practical issue. Attempts to replace metallic devices with ceramics and polymers continue, but in recent years most of these efforts have ended in failure. Considering that the advantages and disadvantages of each material depend on the differences in the chemical bonds that constitute them, it is easy to understand that it is difficult to replace it with another type of material. It is necessary to motivate development based on an understanding of the properties of metals and the reasons why they are used.

Many metallic biomaterials are used for diagnosis and treatment in medicine, and it is no exaggeration to say that advances in materials have led to advances in treatment technology, especially in dentistry and orthopedics. Recently, its uses have been expanding, including as stents in cardiovascular medicine and cerebral artery clips in neurosurgery.

The contents of each chapter in this book are as follows, and each chapter is closely related. However, each chapter can be read and understood independently. Please start by reading the chapter you need.

Chapter 1 Current Status of Metallic Biomaterials includes an overview of biomaterials, the positioning of metallic materials as biomaterials, mechanical and chemical properties of materials, the difference between hard biomaterials and soft biomaterials, history of metallic biomaterials, biomaterials and regenerative medicine, demand and market of medical devices. It consists of metallic biomaterials, predominant property as metallic biomaterials, research and development of metallic biomaterial, and utilization of metals as medical devices, and the positioning of metallic materials as biomaterials for medical devices and an overview of metallic biomaterials.

The purpose of this book is to help you understand the overall picture of this book, and you should be able to gain a considerable amount of knowledge about metallic biomaterials just by reading this chapter. People who have a wrong impression of metallic biomaterials should be able to correct that impression.

Chapter 2 General Property of Metals in Biological Environment covers band structure and metallic bond, structure of metals and alloys, phase transformation and structure, plastic deformation and dislocation, improvement of crystal structure by additive manufacturing, surface structure of metals, concept of corrosion, corrosion reaction, potential-pH diagram, localized corrosion, biological factors affecting corrosion behavior, safety, and biocompatibility. This chapter provides the minimum knowledge of materials engineering and metallic biomaterials necessary to understand the contents of this book. This chapter describes the crystal structure, mechanical properties, surface structure, and chemical properties of metals, as well as the behavior of metals in contact with living tissue or in the human body.

Chapter 3 Evaluation Methods of Metallic Biomaterials includes evaluation of mechanical property, strength and toughness test, fatigue and fretting fatigue test, wear test, joint simulators, test solution of corrosion resistance, polarization test, electrochemical impedance method, dissolution test, tarnish test, corrosion potential measurement, points to note in corrosion tests, characterization of passive film, adsorption of proteins, evaluation of bone formation ability by simulated body fluids, outline of biological evaluation, toxicity evaluation, cell compatibility/functionality evaluation, antithrombotic evaluation, and bacterial adhesion. It consists of biofilm formation evaluation and animal experiments, and explains how to evaluate metallic materials in biological simulated environments and in-body environments. This chapter also provides the minimum necessary content to understand the contents of the subsequent chapters of this book. Proficient techniques are required when conducting evaluations in actual research and development, but in this chapter you can easily learn what methods are available.

Chapter 4 Medical Use of Metals consists of use of metals for medical devices, orthopedics, cardiology, dentistry, endoscopes, surgical robots, and imaging equipment, and describes what metallic materials are used in clinical settings and how they are used. This book focuses on orthopedics, cardiology, and dentistry, where metallic materials are widely used, but many other metallic materials are used in therapeutic instruments, surgical instruments, medical equipment, etc. Readers can learn about the current status of the use of metallic materials.

Chapter 5 Degradation and Current Problem of Metallic Biomaterials consists of biological environment, degradation of materials in the human body, infectious disease, MRI artifact, corrosion, metal allergy, friction wear, fracture, and stress shielding. This chapter details the problems it causes and measures to avoid them. Textbooks on other biomaterials do not have chapters that give such a negative impression. However, the basis of material development is to know the weaknesses and limitations of the target material and to overcome these. This chapter is a unique and characteristic chapter of this book.

Chapter 6 Titanium and Titanium Alloys includes history of application to medicine, mechanical property of commercially pure titanium (cp Ti), crystal structure of titanium alloys, mechanical property of titanium alloys, titanium-zirconium alloys, and corrosion resistance of titanium and titanium alloys. It consists of passive film on titanium, response to the host body, principles of biocompatibility of titanium, tasks of titanium for medical application, and application of titanium to regenerative medicine. Ti material is used as a metallic biomaterial due to its light weight, good corrosion resistance and biocompatibility. With regard to CP Ti and Ti alloys, which are expected to expand in use in the future, the course focuses on materials used for medical purposes, allowing students to systematically learn about the composition and properties of Ti materials. In particular, he discusses why CP Ti and Ti alloys exhibit excellent biocompatibility among metallic materials.

Chapter 7 Cobalt-Based Alloys contains history of cobalt-based alloys, cobalt-based alloys for medical devices, mechanical property of cobalt-based alloys, corrosion resistance of cobalt-based alloys, passive film on cobalt-based alloys, metallosis by cobalt-chromium alloy, low-nickel containing cobalt-chromium alloy, and future prospect. The use of Co-based alloys is expanding for medical purposes. I focused on materials used for medical purposes and systematically explained Co-based alloys. The readers can learn about the composition and properties of Co-based alloys.

Chapter 8 Stainless Steels contains stainless steels for medical devices, history of stainless steels for medical devices, mechanical property of stainless steels for medical devices, magnetism, corrosion resistance, improvement of corrosion resistance by additive manufacturing, reaction with the host body, and development of nickel-free high nitrogen stainless steels. This chapter focuses on stainless steels used in medical applications, and allows students to systematically learn about the composition and properties of stainless steels used in medical applications. You can learn about stainless steel, which is used as a precursor to many medical devices and treatment instruments.

Chapter 9 Other Metals and Functional Alloys explains medical metallic materials other than those mentioned above, especially functional materials. Noble metals and alloys, shape memory and superelastic alloys, bioabsorbable metals, magnet alloys, tantalum and niobium, zirconium alloys, and high entropy alloys are explained. These materials are already used in medical devices but are used in small amounts, or materials that are expected to develop in the future based on their functions. High entropy alloys are materials that are expected to be further developed through future research and development.

Chapter 10 Surface Treatment and Surface Morphology consists of dry process, wet process, surface morphology control, biofunctional surface morphology, cleaning and hydrophilic treatment, time transient of surface treatment, and optimal surface treatment. Surface treatment methods and surface morphogenetic methods for imparting bio-tissue compatibility and bio-functionality to metallic materials are explained by technology and purpose, and are considered research trends and ideal surface treatment methods. This is a field where many research papers are being published one after another, and you can learn how a certain surface treatment method is positioned.

Additive manufacturing is attracting attention as a method of forming metallic materials, and its future development is expected. Many detailed textbooks, handbooks, and reviews have been published, so please refer to them for more information on additive manufacturing. On the other hand, this book describes examples of the use of additive manufacturing to improve the performance of each metallic biomaterial and its results for each material.

In this way, the structure of this book is unique and unparalleled, and I wrote it with the belief that this is the best path to understanding metallic biomaterials. It would be my great pleasure if this book could help you understand metallic biomaterials.

This book is a compilation of the knowledge that the author gained on the job while engaged in educational and research activities, and during this process many people provided advice over the years. I would like to take this opportunity to thank you. I would also like to thank the many researchers and companies listed below for providing diagrams and photographs, and for providing valuable and useful advice regarding the content of this book. I would like to express my gratitude to you.

Peng Chen, Ph.D., Tohoku University

Akihiko Chiba, Ph.D., Tohoku University

Sachiko Hiromoto, Ph.D., National Institute for Materials Science

Hideki Hosoda, Ph.D., Tokyo Institute of Technology

Manabu Ito, Ph.D., M.D., National Hospital Organization

Akio Kishida, Ph.D., Tokyo Medical and Dental University

Takuya Konno, Ph.D., M.D., National Hospital Organization

Norio Maruyama, Ph.D., National Institute for Materials Science

Keiji Moriyama, Ph.D., D.D.S., Tokyo Medical and Dental University

Akiko Nagai, Ph.D., M.D., Aichi Gakuin University

Takayoshi Nakano, Ph.D., Osaka University

Takayuki Narushima, Ph.D., Tohoku University

Mitsuo Niinomi, Ph.D., Tohoku University

Naoyuki Nomura, Ph.D., Tohoku University

Kei Oya, Ph.D., Pharmaceutical and Medical Devices Agency

Yukyo Takada, Ph.D., Tohoku University

Yusuke Tsutsumi, Ph.D., National Institute for Materials Science

Akiko Yamamoto, Ph.D., National Institute for Materials Science

Toru Yamamoto, Ph.D., Hokkaido University

Takayuki Yoneyama, Ph.D., D.D.S., Nihon University

AMTI Force & Motion, Advanced Mechanical Technology, Inc.
Asahi Intec Co. Ltd.
Cordis Japan G.K.
GC Co.
LivaNova Japan K.K.
MANI Inc.
Medtronic Co. Ltd.
Striker Japan Co. Ltd.
Teijin Nakashima Medical, Co. Ltd.

Finally, I would like to dedicate this book to my wife Eiko, who has been my partner for many years.

March 2024

Takao Hanawa, Ph.D.

Contents

Preface iii

Notes on Using This Book xix

1. Current Status of Metallic Biomaterials **1**
- 1.1 Introduction 1
- 1.2 Biomaterials 2
- 1.3 Metals among Biomaterials 4
- 1.4 Mechanical and Chemical Properties of Materials 6
- 1.5 Hard Biomaterials and Soft Biomaterials 8
- 1.6 History of Metallic Biomaterials 9
- 1.7 Biomaterials and Regenerative Medicine 10
- 1.8 Demand and Market of Metallic Biomaterials 13
- 1.9 Predominant Properties for Metallic Biomaterials 14
- 1.10 Research and Development of Metallic Biomaterials 16
- 1.11 Utilization of Metals as Medical Devices 19

References 20

2. General Property of Metals in Biological Environment **22**
- 2.1 Introduction 22
- 2.2 Band Structure and Metallic Bond 23
- 2.3 Structure of Metals and Alloys 25
- 2.4 Phase Transformation and Structure 28
- 2.5 Plastic Deformation and Dislocation 31
  - 2.5.1 Slip Deformation and Dislocation 31
  - 2.5.2 Strengthening 32
    - Solid Solution Strengthening 33
    - Precipitation Strengthening 34
    - Work Strengthening (Work Hardening) 34
    - Boundary Strengthening 35
  - 2.5.3 Twin Deformation 35
- 2.6 Improvement of Crystal Structure by Additive Manufacturing 35
- 2.7 Surface Structure of Metals 36
- 2.8 Concept of Corrosion 37
- 2.9 Corrosion Reaction 38
- 2.10 Potential-pH Diagram 40

2.11 Localized Corrosion 42
2.11.1 Outline 42
2.11.2 Pitting Corrosion 43
2.11.3 Crevice Corrosion 44
2.11.4 Galvanic Corrosion 44
2.11.5 Intergranular Corrosion 45
2.11.6 Stress Corrosion Cracking 45
2.11.7 Progress of Localized Corrosion 45
2.12 Biological Factors Affecting Corrosion Behavior 46
2.12.1 Outline 46
2.12.2 Temperature and pH 46
2.12.3 Calcium Phosphate Precipitation 46
2.12.4 Dissolved Oxygen Concentration 47
2.12.5 Proteins and Amino Acids 47
2.12.6 Cells and Extracellular Matrix 48
2.12.7 Body Fluid Circulation 49
2.12.8 Geometric Structure of Material 50
2.13 Safety 50
2.13.1 Concept of Toxicity 50
2.13.2 Toxicity of Metal Elements 52
2.14 Biocompatibility 54
2.14.1 Definition 54
2.14.2 Bone Formation and Bone Bonding 54
2.14.3 Soft Tissue Adhesion 54
2.14.4 Blood Compatibility 55
References 57

3. Evaluation Methods of Metallic Biomaterials 59
3.1 Introduction 59
3.2 Evaluation of Mechanical Property 59
In Vitro Material Test 60
In Vitro Product Test 60
In Vivo Implantation Test 60
3.3 Strength and Toughness Test 60
3.4 Fatigue and Fretting Fatigue Test 62
3.5 Wear Test 64
3.6 Joint Simulators 65
3.7 Test Solution of Corrosion Resistance 67
3.8 Polarization Test 67
3.8.1 Anodic Polarization Test 67
3.8.2 Tafel Extrapolation Method and Polarization Resistance Method 70
3.9 Electrochemical Impedance Method 71
3.10 Dissolution Test 72
3.11 Tarnish Test 73
3.12 Corrosion Potential Measurement 73
3.13 Tribocorrosion Tests 74

3.14 Points to Note in Corrosion Tests 75
3.15 Characterization of Passive Film 75
3.16 Adsorption of Proteins 77
3.17 Evaluation of Bone Formation Ability by Simulated Body Fluids 78
3.18 Outline of Biological Evaluation 79
3.19 Toxicity Evaluation 80
3.20 Cell Compatibility/Functionality Evaluation 82
3.20.1 Selection of Cell Types 82
3.20.2 Outline of Cell Culture Evaluation 83
Cell Fixation 84
Observation of Cells Using Scanning Electron Microscopy (SEM) 84
Observation of Cells by Staining 84
Fluorescence Observation of Cells 85
Cell Migration 86
Cell Count 86
3.20.3 Hard Tissue Compatibility Evaluation 87
Measurement of Calcification Amount 87
Protein Measurement 88
Gene Expression Analysis 88
3.21 Antithrombotic Evaluation 89
3.22 Bacterial Adhesion/Biofilm Formation Evaluation 90
3.23 Animal Experiment 91
References 92

4. Medical Use of Metals **95**
4.1 Introduction 95
4.2 Use of Metals for Medical Devices 95
4.3 Orthopedics 97
4.3.1 Metals in Orthopedics 97
4.3.2 Artificial Joints 98
4.3.3 Bone Fixators 101
4.3.4 Spinal Fixators and Spacers 102
4.4 Cardiology 105
4.4.1 Catheter and Guidewire 105
4.4.2 Stent and Stent Graft 107
Stent 107
Stent Graft 109
Drug Eluting Stent 110
4.4.3 Cerebral Aneurysm Clip and Embolization Coil 110
Cerebral Aneurysm Clip 111
Embolization Coil 111
4.4.4 Artificial Heart, Pacemaker, and Artificial Valve 112
Pace Maker 112
Implantable Cardioverter Defibrillator 113
Artificial Valve 113

4.5 Dentistry 114
4.5.1 Outline 114
4.5.2 Restorations 114
4.5.3 Prosthodontics 116
4.5.4 Dental Casting Alloys 117
4.5.5 Dental Implant 119
4.5.6 Orthodontics 119
4.5.7 Endodontics and Dental Surgery 120
4.5.8 Adhesion of Polymers to Metals in Dentistry 121
4.6 Endoscope, Surgical Robot, and Imaging Equipment 123
References 123

5. Degradation and Current Problem of Metallic Biomaterials 126
5.1 Introduction 126
5.2 Biological Environment 127
5.3 Degradation of Materials in the Human Body 128
5.4 Infectious Disease 130
5.5 MRI Artifact 132
5.6 Corrosion 133
5.6.1 Corrosion of Medical Devices 133
5.6.2 Example of Corrosion in Dentistry 134
5.6.3 Example of Corrosion in Orthopedics and Cardiology 136
5.7 Metal Allergy 137
5.8 Friction Wear 139
5.8.1 Wear of Medical Devices 139
5.8.2 Wear Mechanism 139
5.8.3 Wear Property of Metals 140
5.9 Fracture 140
5.9.1 Outline 140
5.9.2 Fatigue Fracture 141
5.9.3 Fatigue Fracture in Living Tissue and Simulated Body Fluids 143
5.9.4 Fretting Fatigue 143
5.9.5 Fracture under Single Load 144
5.9.6 Fracture by Human Error 144
5.10 Stress Shielding 145
References 146

6. Titanium and Titanium Alloys 148
6.1 Introduction 148
6.2 History of Application to Medicine 148
6.3 Mechanical Property of Commercially Pure Titanium (CP Ti) 150
6.4 Crystal Structure of Titanium Alloys 152
6.5 Mechanical Property of Titanium Alloys 155
6.6 Titanium-Zirconium Alloys 159
6.7 Corrosion Resistance of CP Ti and Titanium Alloys 160
6.8 Passive Film on Titanium 162

6.9 Response to the Host Body 165
6.10 Principle of Excellent Biocompatibility of Titanium 167
6.10.1 Relationship between Corrosion Resistance and Biocompatibility 167
6.10.2 Property as *n*-type Semiconductor 167
6.10.3 Dissociation of Surface Hydroxyl Groups–Surface Electric Charge 168
6.10.4 Dielectric Constant–Electrostatic Force 168
6.10.5 Calcium Phosphate Formation 170
6.10.6 Band Gap Energy 171
6.11 Tasks of Titanium for Medical Application 173
References 174

7. Cobalt-Based Alloys **180**
7.1 Introduction 180
7.2 History of Cobalt-Based Alloy 180
7.3 Cobalt-Based Alloys for Medical Devices 182
7.4 Mechanical Property of Cobalt-Based Alloys 183
Large SFE 185
Medium SFE 185
Small SFE 186
7.5 Corrosion Resistance of Cobalt-Based Alloys 186
7.6 Passive Film on Cobalt-Based Alloys 188
7.7 Metallosis by Cobalt-Chromium Alloy 189
7.8 Low-Nickel-Containing Cobalt-Chromium Alloy 189
7.9 Future Prospect 190
References 190

8. Stainless Steels **193**
8.1 Introduction 193
8.2 Category 193
8.3 Stainless Steels for Medical Devices 194
8.4 History of Stainless Steels for Medical Devices 197
8.5 Mechanical Property of Stainless Steels for Medical Devices 197
8.6 Magnetism 200
8.7 Corrosion Resistance 201
8.8 Improvement of Corrosion Resistance by Additive Manufacturing 205
8.9 Reaction with the Host Body 206
8.10 Development of Nickel-Free High Nitrogen Stainless Steels 207
References 209

9. Other Metals and Functional Alloys **211**
9.1 Introduction 211
9.2 Noble Metals and Their Alloys 212
9.2.1 Outline 212
9.2.2 Noble Metals 212
9.2.3 Dental Casting Gold Alloys 213

9.2.4 Dental Wrought Alloys 216
9.2.5 Noble Metal Alloys for Metal-Ceramic Restorations 216
9.2.6 Brazing Alloys 218
9.2.7 Silver-Palladium Alloys 218
9.2.8 Dental Amalgam 219
9.2.7 Platinum and Platinum Alloys 219
9.3 Shape Memory and Superelastic Alloys 220
9.3.1 Martensitic Transformation 220
9.3.2 Shape Memory and Superelasticity 223
9.3.3 Nickel-Titanium Alloy 226
Low Temperature Treatment (Work Hardening) 227
Aging Treatment (Precipitation Treatment) 228
Medium Temperature Treatment (Grain Refinement) 228
Training Treatment 228
9.3.4 Corrosion Resistance of Nickel-Titanium Alloy 228
9.3.5 Nickel-Free Shape Memory and Superelastic Alloys 229
9.4 Biodegradable Metals 229
9.4.1 Outline 229
9.4.2 Magnesium Alloys 230
9.4.3 Pure Iron and Zinc Alloy 233
9.5 Magnet Alloys 233
9.6 Tantalum and Niobium 234
9.7 Zirconium Alloys 235
9.7.1 General Property 235
9.7.2 Application to Artificial Joints 237
9.7.3 Zirconium-Based Alloys 237
9.8 High Entropy Alloys 240
References 242

10. Surface Treatment and Surface Morphology **249**
10.1 Introduction 249
10.2 Dry Process 250
10.2.1 Outline 250
10.2.2 Spraying 252
10.2.3 Vapor Deposition 253
10.2.4 Ion Implantation 256
10.2.5 Gas Treatment 257
10.2.6 Blasting 258
10.2.7 Hard Film Coating by PVD 258
10.2.8 Ion Implantation of Nitrogen and Noble Metals 259
10.2.9 Heat Diffusion Treatment 259
10.2.10 Laser Irradiation 260
10.2.11 Thermal Oxidation 260
10.3 Wet Process 261
10.3.1 Outline 261
10.3.2 Electrochemical HA Coating 261

10.3.3 Electrochemical TiO_2 Coating 261
10.3.4 Immersion and Precipitation 262
10.3.5 Acid Etching 263
10.3.6 Immobilization of Biofunctional Molecules 264
10.3.7 Adhesion Improvement with Polymers 266
10.4 Surface Morphology Control 268
10.5 Biofunctional Surface Morphology 270
10.6 Cleaning and Hydrophilic Treatment 271
10.7 Time Transient of Surface Treatment 271
10.8 Optimal Surface Treatment 275
References 276

Appendix: Specifications of Metallic Biomaterials **284**

Index **291**

Notes on Using This Book

1. Metal elements are spelled out as titanium, gold, etc., in chapter and section headings, but they are spelled out as Ti, Au, etc., in the main text. Nonmetallic elements such as oxygen and nitrogen are spelled out, but when they are written as alloying elements, they are written as O or N.
2. Alloy notation is expressed in mass% unless otherwise specified.
3. In principle, industrially pure titanium is expressed as CP Ti. When expressing CP Ti and Ti alloys collectively, they are referred to as Ti or Ti material.
4. Abbreviations are explained when each chapter first appears. If the chapter changes, we will explain it again when it first appears.
5. Metallic materials and metals are used interchangeably. Metals is a generic term for pure metals and alloys. In other words, metallic materials and metals are used interchangeably.
7. Since "bioaffinity" and "biocompatibility" are used with almost the same meaning, they have been unified into "biocompatibility".
8. "Biofunction" is used to refer to properties that do not interfere with biological functions, such as inhibiting nonspecific protein adsorption, inhibiting cell adhesion, promoting bone formation, soft tissue adhesion, and preventing mechanical misalignment with biological tissue.
10. Hydroxyapatite is abbreviated as HA. However, materials that cannot be called HA, such as biological apatite, are written as apatite.
11. International Organization for Standardization standards are written as ISO.
12. American Society for Testing and Materials standards are written as ASTM.

Chapter 1

Current Status of Metallic Biomaterials

1.1 Introduction

Our bodies consist of tissues such as the skin, muscle, bone, and organs. These can be damaged by aging, disease, accidents, etc., and can lose part or all of their form and function. In this case, a conservative treatment with medication is the first choice. If this is difficult to cure, organ or tissue transplantation becomes necessary. However, tissue and organ transplants are always difficult, so in the end repair and regeneration are performed using materials. Many materials are used to reconstruct and regenerate lost human body forms and functions. These materials have supported medical advances and contributed to lifesaving, treatment, and improvement of quality of life (QOL). Materials used in medical procedures such as diagnosis and treatment, as well as materials used in biological research, are generally called "biomaterials". This chapter explains the position and necessity of metals among biomaterials. This chapter includes an overview of biomaterials, the positioning of metals as biomaterials, mechanical and chemical properties of materials, differences between hard biomaterials and soft biomaterials, history of metallic biomaterials, biomaterials and regenerative medicine, demand and market of metallic biomaterials, predominant properties for metallic biomaterials, research and development of metallic biomaterials, and utilization as medical devices, to assist readers understanding the position of metals as biomaterials for medical devices, an overview of metallic biomaterials, and the overall picture of this book. There are excellent textbooks on biomaterials (Wagner et al. 2020). There are also several textbooks and a handbook on metallic biomaterials (Helsen and Breme 1998, Zheng et al. 2017, Niinomi 2019, Wen 2020, ASM Handbook Vol. 23 2023). In addition, there are extensive textbooks on Ti materials in medicine (Brunette et al. 2001) and excellent reviews (Prasad 2017, Niinomi 2018). For dental materials, classic textbooks are well known (Anusavice 2003, Powers and Sakaguchi 2006).

1.2 Biomaterials

When hearing the word "biomaterial", many people probably think of materials created from human tissues or living organisms, such as proteins, sugar chains, lipids, nucleic acids, and cells. In fact, biomaterials such as silk, chitin and chitosan extracted from crab shells, and calcium carbonate derived from seashells and coral are used as biomaterials. Near recently, cells and living tissues have also been used as biomaterials. However, currently, the majority of biomaterials are the three major artificial materials: metallic materials (metals), inorganic materials (ceramics), and organic materials (polymers), in addition to the above biological origin materials.

Figures to the right on Fig. 1.1 show examples of medical devices using biomaterials. The term "biomaterials" was once used as materials only for medical devices that are completely implanted into the body and used for treatment, such as artificial bones, artificial joints, spinal fixation devices, intraocular lenses, artificial skins, stents, artificial valves, etc. Blood is also a living tissue, so syringes and artificial dialysis membranes are also biomaterials. Currently, nanometer-sized carriers required in drug delivery systems (DDS) used in cancer treatment and gene therapy are also biomaterials. The origin of regenerative medicine is "tissue engineering" using scaffold materials, stem cells, and growth factors, and biomaterials are used as scaffold materials and cell growth factors. Furthermore, many biomaterials are used in parts of inspection and diagnostic equipment that come into contact with blood and body fluids. On the other hand, materials used in biological research such as cell culture vessels that come into contact with living tissue, cells, and biomolecules also

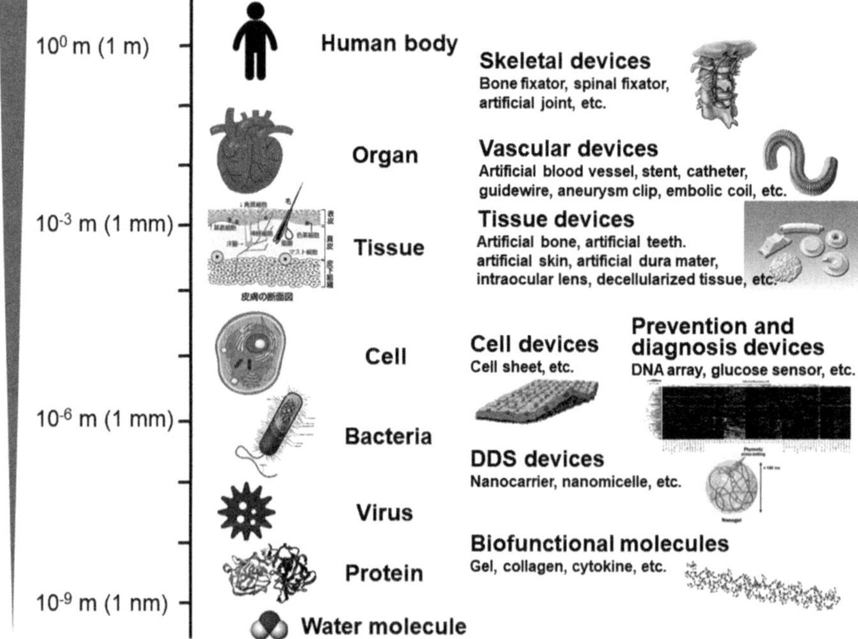

Fig. 1.1. Spatial hierarchy of human components and medical devices. The science and engineering underlying research and development of metallic biomaterials is relevant at all size levels.

fall under the category of biomaterials. As described above, the scope of biomaterials is diverse, and its definition changes over time. In a narrow sense, it is "materials used in contact with living tissues other than normal skin," but it can also be defined more broadly as "materials used in general medical practice, including prevention, diagnosis, and treatment, and biological research." In this way, biomaterials cover a wide range of fields, and their research and development includes not only materials science and engineering, but also surface and interface science and engineering, electronics, mechanical engineering (material mechanics), cell biology, histology, molecular biology, bacteriology, immunology, clinical medicine, and clinical dentistry (Fig. 1.2). Therefore, for research and development of biomaterials, knowledge and experimental techniques of the above fields are necessary.

Figure 1.1 also shows the components of the human body according to their size. Biological tissues and organs consist of cells, proteins, sugars, nucleic acids, etc. In addition to the above, tissues such as bones, cartilage, and teeth are composed of calcium phosphate such as apatite. Furthermore, enzymes and hormones that control biological functions are organic molecules. In this way, by disassembly of the constituent elements of the body, we arrive at inorganic and organic molecules. In other words, the basis of research and development of biomaterials requires researches on inorganic and organic molecules. Even now, the functions of most of the molecules that make up the human body are still unknown. Advances in materials have led to advances in treatment techniques, especially in dentistry and orthopedics. Furthermore, although it was thought that artificial materials would be weeded out due to advances in regenerative medicine, it has become clear that it will take a considerably long time for this to become a reality. For this reason, the importance of artificial materials is being recognized once again.

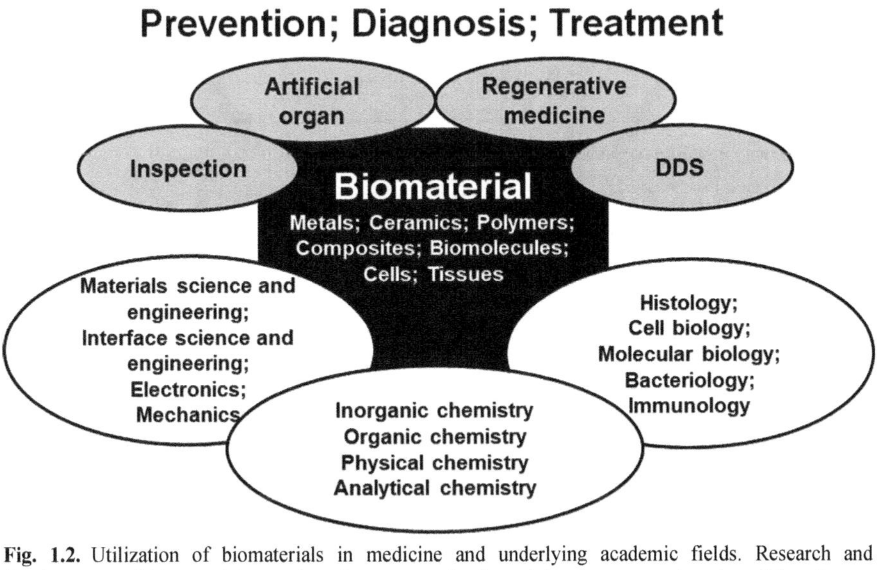

Fig. 1.2. Utilization of biomaterials in medicine and underlying academic fields. Research and development of biomaterials are based on many fundamental sciences, engineering, life sciences, medicine, and dentistry, and is interdisciplinary field.

1.3 Metals among Biomaterials

Artificial materials can be generally classified into metals, ceramics, and polymers. Metals as materials have a long history, and the foundations of today's materials science and engineering were developed through research into metals. However, the mass of people think that metals are "unfavorable materials" as biomaterials because of the environmental pollution and health hazard caused by heavy metals and their derivatives. When using metals as medical devices, improving safety is the first priority, and therefore efforts have been focused on improving corrosion resistance and preventing fracture in the body. Furthermore, metals are typically artificial materials and are recognized to show no biofunction. Rapid technological innovation over the last half century, with improvements in the fracture toughness and electronic function of ceramics, and the development and diversification of synthesized polymers, has enabled a wide range of applications of them to medical devices. In particular, the excellent tissue compatibility and biofunction of ceramics and polymers hold great promise as biomaterials, and many devices consisting of metals have been replaced by ceramics and polymers over the past 40 yr (Fig. 1.3). However, in spite of this event, there is still a large demand for metals due to their high fracture toughness, long-term durability, price, etc., and modern society cannot exist without metals. This situation is exactly the same in medical devices, where materials with excellent biocompatibility and biofunction are attracting attention; however, the necessity of metals remains unwavering. Components that can use ceramics and

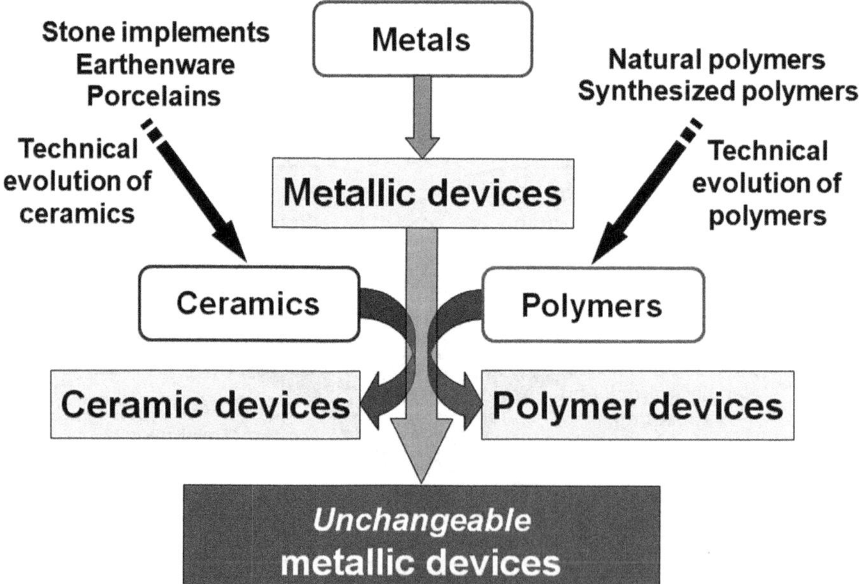

Fig. 1.3. Substitution of devices consisting of metals by ceramics and polymers due to their technological innovation. Each material is used in the right place according to their advantages. Components that do not need to be metal are already being replaced with ceramics and polymers. Currently, equipment and parts that use metals must be made of metals, so metals are used. This is not limited to medical devices, but applies to all of our society.

polymers have already been replaced with these materials; therefore, it is difficult to replace components that currently use metals with ceramics and polymers. Metals are still used in many medical devices due to their excellent strength and toughness, and it is clear that metals play an extremely important role in medicine, as many medical implants are made of metals. Therefore, it is certain that metals will continue to be used in medicine into the future. This is similar to the need for metals in all fields, from everyday household goods to structures and transportation machinery.

Figure 1.4 summarizes the types, advantages, and devices consisting of each material. Each material is used as a material for many medical devices, taking advantage of its own merits. On the other hand, Fig. 1.5 shows the advantages and disadvantages of each material, the expecting degree as research target for biomaterials and degree of practicality as "implant" devices.[1] The tissues and organs of the human body basically consist of polymers, and the enzymes, sugar chains, lipids, and nucleic acids that govern biofunctions are also polymers. Therefore, if we can synthesize molecules that mimic the polymers that exist in the human body, we can create molecules that have biological functions. Furthermore, the basic inorganic component of human hard tissues (bones, cartilage, and teeth) is apatite, which is a form of calcium phosphate, and calcium phosphate ceramics play an important

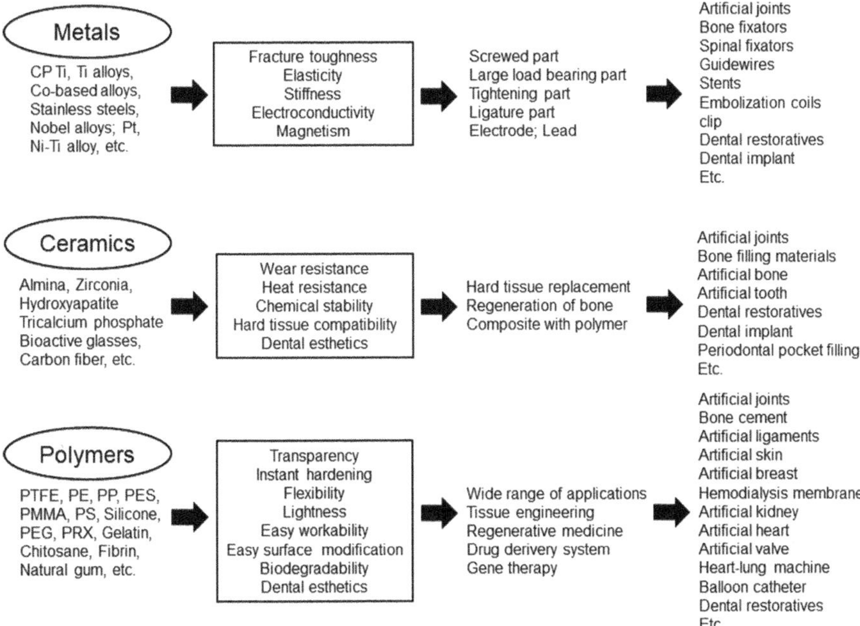

Fig. 1.4. Types, advantages, and medical devices of metals, ceramics, and polymers. Each material has its own advantages, and the right materials are used in the right places for applications where those advantages can be demonstrated.

[1] What is being focused on here are medical devices that are implanted inside the body, and as many people have seen, polymer materials are often used in medical devices used outside the body for diagnosis and treatment.

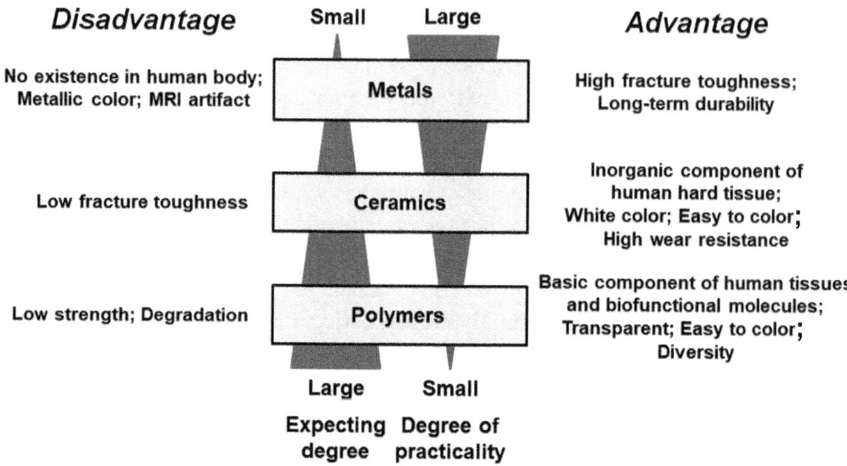

Fig. 1.5. Expecting degree as research target for biomaterials and degree of practicality as implant materials of metals, ceramics, and polymers, based on their advantages and disadvantages. Metals are most commonly used as implant materials because of their high fracture toughness and durability.

role in bone formation and osseointegration[2] (see Section 6.9). Therefore, it is being actively researched as a typical inorganic material that promotes bone formation. On the other hand, although many metal elements always exist in our bodies, metallic materials do not exist. In other words, there is no model for developing metallic materials that exhibit biological functions within the human body. This makes metals less attractive as biomaterial research subjects, leading to the misunderstanding that it is better to avoid using metals as biomaterials as much as possible.

However, the proportion of metallic materials used in commercial implants is high, with over 70% of implants being made of metals. In other words, just under 30% of implants are made of ceramic or polymer. When it comes to orthopedic implants, over 95% are made of metals.[3]

1.4 Mechanical and Chemical Properties of Materials

Table 1.1 summarizes the advantages and disadvantages of metals, ceramics, and polymers as biomaterials. All materials have advantages and disadvantages, and there is no material that has only advantages and no disadvantages. The advantages of metals are high strength, high ductility, and high fracture toughness values. This is also clear from the comparison of stress-strain curves shown in Fig. 1.6 (see Section 3.3 and Fig. 3.1). This stress-strain curve shows that only metals have both high strength and high ductility. The serious disadvantages in practical use are esthetic problems due to metallic luster as dental restorations and MRI artifacts due

[2] Definition is as follows. Formation of a direct interface between an implant and bone, without intervening soft tissue. No scar tissue, cartilage or ligament fibers are present between the bone and implant surface. The direct contact of bone and implant surface can be verified microscopically.

[3] Calculated based on statics from the Ministry of Health, Labor and Welfare, Japan.

Table 1.1. Comparison of physical and chemical properties among metals, ceramics, and polymers.[6]

Property	Metals	Ceramics	Polymers
Strength	Excellent (Tensile)	Excellent (Compressive)	Poor (Tensile)
Plastic deformability	Excellent	Poor	Excellent
Hardness	Good	Excellent	Fair
Fracture toughness	Excellent	Poor	Poor
Creep at body temperature	Excellent	Excellent	Poor
Wear resistance	Good	Excellent	Poor
Lightness	Poor	Good	Excellent
Heat resistance	Good	Excellent	Poor
Chemical stability	Fair	Excellent	Fair
Dental esthetics	Poor	Excellent	Excellent
MRI artifact	Poor	Excellent	Excellent

to high magnetic susceptibility (see Section 5.5). The advantages of ceramics are that chemical stability, osteoconductivity (bone formation ability), bone replacement properties, etc., can be selected depending on the type, and can be colored in the same as teeth in dentistry. The disadvantage is their low fracture toughness. Because the value is small and easy to fracture, there is a limit to the size of parts that are subject to large loads and implants in the body. The advantages of polymers are light weight, transparency, flexibility, etc., and a variety of materials can be selected. The disadvantages of polymers are low strength and creep[4] at body temperature, so gradually deform under load in the human body. For this reason, most of bone fixators, stem of artificial joint, orthodontic wires, partial denture clasps, etc., cannot be made from polymers. In addition, there remains a problem regarding long-term stability in the body. On the other hand, in dental treatment, the metallic luster of metals is a fatal drawback from an esthetic point of view. Composite resins[5] and zirconia ceramics are now being used for restorations and prosthetics in areas that are visible from the outside of the oral cavity. Doctors and patients often prioritize esthetics. Perhaps the most sought-after product to switch from metal to polymer is orthodontic wire. If this could be done using polymeric materials, it would revolutionize orthodontic treatment. Unfortunately, only metals can maintain elasticity in the oral cavity environment for long periods of time without deteriorating due to creep at the body temperature. For this purpose, a method has been adopted in which the metal wire is coated with a white polymer.

These properties of each material are dependent on the chemical bonds that make up the materials as solid state. As shown in Fig. 1.7, metals form aggregates through metallic bonds (see Section 2.2), and ceramics form aggregates through ionic or

[4] Creep is a phenomenon in which a material gradually deforms over a long period of time under a load, and occurs in polymers at room temperature or body temperature.

[5] Composite materials made by resins dispersing glass particles.

[6] Note that the rankings of excellent, good, fair, and poor are relative comparisons between the three materials.

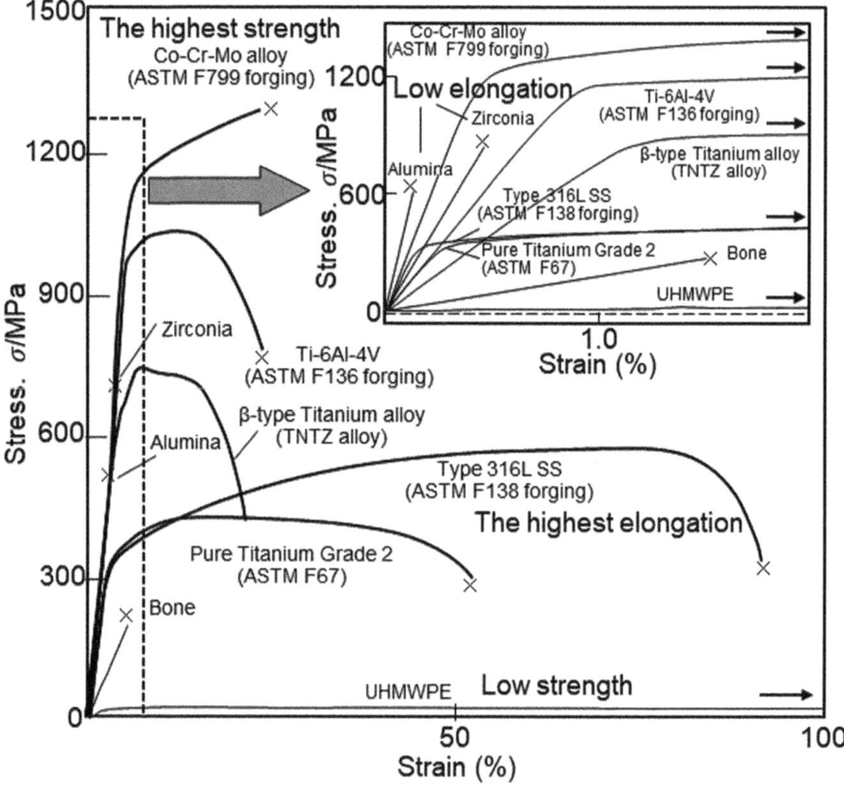

Fig. 1.6. Stress-strain curves of typical metals, ceramics, polymer (Provided by Dr. Takayoshi Nakano, Osaka University). The dashed area expands to the upper right. UHMWPE: ultra-high molecular weight polyethylene. Metals have high strength and high elongation, while ceramics have low elongation and polymers have low strength.

covalent bonds. In polymers, molecular chains formed by covalent bonds are weakly bonded to each other by van der Waals forces or hydrogen bonds. In this book, materials composed of metallic bonds are defined as metallic materials (metals). Furthermore, metals generally become polycrystalline during normal manufacturing processes. Differences in these chemical bonds result in unique mechanical and chemical properties, as shown in Table 1.1. Therefore, it is difficult to change these fundamental properties, and the use of each material is selected to take its advantage. In addition, rough comparison of properties among CP Ti, and Ti alloy, Co-based alloy, and stainless steel as predominant metallic biomaterials is summarized in Table 1.2 (see Chapters 6, 7, and 8).

1.5 Hard Biomaterials and Soft Biomaterials

Many biomaterial researchers are based on polymer science. Therefore, in biomaterials research, so-called "soft materials" that exhibit functions in aqueous

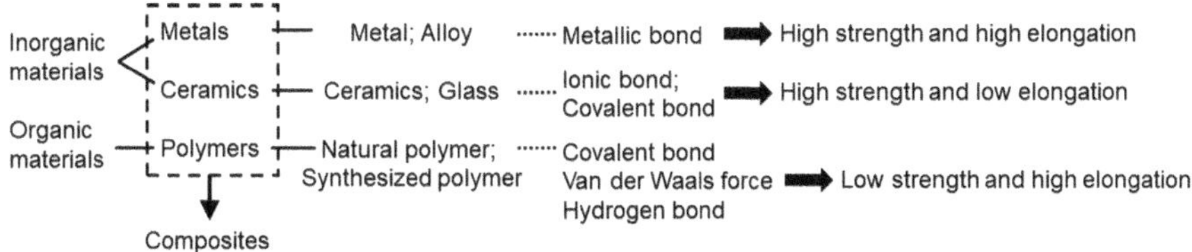

Fig. 1.7. Category of materials and the types of chemical bonds that make them up. Strength and elongation of them are governed by their chemical bonds. Therefore, it is difficult to change their basic property.

Table 1.2. Comparison of properties of main metallic biomaterials.[7]

Materials		Mechnaical property		Workability		Corrosion resistance
		Tensile strength	Wear resistance	Plasticity	Machinability	Pitting
Stainless steel	Type316L	Good	Excellent	Excellent	Excellent	Poor
Co-Cr-Mo alloy	Cast	Good	Good	Poor	Poor	Good
	Anealed	Excellent	Good	Good	Good	Fair
Ti; Ti alloy	CP Ti	Excellent	Excellent	Fair	Fair	Excellent
	Ti-6Al-4V	Excellent	Excellent	Fair	Excellent	Excellent

solutions such as body fluids are being actively studied: functional molecules, supermolecules, gels, and nano-carriers for regenerative medicine, gene therapy, and drug delivery systems. Soft materials basically perform their functions in aqueous solutions (body fluids). On the other hand, metals, ceramics, and solid polymers are classified as "hard materials" that are used in a solid state in contact with living tissues (Fig. 1.8). In addition, hard materials are used for medical equipment and machines that are used outside the human body. In this regard, biomaterials can be roughly classified into soft biomaterials and hard biomaterials, and metals belong to the hard biomaterial group. However, calcium phosphates, which replace bone by dissolution in the body, may be positioned between soft and hard biomaterials.

1.6 History of Metallic Biomaterials

The main history of metals for medical devices is summarized in Table 1.3. Metals were first used as dental materials, with Au wire being used in Egypt at least 2,500 yr ago. Furthermore, for filling restorations in dentistry, Au foil and Sn with a low melting point are used, followed by Ag amalgam. Co–Cr alloys have been developed for denture bases, and casting Au alloys have been developed for dental restoration. In orthopedics, wires were used as bone fixators, and stainless steel, which is relatively safe, became mainstream after using Ni-plated steel plates and

[7] Note that the rankings of excellent, good, fair, and poor are relative comparisons between the three materials.

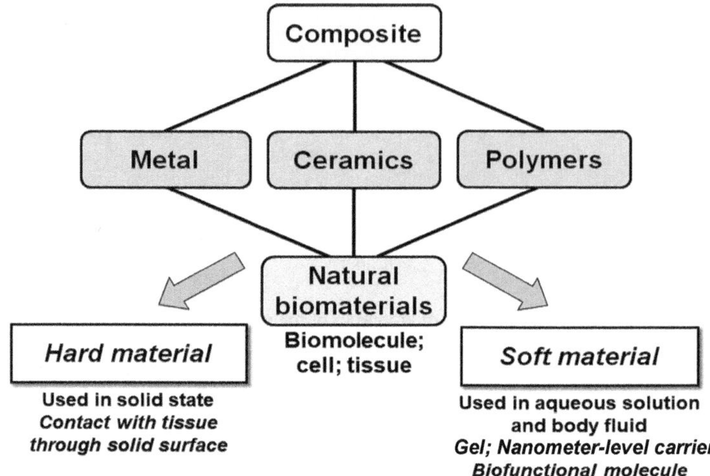

Fig. 1.8. Categorization of biomaterials into hard materials and soft materials. Metals and ceramics belong to hard materials, while polymers belong to both hard and soft materials. Both hard and soft materials are important as biomaterials.

V-containing steel. Since then, the use of Ti alloys has increased, and now Ti-6Al-4V alloys developed for aerospace applications are diverted to all types of implants. In this way, progress in metals for medical devices has depended on the development of the metallic materials themselves.

Current metallic biomaterials are classified into three groups as follows: metals and alloys developed for other purposes are used for medical devices without any change, alloys developed for other purposes were improved to use in medical devices (for example, type 316L stainless steel, Ti-6Al-4V ELI alloy, etc.), and alloys originally developed for biomedical use (Co-based alloys, Ti-6Al-7Nb alloy, Zr alloys, etc.). New alloys are continuously developed to improve their properties and add functions. On the other hand, surface treatment and modification techniques to add biocompatibility and biofunction are also creating a new history in medical materials. Details of history of Ti alloys, Co-based alloys, and stainless steels are explained in the later chapters for each metal and alloy (see Chapters 6, 7, and 8).

1.7 Biomaterials and Regenerative Medicine

Treatments using regenerative medicine have been attracting attention in recent years, but expectations have grown too high and there's a misconception that regenerative medicine will solve all medical problems of humans. Some researchers include treatments using artificial materials to it, so the definition of regenerative medicine is expanding, and making its definition unclear. When regenerative medicine is defined as "treatment that uses stem cells to regenerate living tissue," current regenerative medicine research can be roughly divided into the following three types, as shown in Fig. 1.9.

(A) Regenerative medicine using only stem cells: The main focus is on cell development and research on cell growth factors and function expression factors.

Table 1.3. Main history of metallic biomaterials.

Year	Material	Purpose	Place of invention
Around BC700	Au strip	Dental bridge Partial denture base	Eritrea
Around BC500	Au wire	Fastening restorative	Egypt; Phoenicia
Around BC400	Au strip	Dental crown and bridge	Roma
Around BC400	Au wire	Bone fixator	Greece
695	Amalgam	Dental restorative	China (Tang)
Around 1480	Au foil	Dental filling	Italy
After 1500	Au wire; Ag wires	Bonding artificial tooth	All over Europe
1562	Au plate	Cleft palate restorative	All over Europe
After 1600	Au wire; Fe wire; bronze wire	Laceration suture material	All over Europe
After 1700	Fe wire; Ag wire; Bronze wire	Bone fixator	All over Europe
After 1700	Sn	Dental filling restorative	France
After 1800	Ag amalgam	Dental filling restorative	France
1886	Ni-plated steel plate	Bone plate and screw	UK
1896	Ag-Sn amalgam	Dental filling restorative	USA
1910	Ag	Hemoclip	
1920	V containing steel	Bone plate and screw	USA
1926	Au alloy	Dental casting restorative	USA
Around 1926	Type 302 stainless steel	Bone fixator	USA
1929	Co–Cr–Mo alloy	Partial denture base	USA
Late 1930s	Type 316 stainless steel; Co–Cr–Mo alloy	Bone fixator	USA
1956	Type 316L stainless steel	Artificial hip joint	USA
1956	Co–Cr–Mo alloy	Artificial hip joint	USA
1960	Co–Cr–Mo alloy	Head of artificial hip joint	USA
1966	Stainless steel	Aneurysm clip	
1960s	CP Ti	Artificial joint	Sweden
1970s	Ti–6Al–4V alloy	Artificial joint; Bone fixator	
1982	CP Ti	Dental casting restorative	Japan
1986	Type 316L Stainless steel	Stent	USA
1995	CP Ti	Aneurysm clip	

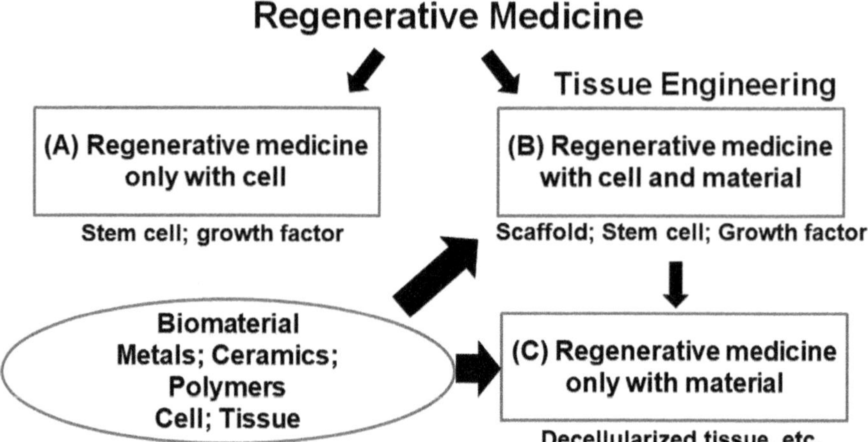

Fig. 1.9. Category of regenerative medicine and the contribution of biomaterials. Biomaterials play important roles for regenerative medicine. It is difficult to construct medical devices consisting of metals only by regenerative medicine with stem cells at present.

(B) Regenerative medicine using stem cells and materials: The origin of regenerative medicine is tissue engineering using cells and scaffold materials, which requires research on cells, scaffold materials, and cell growth factors.

(C) Regenerative medicine using only materials: Regenerative medicine using only materials such as decellularized tissue is being researched.

Artificial materials are contributing to regenerative medicine (B) as scaffolding materials. Recently, there has been a growing misconception that only (A) is regenerative medicine, "regenerative medicine equals cell research", but it must be said that this ignores the time axis of research and development or the cost of treatment. There are only a limited number of tissues that can be regenerated without scaffold materials, and it will be difficult to regenerate all tissues and organs using cells alone without materials in the near future. In particular, treatments that rely primarily on metals, such as joint reconstruction, tooth restoration and prosthetics, bone fracture fixation, spinal fixation, and vasodilation, are difficult to achieve only through regenerative medicine, while currently only a portion of these treatments can be regenerated. Regenerative medicine treatment uses tissue as a starting material, so the regenerated tissue has biofunction. If autologous cells are used, there is no rejection reaction, so it is a technology that is expected to advance. However, regenerative medicine technology is still under development and requires long-term hospital treatment in many cases, so challenges remain in its application to the elderly and patients wishing to return to society as soon as possible. On the other hand, treatment using artificial materials enables early functional reconstruction and has a long track record. Therefore, regenerative medicine and treatments using artificial materials, especially metals, will remain inseparable and inviolable for the time being, and advances in regenerative medicine will not eliminate treatments using artificial materials (Fig. 1.10).

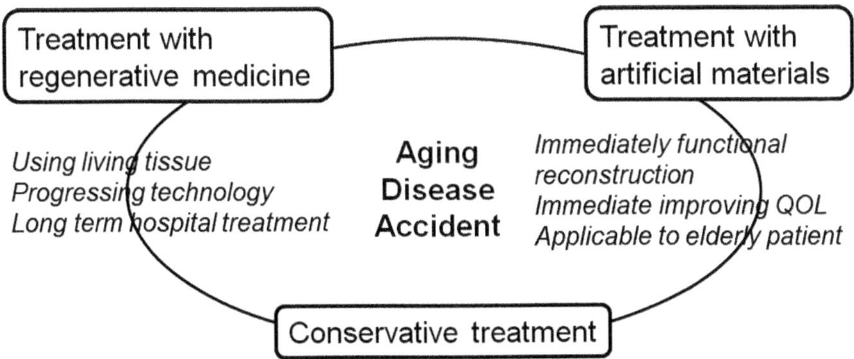

Fig. 1.10. Treatments using regenerative medicine and artificial materials according to the case and patient's wishes. Metallic biomaterials strongly contribute to treatments with artificial materials. This situation will continue into the future.

At present, biodegradable polymers, biopolymers, calcium phosphate ceramics, and composite materials have been proposed as scaffold materials used in regenerative medicine, while metals have been considered to be unrelated to regenerative medicine. However, metal is an effective material for ensuring a certain level of size and durability for regenerated organs, and its use as a scaffold material is already being attempted. Since the metal remains in the body semi-permanently, CP Ti is used because it has relatively high tissue compatibility. Many shapes can now be manufactured for use in regenerative medicine, such as Ti meshes, fibers, and sheets as shown in Fig. 1.11, and even more can be manufactured through additive manufacturing (AM). The use of metals as scaffolding materials is likely to expand in the future, so those involved in regenerative medicine need to know the basics required when using metallic biomaterials *in vivo*.

1.8 Demand and Market of Metallic Biomaterials

The global medical devices' market size was valued at $512.29 billion in 2022 and is projected to grow from $536.12 billion in 2023 to $799.67 billion by 2030 (Fortune Business Insights 2023). The global medical devices market was worth $448 billion in 2020 and is forecasted to reach $671.49 billion by 2027, growing at a compound annual growth rate of 5.2 percent. Medical devices refer to an apparatus, instrument, appliance, or machine for prevention, diagnosis, treatment, monitoring, or alleviation of disease. These devices offer numerous advantages to patients by helping medical service provider in diagnosis and treatment of patients; in addition, they assist patients to improve their quality of life. Growth factors are as follows: the increasing prevalence of chronic diseases that include cancer, unhealthy lifestyle and eating habits also attracts other types of critical diseases, rising trend for medical wearable devices, and integration of artificial intelligence (AI) in the medical devices such as remote patient monitoring devices, wearable medical equipment, electronic health records (EHR), and many more threats for data breaches and hack of critical information through these devices (MPO 2023). According to AdvaMed, the U.S. occupies about 40% of the global medical device market. In segmenting the

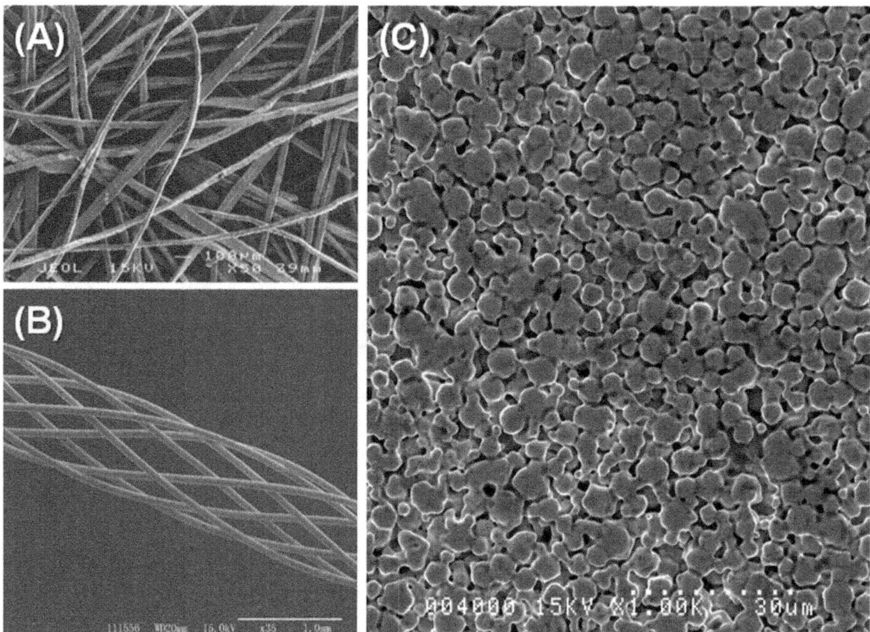

Fig. 1.11. (A) Fiber, (B) mesh, and (C) porous membrane sheets consist of CP Ti. These flexible and functional titanium materials may be effective to apply metals to regenerative medicine.

U.S. market share, Fortune Business Insights found that *in vitro* diagnostics (IVD), cardiovascular devices and orthopedic devices are the largest segments. The report expects the IVD segment will grow at a higher compound annual growth rate (CAGR) due to the increased use of real-time diagnostics tests for the diagnosis of diabetes, cancer, and HIV/AIDS. The report also notes an uptick in the market for portable and wearable devices for treatment of chronic conditions due to a shift in preference among the elderly for home healthcare services following the COVID-19 pandemic (Patel 2022). As described above, the demand for medical devices continues to increase, and metallic materials occupy an important position as materials for such devices.

1.9 Predominant Properties for Metallic Biomaterials

What is required of metallic biomaterials, which are hard materials for medical purposes, is that the dimension of the material in the solid state does not change, with the exception of biodegradable metals such as Mg alloys. The following properties are required:

(1) Not to be significantly deformed during use.

(2) Not to fracture during use.

(3) To be used as a solid state for long time.

In other words, high strength, fracture toughness, fatigue strength, corrosion resistance, etc., are required.

When hard materials are used as biomaterials, their solid surfaces come into contact with living tissue and function in the solid state. This function also includes mechanical functions. The abiotic-biotic interface between a solid surface and a living tissue tends to be clear, and inhibit mass transfer and the conduction of biological functions (Fig. 1.12). Therefore, much research has been conducted to transform this clear interface into an intelligent interface that is unclear and assist mass transfer and conduct biological functions. These studies include not only those that create functional surfaces based on interfacial chemistry, but also those that exhibit mechanical functions. Since metals are artificial materials, there are many issues in terms of biocompatibility and biofunction. Therefore, resolving this issue is essential for significantly improving treatment effectiveness and efficiency, reducing the burden on patients, ensuring minimal invasion, and improving QOL. In other words, in addition to the above properties, the properties required for hard biomaterials are:

(4) Tissue compatibility and biofunction such as bone formation, soft tissue adhesion, antithrombotic properties, and non-biofilm formation.

(5) During the healing period of living tissue, the tissue exhibits rigidity that does not apply mechanical loads, and after healing, it does not damage or destroy living tissue due to deformation and frictional wear similar to living tissue.

The properties of (4) are interfacial and can be achieved mainly through surface treatment. The properties of (5) are mechanical, and are primarily properties that can be achieved through material development, alloy design and manufacturing process for metals.

On the other hand, it is not possible to add biofunctions to metals during their manufacturing processes, such as melting, casting, forging, working, and heat treatment. This is the greatest weakness of metals as biomaterials. Therefore, surface treatment and surface modification are required to add biocompatibility and biofunction to metals (see Chapter 10).

Of course, biomaterials must be safe for the human body. Metallic biomaterials that come into contact with living tissue do not exhibit toxicity as they are, because there is a risk that they will become toxic if they are dissolved as metal ions through corrosion or become wear debris due to friction wear (see Figs. 2.27 and 5.1). Therefore, high corrosion resistance is absolutely necessary for metallic biomaterials. In addition, various properties are required depending on the application, such as strength, toughness, elasticity, rigidity, flexibility, lightness, *in vivo* activity, *in vivo* inertness, biodegradability, X-ray radiopaque, etc.

Table 1.4 summarizes the requirements for metallic biomaterials from the clinical field of medicine and dentistry. As mentioned above, metals are essential for medical devices, and as a practical matter, metallic medical devices are required to have a high level of biological function.

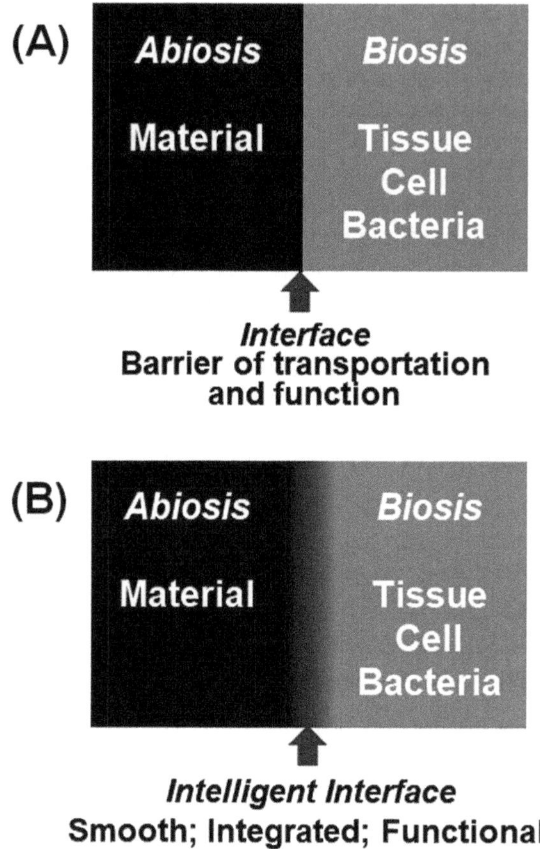

Fig. 1.12. (A) Clear interface formed between material and biological tissue and (B) intelligent interface that gradually transitions between material and biological tissue. Researchers in the field of biomaterials are making the best effort to create intelligent interfaces using surface treatment techniques.

1.10 Research and Development of Metallic Biomaterials

The research and development of biomaterials differs greatly from that of other materials because biological evaluation using cells and animals is essential, and approval by a national regulation agency[8] may be required depending on the intended use. For this reason, biological evaluations occupy a large proportion of the research process, but on the other hand, evaluations from a materials engineering perspective are sometimes kept to a minimum on research level, and the biocompatibility and biofunction of newly developed materials are evaluated through cell and animal experiments. In other words, this is a field in which the success of researches through cell and animal experiments can be advertised. Of course, materials whose durability over the period of use is not guaranteed will be excluded at the stage of practical research. It is essential to ensure durability and safety, that is, mechanical properties

[8] FDA in the United States.

Table 1.4. Requirements for metallic biomaterials from the clinical field of medicine and dentistry.

Required property	**Applicable medical devices**	**Effect**
Free of toxic element	All implants	Safety
High corrosion resistance	All implants	Safety; Durability
High fatigue strength	All implants	Durability
Low elastic modulus	Bone fixator; Stem of artificial joint; Spinal rod	Prevention of osteolysis by stress shielding
Superelasticity; Shape memory effect	Multi purposes	Mechanical compatibility
High wear resistance	Artificial joint	Prevention of wear debris generation
Biodegradability	Stent; Bone fixator	Elimination of devices after healing
Bone formation; Bone bonding	Stem of artificial hip joint; dental implant	Fixation of implant device
Prevention of bone formation	Bone fixator	Prevention of re-fracture during retrieval
Soft tissue adhesion	Dental implant; Orthodontic implant anchor; Transdermal device; Screw of external bone fixator; Housing of pace maker	Inhibition of infection by bacterial invasion; Fixation of device in soft tissue
Antithrombogenicity	Device contacting blood	Inhibition of thrombus formation
Antibacterial property	All implants; surgical instrument	Prevention of infectious diseases
Decreasing MRI artifact	All implants; surgical instrument	Ensuring diagnosticity

and corrosion resistance, before biological evaluation, and as mentioned above, biological evaluation alone is not enough.

Research and development of metallic biomaterials can be classified as follows.

[1] Design of new alloy compositions.

[2] Development of working and heat treatment technology. AM technology is classified here.

[3] Development of new surface treatment and surface modification technologies.

- Composite with ceramics and ceramic coating.
- Immobilization of functional molecules and biomolecules.
- Composite with polymers.

[4] Development of surface morphology. Nanometer/micrometer-level periodic structure.

[5] Evaluation of mechanical properties.

[6] Evaluation of corrosion resistance.

[7] Safety/toxicity evaluation.

[8] Evaluation of biocompatibility and biofunction.

[9] Development of *in vitro* evaluation technology.

New material development is carried out by developing alloys in [1], manufacturing process development in [2], surface treatment technology in [3], and morphological control technology in [4]. In general, if a metallic material does not have high strength and ductility, it has no value as the metallic material, so [5] is required when a new material is developed. In addition, when used for medical purposes, the corrosion resistance in [6] must also be confirmed. If these goals are achieved, the safety and biocompatibility of [7] and [8] will be confirmed. In recent years, research on the compatibility of metals with living tissues and biofunction has become active, but research on mechanical properties and corrosion resistance, which are important for metals, is always conducted in parallel. In addition, performance evaluation is essential for material development, and in the case of biomaterials, it is necessary to develop *in vitro* evaluation techniques as described in [9], especially *in vitro* evaluation techniques that can reduce animal experiments.

As shown in Fig. 1.13, research and development aimed at practical application involves the development of new materials and surfaces, evaluation and verification, safety testing, clinical trials, and regulatory approval. Even if it does not reach practical application, if it can derive a general theory, universal principle, and general-purpose technology by thoroughly investigating each research process in the

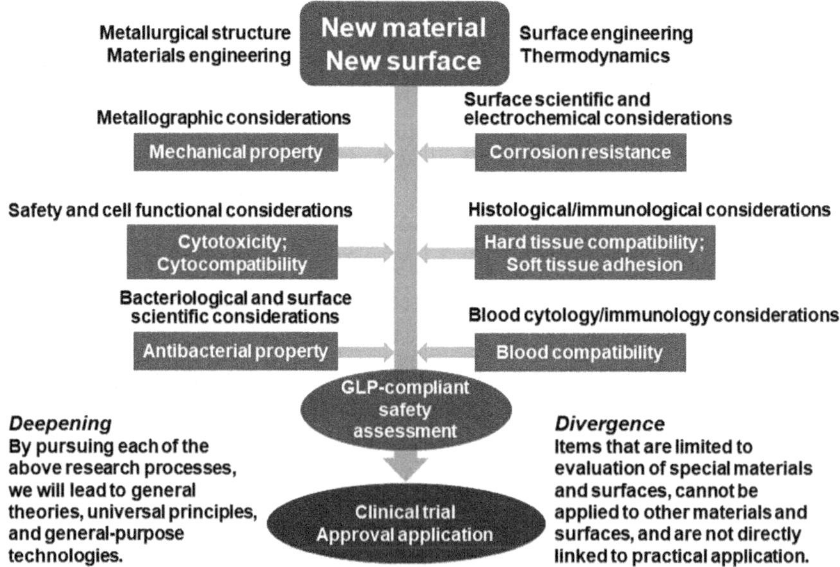

Fig. 1.13. Research process aimed at practical application and deepening and divergence of research on biomaterials. All researches and development must contribute to deepening of the field of biomaterials that may contribute to materials science and engineering, medical and dental treatments, and even life science.

design, manufacturing process, and evaluation process, this research can contribute to biomaterial science. On the other hand, if the research is limited to evaluating a special material or surface, cannot be applied to other materials or surfaces, and is not directly connected to practical application, then this research is divergent. In any case, it is important to have an attitude of pursuing principles in each process.

The development of materials, not just biomaterials, is carried out through design, manufacturing processes, and evaluation. It is often the case that only biocompatibility and biofunction are emphasized, without any research being conducted on mechanical properties and durability. Unless all the properties that are actually required, including durability and safety evaluations, are evaluated, we cannot talk about the science of the material itself, and we cannot feed these back into the design to create even better materials. The basis of materials research is knowing the defects and limitations of materials and improving them. All materials have advantages and disadvantages, and the appropriate materials should be used as the appropriate devices to take advantage of those characteristics. It is not possible to improve the performance of a material without sufficient characterization of the material and without discussing the relationship between biological evaluation and material properties.

Material design, manufacturing process, and biological evaluation of biomaterials utilize science and technology from various fields, and there is no academic field called "biomaterials science" at present. In practical sciences such as biomaterials, new science may arise in the process of elucidating the mechanisms from developed technologies. There is a misconception that technology is created deductively based on the foundation of science, while with biomaterials it is also possible to take an inductive approach to discover unified theories and general principles from individual technologies.

Investigation of surface property including electronic property of materials will be essential to better understand the interface phenomena between materials and host bodies using materials informatics (MI) and materials digital transformation (Material DX), because all biological and tissue reactions start from an electronic transfer of the surface (Hanawa 2022). However, the progress of MI and DX in corrosion science and engineering, typical surface reaction of metals, is quite slow. Advances in this field are essential for predicting the biocompatibility and biofunction of materials to specify reactions strictly at the electronic level.

1.11 Utilization of Metals as Medical Devices

The development process for medical devices leading to commercialization is not necessarily a straight path; it is possible to look back and revise the design at any stage of the process, and commercialization is achieved through repeated development, verification, and improvement with a clear goal. In addition, the products are numerous and diverse, and there are various development patterns depending on the type of equipment and class. However, in order to put any of these patterns into practical use, it is ultimately necessary to obtain manufacturing and sales approval from the manufacturer and commercialize it, and to deliver better medical devices to patients faster. In order to help improve the quality of medical care, it is important to be aware of commercialization strategies from the early stages of development and proceed with research and development with a sense of speed. The practical application of medical devices can be broadly divided into the following three categories.

- New medical devices: Distinctly different medical devices. The structure, method of use, efficacy, effectiveness, or performance are different from those of medical devices that have already been approved.
- Improved medical equipment: It is a medical device that does not fall under either a new medical device or a generic medical device. Items that are not substantially equivalent to existing equipments in structure, method of use, efficacy, effect, or performance.
- Generic medical devices: The structure, method of use, efficacy or effect, and performance are the same as those of already approved medical devices. It is a medical device that recognized that product or performance is substantially equivalent.

There are excellent guides on the practical application of medical devices (Zenios et al. 2010). Before it can be put into practical use, it is necessary to work together with the national regulatory authority (in the case of the United States, the FDA) and the manufacturer of the devices that are planning to sell it, based on the regulatory science and medical economics.

References

Anusavice, K.J. 2003. Phillips' Science of Dental Materials, 11th Ed. Sanders, St. Louis, MO, USA.

ASM Handbook, Vol. 23. 2023. Materials for Medical Devices. ASM International, Materials Park, OH, USA.

MPO. 2023. Breaking news, Medical devices market to top $671.49 billion by 2027, Medical Product Outsourcing. https://www.mpo-mag.com/contents/view_breaking-news/2021-09-16/medical-devices-market-to-top-67149-billion-by-2027/.

Brunette, D.M., P. Tenvall, M. Textor and P. Thomsen [eds.]. 2001. Titanium in Medicine. Springer, Berlin, Germany.

Hanawa, T. 2022. Biocompatibility of titanium from the viewpoint of its surface. Sci. Technol. Adv. Mater. 23: 457–472.

Helsen, J.A. and H.J. Breme [eds.]. 1998. Metals as Biomaterials. John Wiley & Sons, West Sussex, UK.

Firtune Buisiness Insights. 2023. Medical device/medical device market. https://www.fortunebusinessinsights.com/industry-reports/medical-devices-market-100085.

Niinomi, M. 2018. Recent progress in research and development of metallic structural biomaterials with mainly focusing on mechanical biocompatibility. Mater. Trans. 59: 1–13.

Niinomi, M. [ed.]. 2019. Metals for Medical Devices, 2nd Ed. Woodhead, Elsevier, Cambridge, MA, USA.

Patel, R. 2022. Report: Medical device market expected to grow over next seven years. Knobblemedical, http://knobbemedical.com/medicaldeviceblog/article/report-medical-device-market-expected-to-grow-over-next-seven-years/.

Powers, J.M. and R.L. Sakaguchi [eds.]. 2006. Craig's Restorative Dental Materials, 20th ed. Mosly, St. Louis, MO, USA.

Prasad, K., O. Bazaka, M. Chua, M. Rochford, L. Fedrick, J. Spoor et al. 2017. Metallic biomaterials: current challenges and opportunities. Materials 10: 884.
Wagner, W.R., S.E. Sakiyama-Elbert, G. Zhang and M.J. Yaszemski [eds.]. 2020. Biomaterials Science—An Introduction to Materials in Medicine, 4th Ed. Academic Press, Elsevier, San Diego, CA, USA.
Wen, C. [ed.]. 2020. Metallic Biomaterials Processing and Medical Device Manufacturing. Woodhead, Elsevier, Sawston, Cambridge, UK.
Zenios, S., S. Makower and P. Yock [eds.]. 2010. Biodesign—The Process of innovating Medical Technologies. Cambridge University Press, New York, NY, USA.
Zheng, Y., X. Xu, Z. Xu, J.Q. Wang and H. Cai. 2017. Metallic Biomaterials, New Directions and Technologies. Wiley, Hoboken, NJ, USA.

CHAPTER 2

General Property of Metals in Biological Environment

2.1 Introduction

Metals have advantages that cannot be obtained from other materials, such as high strength, toughness, an appropriate balance of rigidity and elasticity, and durability, so they are widely used as essential materials for medical devices that require these properties. Since metals are basically aggregates consisting of metallic bonds, they exhibit different properties from ceramics and polymers, which consist of ionic and covalent bonds. In addition, the characteristics of metals is that their mechanical properties are governed by metastable phases, defects, etc., and even alloys with the same composition can show variety of properties due to the manufacturing process such as working and heat treatment. On the other hand, it is often misunderstood that the surface condition of metallic biomaterials does not change during normal use. This is based on the misconception that Au is often used in biological research and that Au's inertness is common to all metals. In biological environments where proteins and cells come into contact, the surface conditions of many metals change irreversibly. In order to handle metals in a biological environment, it is necessary to correctly understand their change in surface structure and composition. This knowledge is also essential for creating surfaces that promote biocompatibility and biofunction. In this chapter, the minimum essentials for correctly handling metallic biomaterials are explained, divided into mechanical property, surface property, and biological property. If you would like to learn more detailed principles regarding the properties of metals, refer to textbooks (Callister and Rethwisch 2015) as an introduction to the structure and properties of metals. In addition, many specialized handbooks have been published on crystal[1] structure, phase transformation, mechanical properties, corrosion resistance, etc. (ASM Handbook Series 2023).

[1] A crystal is a solid in which atoms are arranged regularly over a long range.

2.2 Band Structure and Metallic Bond

Schematic illustrations of orbital splitting in the production of molecules from hydrogen and helium atoms are shown in Fig. 2.1A. In molecules with bonded atoms, there are electron orbitals with different electron energies for the same number of bonded atoms. In both hydrogen and helium, two atoms combine to form a hydrogen molecule and a helium molecule. Since only two electrons can occupy in one orbital, hydrogen molecules form low-energy bonding molecular orbitals occupied with two electrons and non-bonding molecular orbitals empty of electrons. In contrast, in a helium molecule, both bond orbitals are occupied with four electrons. In Fig. 2.1B, it shows the orbits of a Li_2 molecule with two lithium atoms and a Li_3 molecule with three lithium atoms. Two molecular orbitals are formed in Li_2, and three molecular orbitals are formed in Li_3. Electrons occupy orbits of lower energy.

Molecular orbital formation of 2s electrons in lithium atom is shown in Fig. 2.2A. As the number of bonded atoms increases, the number of electron orbitals increases. Therefore, when a solid metal is formed, a huge number of atoms bond together, resulting in the formation of a huge number of electron orbitals. Therefore, the difference in energy between each electron orbit becomes extremely small, and it appears as if the electron orbits have continuous energy. This is called the "electron orbital band". Continuous change in energy level due to distance between atoms is shown in Fig. 2.2B. This figure shows the band formation and the overlap of the 2s and 2p orbital bands. On the contrary, splitting of intraatomic electron orbital and orbital band formation during crystal growth from atomic groups is shown in Fig. 2.2C. Electrons can basically only move within a band. If the band gap energy (E_g) is large, electrons cannot move between bands. Depending on the mode of electron transfer, band structure, and E_g, solid materials can be classified into metals, insulators, and semiconductors, as shown in Fig. 2.3A. In the case of metals, the highest energy band is occupied with electrons only up to the middle energy and

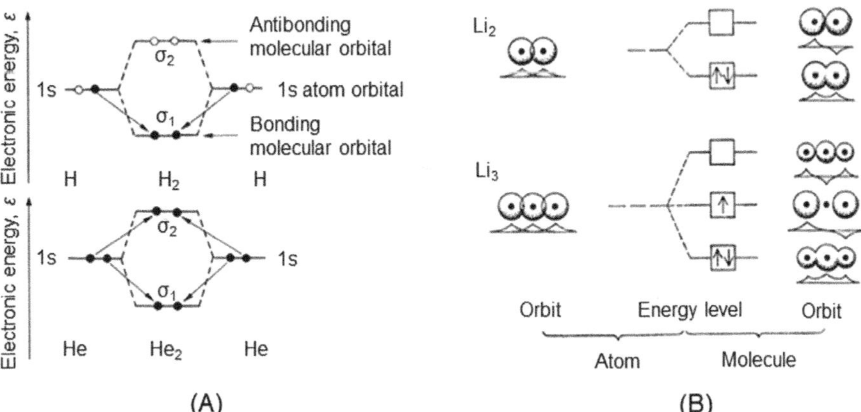

Fig. 2.1. Schematic illustrations of orbital splitting in the production of molecules from hydrogen and helium atoms (A) and orbitals and energy levels of lithium atoms and lithium molecules, Li_2 and Li_3 (B). Electron orbits are created for the number of atoms that combine to form a molecule. Only two electrons can fit into each electron orbit, and basically the orbits with the lowest energy fill up first.

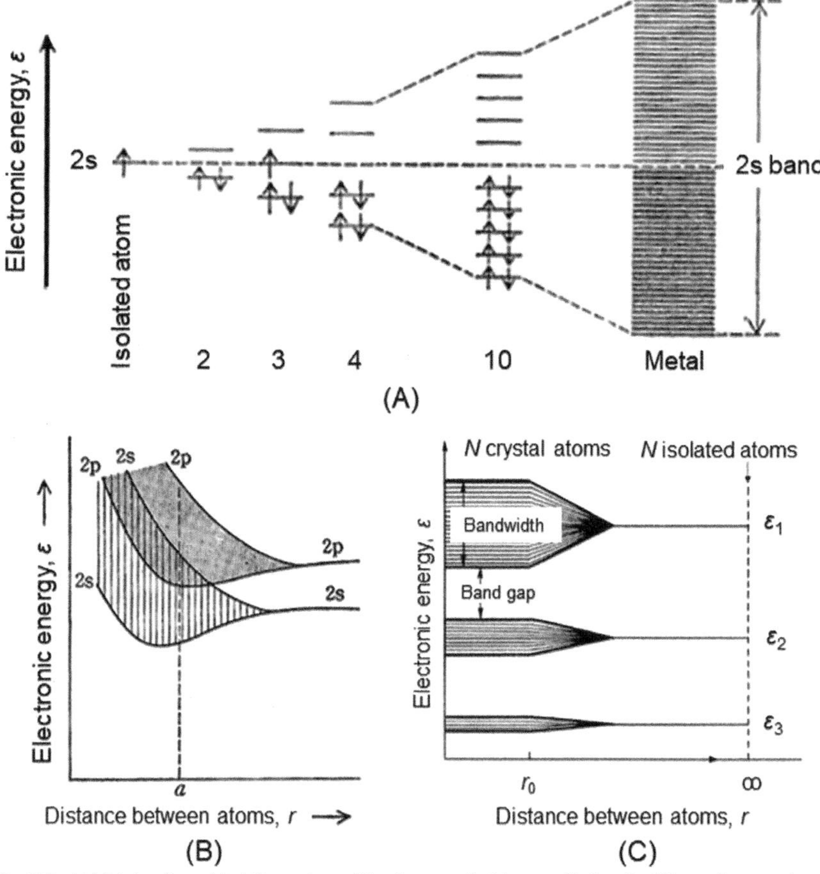

Fig. 2.2. (A) Molecular orbital formation of 2s electrons in Li atom (2s band), (B) continuous change in energy level due to distance between atoms, and (C) splitting of intraatomic electron orbital and orbital band formation during crystal growth from atomic groups. r_0: distance between atoms in crystal. ε_1, ε_2, and ε_2: electronic orbital level in isolated atom. Since solids have a huge number of atoms bonded together, the energy of the huge number of electron orbits that are generated is almost continuous, forming bands in which electrons can move freely.

the high energy side is empty, allowing electrons to move freely within the band. The upper limit of the energy at which the ground state is occupied with electrons is called the "Fermi level energy (E_F)." For an insulator, the lower energy band is completely filled and the higher energy band is empty. However, because the E_g is large, electrons cannot move. In the case of semiconductors, the E_g is small, so if the conditions are proper, electrons can move from a low energy band to a high energy band by external stimulation. Conversely, electrons can also move from higher bands to lower bands. Conceptual diagram of electronic band level occupancy in metallic Na, metallic Cu, and metallic Fe, is shown in Fig. 2.3B. Electrons can move freely in the bands including E_F of metals. As another example, schematic diagram of the density of states-energy curves of the 3s and 3p bands of metallic Mg occupied with electrons up to the E_F is shown in Fig. 2.3C. In this way, in metals, electrons can

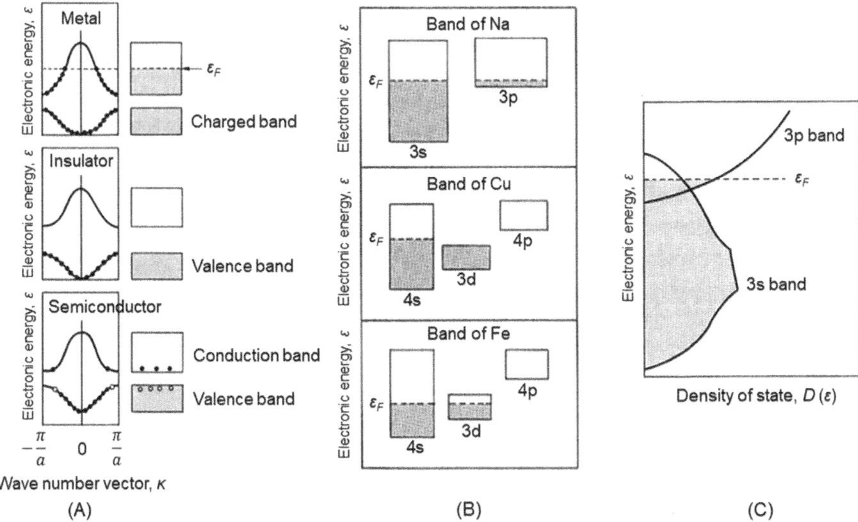

Fig. 2.3. (A) Classification of metals, insulators, and semiconductors based on simple energy band structure and differences in electron band occupancy. Solid circle: Level occupied electron. White circles: level unoccupied electrons. (B) Conceptual diagram of electronic band level occupancy in metallic sodium, metallic copper, and metallic iron. (C) Schematic diagram of the density of states-energy curves of the 3s and 3p bands of magnesium metal. The band is filled with electrons up to the Fermi level in the ground state. Electrons can easily move to an energy region above the Fermi level by external physical stimulation.

move freely within the band where the E_F exists. This is a "free electron". For details on the theory of molecular orbital formation and electron energy band, refer to many excellent textbooks (Abrikosov 2017, Brandt and Chudinov 1975, Ziman 1969).

Metals consist of metallic bond in general (Fig. 2.4). In a metallic bond, atoms alternately emit electrons from their outermost shells to stabilize themselves, and try to balance their charges with equivalent charges, exchanging electrons with neighboring atoms and sharing electrons. The shared electrons become free electrons and move freely in the metal crystals. The characteristics of metals is the property of the crystal consisting of metallic bond. In other words, metals generally refer to polycrystalline consisting of metallic bonds.[2]

2.3 Structure of Metals and Alloys

Metals exhibit great plasticity because, even if atoms are slipped and the metallic bonds are once destroyed, the metallic bonds are immediately regenerated by the action of free electrons. Unlike ionic and covalent bonds, metallic bonds do not show a clear anisotropy in their bonding force. Practically important metals are solids with a relatively simple atomic arrangement (crystal structure), having a body-centered cubic (bcc), face-centered cubic (fcc), or hexagonal closed packing (hcp) (Fig. 2.5).

[2] When an aggregate solid of metallic bonds is a metal, it can be said that a material with Fermi level energy is a metal.

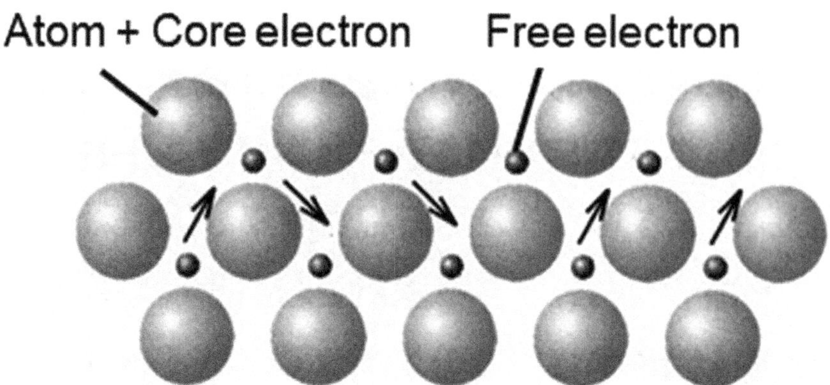

Fig. 2.4. Schematic diagram of metallic bond. Atoms alternately emit electrons from their outermost shells to stabilize themselves, and try to balance their charges with equivalent charges, exchanging electrons with neighboring atoms and sharing electrons. The shared electrons become free electrons and move freely in the metal crystals. The characteristics of metallic materials is the property of the crystal consisting of metallic bond.

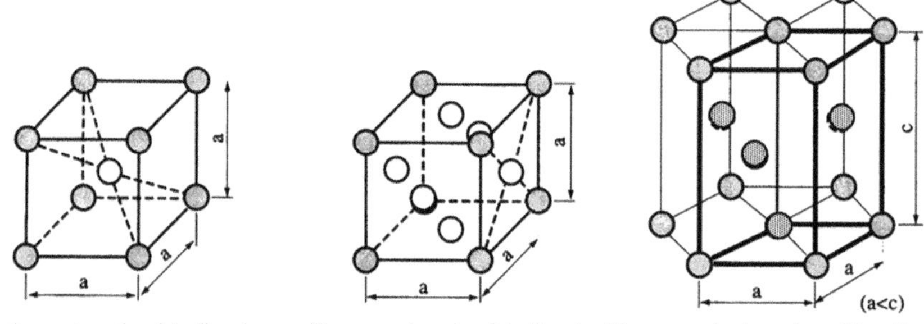

Fig. 2.5. Types of crystal structures of metallic materials. Symbols, a and c are values called lattice constants and represent the size of the crystal lattice. These crystal structure differences govern the mechanical properties of pure metals and alloys. As the temperature increases, the crystal structure changes to a different structure. For example, Ti is hcp at room temperature, but transforms to bcc at temperatures above 882°C.

Among pure metals, at room temperature, Fe, Cr, Mo, W, Nb, Ta, etc. have bcc structures, Au, Ag, Pt, Cu, Ni, Al, etc. have fcc structures, and Ti, Co, Mg, Zn, Cd, etc., have hcp structures.

Metals are usually used as alloys rather than pure metals. An alloy is "a material that consists of two or more types of elements, including at least one metal element, and exhibits metallic properties." In other words, although not all of the constituent elements need to be metal elements, it generally refers to a mixture of two or more metal elements and consists of metallic bonds. Commercially pure Ti (CP Ti) can be said to be an alloy of Ti containing impurity elements. On the other hand, Fe usually contains a large amount of C as an impurity element, and its properties vary greatly depending on the amount of C, so it is used as Fe–C alloys (this is called steel). All metals, including CP Ti and Fe, always contain impurities, and

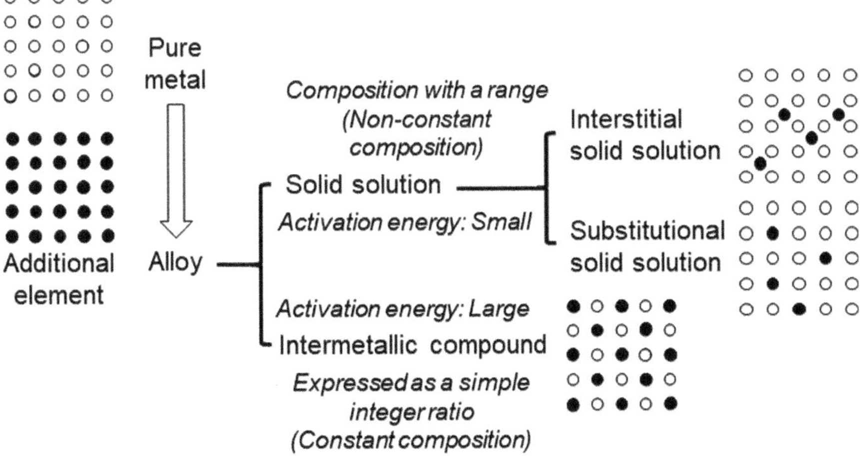

Fig. 2.6. Classification of alloys by structure (solid solutions and intermetallic compounds) and characteristics of metals manifested by metallic bond. Many alloys used in medical devices, such as Ti alloys, Cot-based alloys, and stainless steels, are used in solid solution. Ni-Ti shape memory and superelastic alloy is an intermetallic compound. Activation energy between solvent element and solute element and the compositions governs to form solid solution or intermetallic compound.

there is no genuine pure metal. Alloying produces effects such as decreasing the melting point, increasing strength, and improving corrosion resistance. Alloy compositions are expressed in mass% unless otherwise specified, starting with the alloy component with the highest concentration. For example, Ti–6Al–4V alloy is a 90mass%Ti–6mass%Al–4mass%V alloy. Also, as in the case of Co–Cr–Mo alloy, some compositions are often represented by only the constituent elements.

The crystal structure of an alloy is classified into "solid solution" and "intermetallic compound", as shown in Fig. 2.6, depending on the arrangement of the constituent elements. A solid solution is a phase that is mixed at the atomic level in a solid. The atoms that are present in large amounts are called solvent atoms; the atoms that are contained in small amounts are called solute atoms. There are two ways to mix solute atoms to form a solid solution: interstitial and substitutional, as shown in Fig. 2.6. The interstitial type occurs when solute atoms are extremely small and enter the spaces among solvent atoms and occur when the atomic radii differ greatly, such as in Fe–C alloys. However, most solid solutions are substitutional, in which solute atoms replace solvent atoms. Substitutional solid solutions are usually disordered lattice, but sometimes the solute atoms are arranged regularly. Such solid solutions are called ordered lattice or super lattice. In Au–Cu alloys, this ordered lattice is formed depending on the conditions, and heat treatment is performed through ordered-disorder transformation (see Subsection 9.2.3). An intermediate phase different from the solid solutions described above appears in the composition between each solid solution. In this intermediate phase, when the number of constituent atoms have a simple integer ratio and each metal atom is in a fixed position, the phase is called

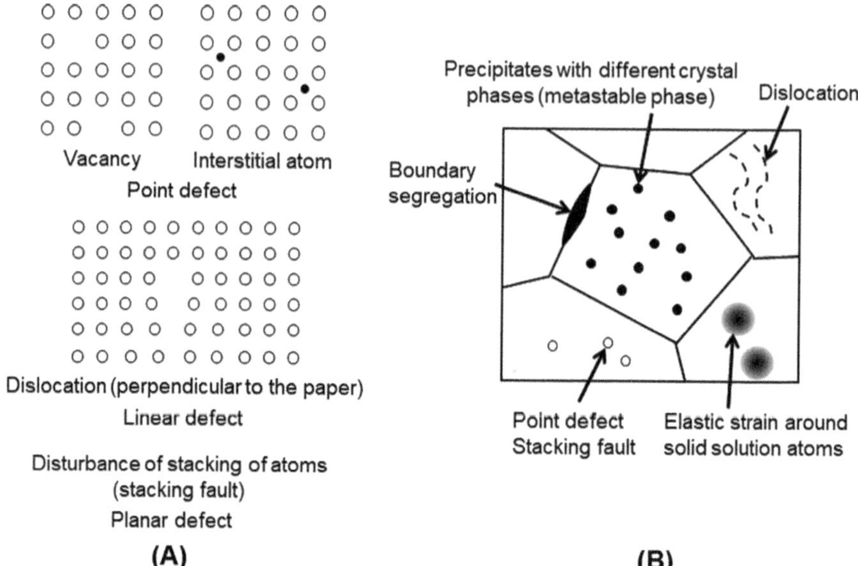

Fig. 2.7. (A) Defects and (B) structural model in crystals of metallic materials. Common crystals always contain many defects that govern the mechanical property of the materials. In particular, the strength is determined by the control of the motion of dislocations.

intermetallic compound. Intermetallic compounds have complex crystal structures and are difficult to deform, hard, brittle, and in many cases heat resistant. Ni–Ti alloy, which exhibits shape memory effect and superelasticity, is an intermetallic compound represented by NiTi. Intermetallic compounds can be expressed as a ratio of the number of atoms, such as AxBy. Examples include Ag_3Sn, $CuAl_2$, Mg_2Si, and ZnS.

In practical metals, perfect crystals do not exist, and defects are inevitably introduced during the manufacturing process as shown in Fig. 2.7A. Therefore, as shown in Fig. 2.7B, crystals always contain defects, and in many cases, another metastable crystal phase (non-equilibrium phase) exists within the crystal grains. Figure 2.8 shows the positions on the periodic table of the constituent elements of Ti alloys, Co-based alloys, stainless steels, and Au alloys used for medical devices and dental restorations. These alloys are composed of elements located relatively close together to form a solid solution, and these elements were selected empirically. Intermetallic compounds are formed between elements located far apart in the periodic table.

2.4 Phase Transformation and Structure

Generally, substances have three states: gas (gas phase), liquid (liquid phase), and solid (solid phase). Metals are no exception; when a solid is heated, it becomes a liquid, and when heated further, it becomes a gas. This change in state (phase) is called "transformation". In metals, the transformation from solid to liquid or from liquid to solid is clearly recognized, while in addition to this, when a solid is

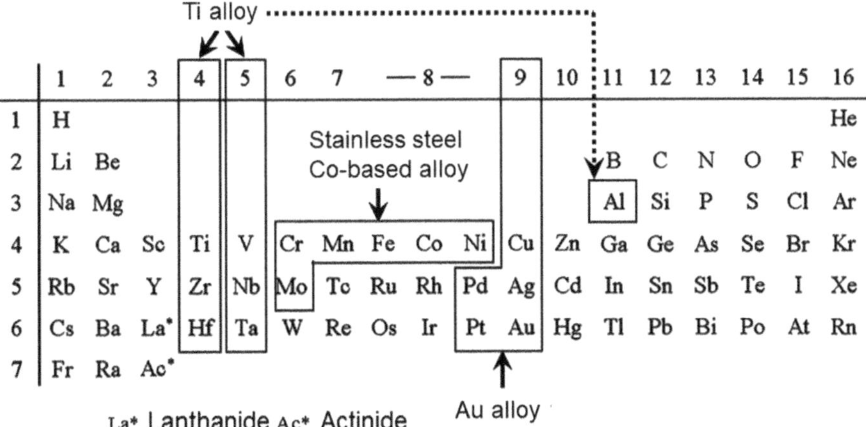

Fig. 2.8. Constituent elements of Ti alloys, Co-based alloys, stainless steels, and Au alloys on the periodic table. These practical alloys are used as solid solution phases. In other words, the component elements and compositions were determined to form solid solutions empirically.

heated, one crystal structure changes to another without any visible change. Phase transformation is extremely important for metals. Even with pure metals, in addition to transformation between the liquid phase and the solid phase, i.e. melting or solidification, phase transformation usually occurs within the solid phase as well. For example, CP Ti in the α phase of a hcp lattice at low temperatures transforms into the β phase of a bcc lattice above 882°C, and becomes a liquid phase at 1670°C. Figure 2.9 shows the Fe–C system equilibrium phase diagram. Particularly important phases in steel are the ferrite (α) phase with a bcc lattice and the austenite phase (γ) phase with an fcc lattice. There is a martensitic phase exhibiting an acicular structure with a bcc lattice. Martensitic transformation is a phase transformation that does not involve atomic diffusion, observed in Fe alloys such as stainless steel, Ti alloys, etc., and the crystal structure changes by chaining each atom's movement in a fixed direction within one atomic distance. The shape memory effect seen in Ni–Ti alloys is caused by martensitic transformation (see Subsection 9.3). In the case of alloys, the transformation from one phase to another does not occur all at once at a certain temperature, but a mixed phase region with a temperature range appears. An equilibrium phase diagram shows the phases that exist in an equilibrium state at a certain composition and temperature. However, since the practical phase transformation occurs in a non-equilibrium state, the transformation does not necessarily follow the equilibrium phase diagram. Therefore, a non-equilibrium phase diagram is also required. Heat treatment actively utilizes the precipitation of non-equilibrium phases. Phase transformation refers to passing through a line on a phase diagram due to temperature change, and by performing heat treatment using phase transformation, mechanical properties can be significantly improved. For example, Ti alloys can be classified into a few types depending on their phase diagrams. Phase diagrams are essential for predicting the design, mechanical properties, and heat treatment effects of alloys, and it is impossible to discuss the mechanical properties of alloys without phase diagrams. Manufacturing processes such as working and heat

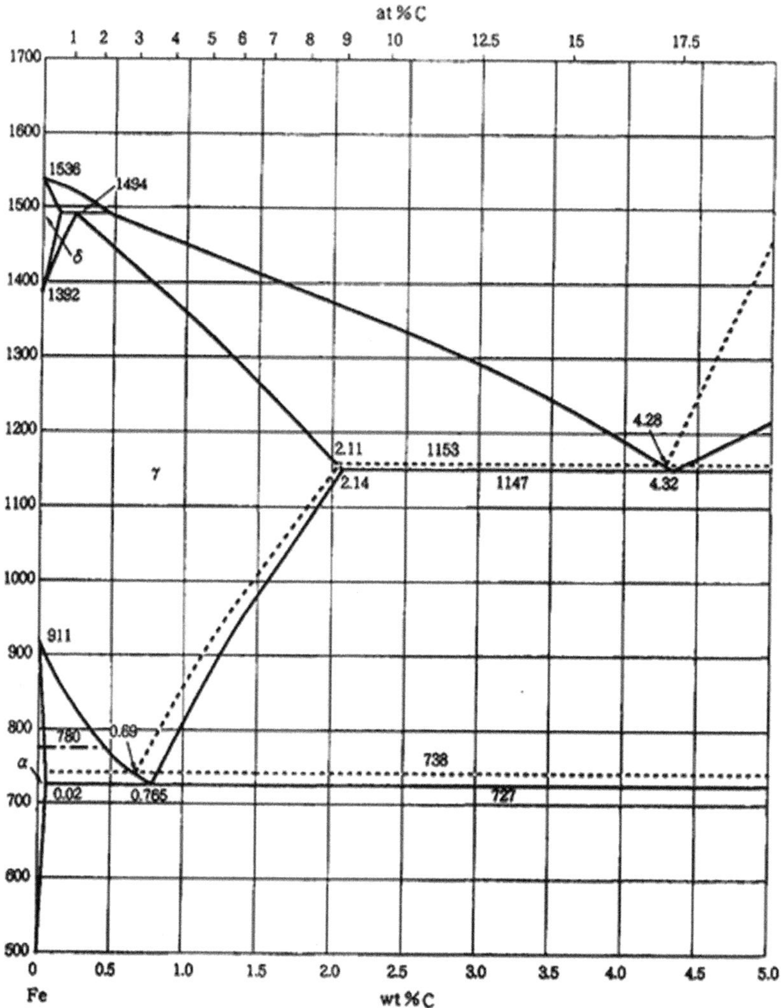

Fig. 2.9. Fe-C binary system equilibrium phase diagram. The dashed line is the so-called Fe-graphite stable system. Equilibrium phases are determined by both temperature and composition. There is unequilibrium phase not shown in equilibrium diagram, such as martensitic phase.

treatment are extremely important for metals. This manufacturing process results in the introduction of defects, precipitation of metastable phases, and grain refinement, which govern the mechanical properties (Fig. 2.10). A feature of metals is that even if they have the same composition, it is possible to create materials with many different properties by changing the manufacturing process such as working and heat treatment. In other words, when deforming or heating a metal, it is necessary to confirm whether these changes occur.

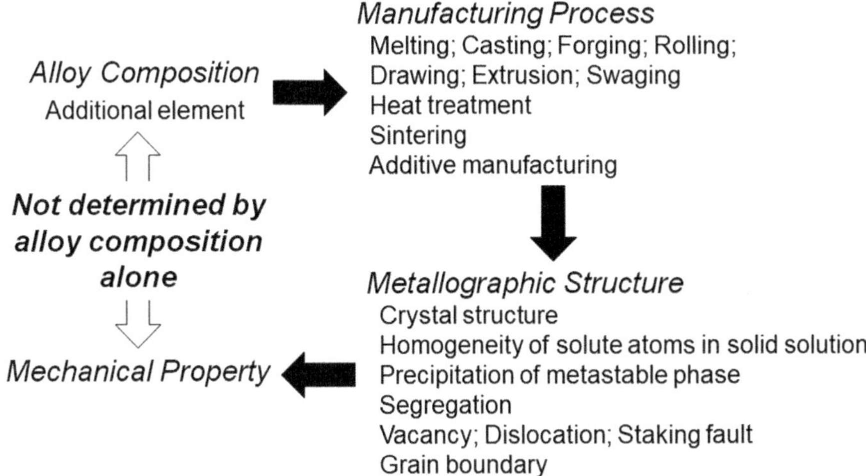

Fig. 2.10. The influence of the manufacturing process of metals on the crystal structure that controls mechanical properties. Mechanical property is strongly influenced by metallographic structure that is governed by manufacturing process. Therefore, mechanical property of the metals is not determined by their compositions unitarily.

2.5 Plastic Deformation and Dislocation

2.5.1 Slip Deformation and Dislocation

When an external force is applied to a single crystal, its components generate shear stress along various atomic planes, acting to cause displacement along the atomic planes. In the case of metal crystals, the force required to separate the bonds all at once between atoms is much greater than the practically observed force required to cause a displacement in the atomic planes. In other words, the force required to break the bonds all at once between atoms is much greater than the practical force required to cause a displacement in the atomic planes (Fig. 2.11A). The direction of this slip is called the slip direction, and this is determined by the crystal structure. The larger the atomic density of the plane, the larger the distance between the planes, and the relative slip between the atomic planes is likely to occur. Conversely, in the direction where the interatomic distance is small, the bonds between atoms are strong and it is difficult for them to separate from each other. In other words, slip occurs in the direction of maximum atomic density on the plane of maximum atomic density. When a single-crystal specimen slips due to deformation, a step is created where the slip plane intersects the specimen surface. This is called a slip line, shown in the picture in Fig. 2.11. This deformation is called "slip deformation".

When an external force is applied to a metal crystal, the force causes to relatively shift the positions of the atoms along the slip plane. If the shear stress is calculated assuming that all atoms are completely displaced along the slip plane, it will be about 1000 times the practical value. In order to explain this contradiction, the idea was introduced that instead of the entire atomic plane slipping at the same time, the atoms shift one by one in sequence. When shear stress is applied to a crystal as shown in

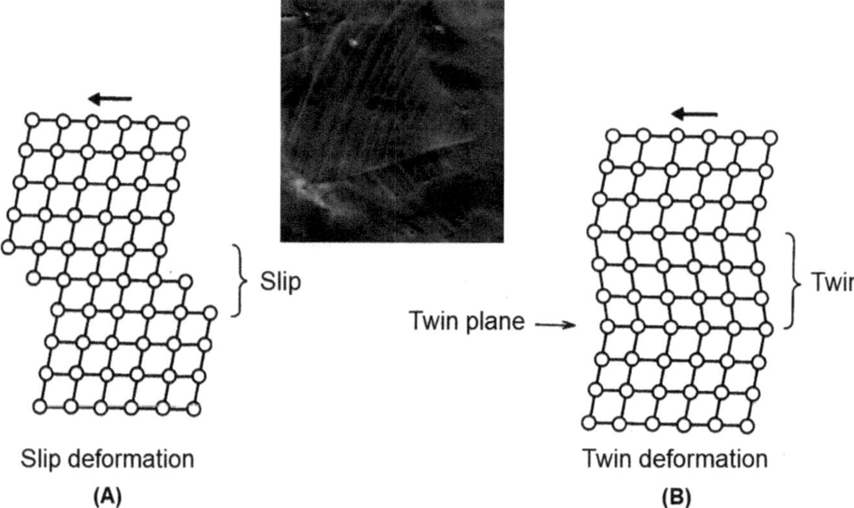

Fig. 2.11. Changes in atomic arrangement due to slip deformation (A) and twin deformation (B) for plastic deformation. Slip deformation occurs by the motion of dislocations. Therefore, metals can be strengthened due to the control of the motion of dislocations. Shape memory and superelastic alloys plastically deform by twin deformation. The scanning electron micrograph between both model (A) and (B) shows step lines formed by slip deformation.

Fig. 2.12A, elastic deformation occurs as shown in Fig. 2.12B. When a larger force is applied, slipping occurs on the slip plane, and when it slips halfway, as shown in Fig. 2.12C, there are places where the vertical atomic planes are interrupted midway above and below the slipping surface. This interrupted part is called a "dislocation." Dislocations generate on the slip plane at the boundary between the slip region and the non-slip region, so rather than just one atom being displaced inside the crystal, the state shown in Fig. 2.12C, continues perpendicular to the plane of the paper. In other words, in the case of slip deformation, dislocations move when plastic deformation occurs, and the atoms eventually shift relative to each other, as shown in Fig. 2.12D. Conversely, if dislocations cannot move, plastic deformation due to slip will not occur.

2.5.2 Strengthening

From the above, metals can be made stronger by suppressing the movement of dislocations. There are several ways to do this:

(A) Eliminate dislocations.

(B) Create a state where a large force is required to move the dislocation.

(C) Reduce the distance that dislocations can travel.

Since it is not possible to eliminate dislocations in ordinary metals, the following methods are used to strengthen metals, aiming at B and C above.

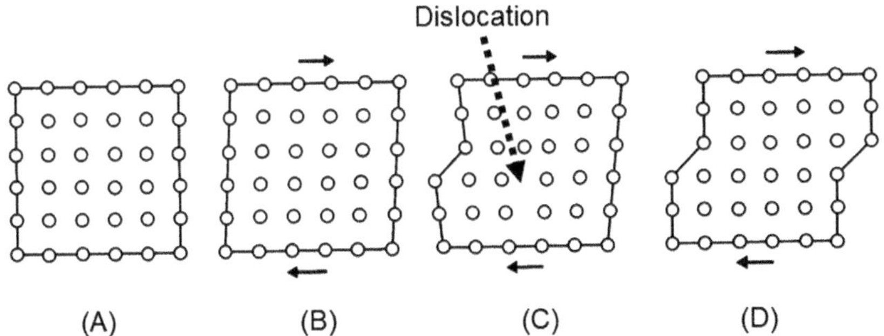

Fig. 2.12. Slip deformation process due to dislocation movement. The arrows indicate the direction of shear stress. The motion of dislocation generates slip deformation or plastic deformation of crystals.

Solid Solution Strengthening

When solute atoms are dissolved in a crystal as shown in Fig. 2.13, the atomic arrangement is disordered due to the difference in the size of the atoms, resulting in an elastic strain field. Depending on the size of the solute atoms, it exerts an attractive force or a repulsive force on the dislocation. This makes the movement of dislocations difficult and strengthens the crystal. Fixed dislocations are released from fixation and become movable by external force or heat.

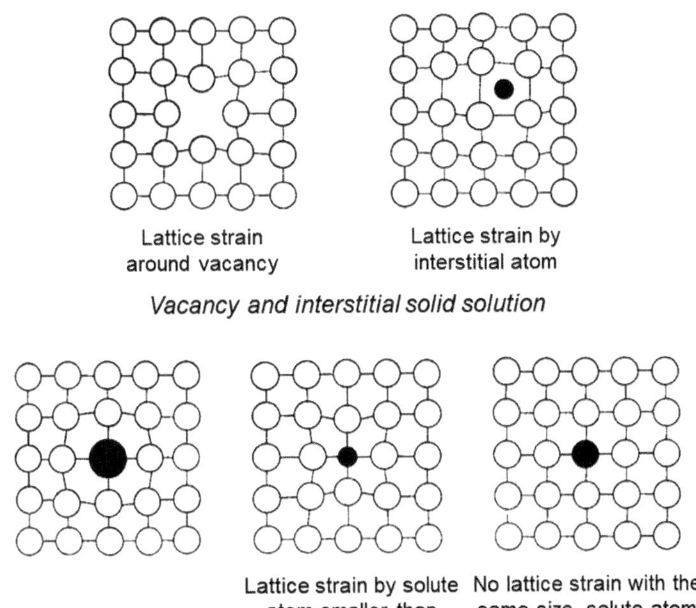

Fig. 2.13. Mechanism of solid solution strengthening by crystal lattice strain due to defects and substitutional solute atoms. In the case that solute and solvent atoms have almost the same size, the alloy is not strengthened by alloying.

Precipitation Strengthening

When precipitates form in the crystal, two phenomena occur as shown in Fig. 2.14. One is when the precipitate is sheared, as shown in Fig. 2.14A, and extra force is required to shear the particles. The other case is when the particle is strong and not sheared (Fig. 2.14B). In this case, the dislocation lines wrap around the particle and overhang (Fig. 2.14B-3), and eventually the dislocation lines surround the particle. It moves forward leaving behind a ring (Fig. 2.14B-4). In this case, an extra force is required to make the dislocation lines stretch out. In both cases, the metal is strengthened. This is precipitation strengthening. In order to form a precipitate in a crystal, first heated to form a uniform solid solution crystal, then rapidly cooled and held at a certain temperature, and finally microscopic crystals of other phases that should appear at room temperature (precipitation).

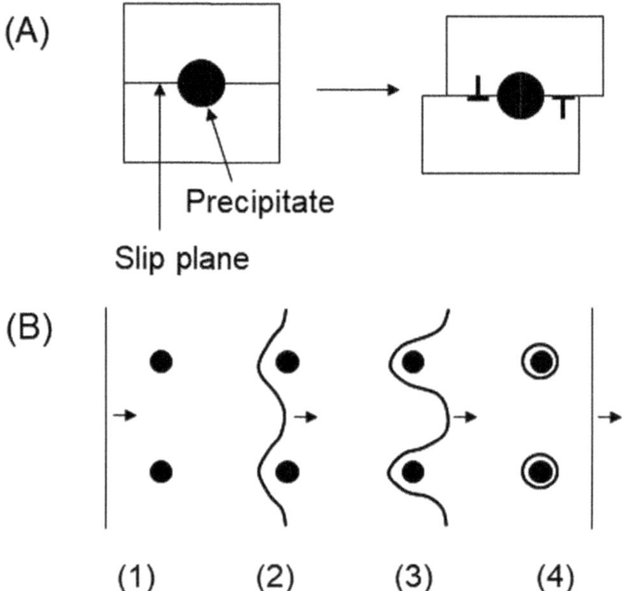

Fig. 2.14. Mechanism of strengthening of metals by precipitation of metastable phases (microcrystals) that act as barriers to dislocation movement. The precipitates are usually unequilibrium phase crystal that are generated by alloying and heat treatments.

Work Strengthening (Work Hardening)

When stress is applied, dislocations are created one after another and multiply. Inside an actual crystal, there are various resistances to the movement of dislocations. This resistance includes dislocations of the same sign, foreign matter within the crystal, and boundaries between crystals (grain boundaries). When this resistance is encountered, the movement of dislocations stops. When dislocations stop, the multiplied dislocations stop one after another at a certain distance and accumulate, making the metal stronger. This is the strengthening of metal through work hardening.

Metal products can be strengthened through cold working. Work hardening increases the strength of the material, but it also makes the material brittle.

Boundary Strengthening

Metals are polycrystalline, and the movement of dislocations is stopped and accumulated at grain boundaries. In order to continue deformation, new dislocations must be created from the crystal or from the grain boundaries. In order to activate boundary strengthening, the refinement of crystal grains is effective because it increases the probability for dislocation to reach grain boundaries.

Apart from the method of preventing dislocation movement explained above, other ways to strengthen metals include dispersion strengthening, which involves dispersing oxide particles or fibers, and composite strengthening, which involves combining the metals with other alloys, ceramics, etc.

2.5.3 Twin Deformation

Twin deformation is a mechanism for plastic deformation that does not involve slip. As shown in Fig. 2.11B, a twin is a part of a crystal that has an atomic arrangement that is mirror-symmetric with the original crystal, with specific planes as boundaries. The boundary plane is called the twin plane. Twin is formed by shear movement of atoms. In slip deformation, the orientation of the crystal in the slipped and non-slipping parts does not change, while in twin deformation, the orientation of the crystal differs on both sides of the twin plane. Twin deformation is important for understanding the mechanism of shape memory effect and superelasticity in Ni–Ti alloys (see Section 9.3).

2.6 Improvement of Crystal Structure by Additive Manufacturing

Additive Manufacturing (AM), a type of 3D printing, is a rapidly expanding technology in many fields. AM is a process in which raw materials are supplied, melted, and solidified from digital 3D data using energy sources such as lasers, electron beams, and plasma to form products layer by layer (ASM Handbook Vol. 24 and 24A 2023). Compared to traditional manufacturing processes, AM can create extremely complex parts from CAD models in less time and with higher yields. Currently, many studies are being conducted to compare the mechanical properties, corrosion behavior, and microstructure of metals fabricated by AM and conventional processes (Ko et al. 2021). In all AM processes, the final microstructure, mechanical properties, and corrosion behavior are strongly dependent on the building conditions, and it is possible to build unique microstructures through AM processes. The average grain size of metals is 30–60 μm for ordinary wrought materials, whereas the average grain size of type 316L stainless steel formed by selective laser melting (SLM) is extremely fine, 10 μm. Moreover, it is possible to improve not only the composition, distribution, and size of the metastable phase of the built body, but also the electrochemical property (Sander et al. 2018).

AM enables the production of complex, net-shape geometries. Additionally, in AM of metal and ceramics, the microstructure and texture of the product, which has received less attention, can be arbitrarily controlled by selecting appropriate process parameters, thereby enabling unprecedented superior properties. One of the unique characteristics of AM is that the texture can be varied as a function of position within the product by controlling the scan strategy. The crystallographic "multiplicity" of the preferential crystal growth direction is important to understand the evolution behavior of the texture in such materials (Hagihara and Naknao 2022).

2.7 Surface Structure of Metals

At the surface, surrounding molecules are adsorbed, creating a stable state to decrease energy. When oxygen is present, oxygen atoms and metal atoms chemically bond that cause an oxide layer on the surface. In metals, the surface concentrations of constituent elements easily change depending on the environment, so the surface composition at the nanometer level is different from the bulk composition, compared with ceramics and polymers. Surface hydroxyl groups are always present on the surface oxides, and water is adsorbed on top of them (Fig. 2.15).

Some kind of reaction film is always formed on the surface of metals as corrosion progresses. Among the reaction films, "passive films" are important for metallic biomaterials. When a reaction film formed in an aqueous solution has extremely low solubility, no pores, and good adhesion to the substrate, it becomes a corrosion-resistant film or "passive film". The passive film is extremely thin (1–5 nm) and transparent, so it cannot be seen with the naked eye. Generally, the

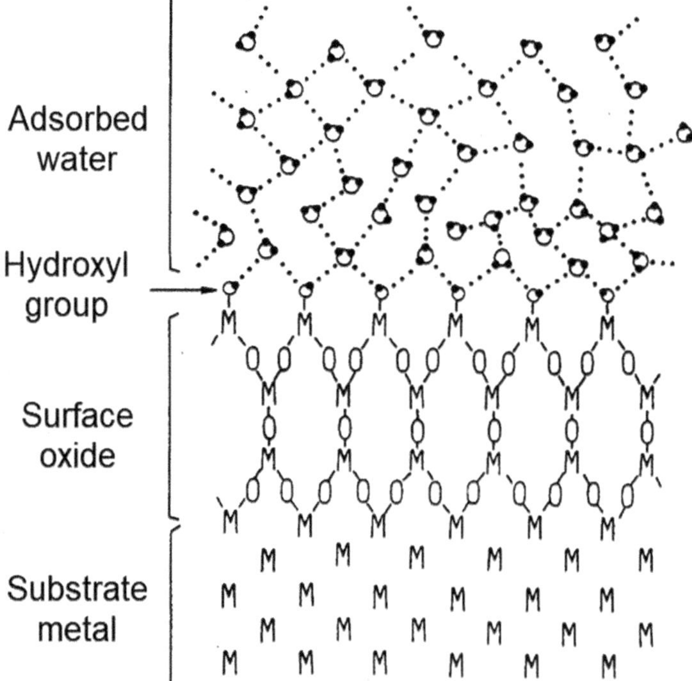

Fig. 2.15. Schematic model of surface structure of metals. Metals usually covered by metal oxide that is covered by hydroxyl groups. Bare metal substrate does not appear on the surface.

Immediate regeneration after rupture

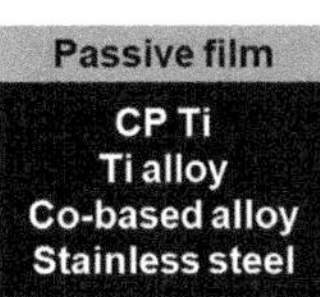

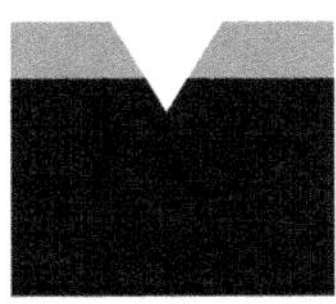

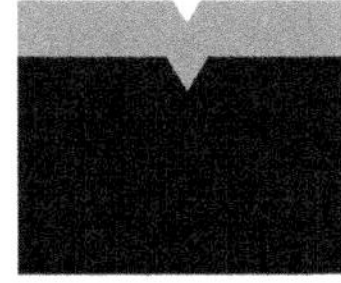

Fig. 2.16. Passive films on passive metals such as CP Ti, Ti alloys, Co-based alloys, and stainless steels and their regeneration after rupture. In the case of CP Ti, regeneration begins at 10^{-8} s after rupture and regeneration completes at 10^{-2} s after rupture. Composition of passive film on CP Ti consists of non-stoichiometric TiO_2 containing Ti^{2+}, Ti^{3+}, OH^-, and H_2O. The passive film is a kind of oxide formed on metal substrate shown in Fig. 2.15 and protect metals against corrosion.

formation rate of passive films is extremely high, so the film tends to become amorphous (non-crystalline). Amorphous films have no grain boundaries and have few structural defects, so they have excellent corrosion resistance. Surfaces of some metallic biomaterials such as CP Ti, Ti alloys, Co–Cr alloys, and stainless steels are covered with a passive film in normal living bodies, which prevents the corrosion and makes them look like noble metals (Fig. 2.16) (see Section 3.14). This state in which the surface becomes apparently chemically stable due to the passive film is called "passivity". Even in the atmosphere, oxidation progresses due to the moisture in the air; CP Ti and Ti alloys, in the product state as biomaterials, are always covered with passive films and become passivated. The passive film is extremely thin and easily destroyed, but it quickly repairs itself and maintains corrosion resistance (see Section 5.8). Although the passive film is apparently stable, microscopically it undergoes repeated partial dissolution and re-precipitation, and its composition changes over time depending on the environment (Kelly 1982). When using metals in environments where they contact with living tissue or blood, it is important to be aware that these surfaces change. Normally, Au can be reused by cleaning it with acid after use in a biological environment, whereas with CP Ti it is impossible to chemically return it to its original condition, and the only way to return to the original clean surface is to mechanically create a new surface by polishing.

2.8 Concept of Corrosion

Corrosion is a phenomenon in which metals are deteriorated and damaged by chemical or electrochemical reactions, and is a reaction that both releases metal ions and forms some kind of reaction film or layer (corrosion product) on the surface. The passive film described above is a kind of corrosion product. Metal elements rarely exist as single metals in nature, and with the exception of Au, they are usually mined as ores in the form of oxides, hydroxides, and sulfides. The ores are turned into metals through a reduction reaction called smelting. When metals are left in their natural state, they will eventually dissolve or oxidize through corrosion, return to their original oxide state, and return to earth (Fig. 2.17). Corrosion is a process in which metal products dissolve, release metal ions, and form oxides. This occurs because metal elements are more stable when they form compounds such as oxides, and metal products are destined to corrode eventually if left untreated. However, it is possible to reduce the corrosion rate to near zero. Practical corrosion resistant alloys

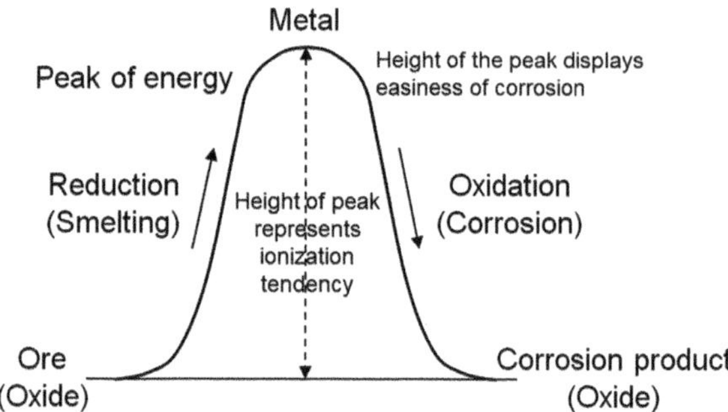

Fig. 2.17. Principles of corrosion of metals. Metals made from oxides as ores will corrode sooner or later and revert to oxides as corrosion products. Easiness of corrosion is determined by chemical energy of metallic state (height of peak), listed in Table 2.1.

have succeeded in extremely slowing down the corrosion rate. Regarding corrosion of metals, many textbooks have been published (Revie and Uhlig 2008, McCafferty 2010, Perez 2016, Predeferri 2018), so refer the detail to them.

Oxidation-reduction potentials versus hydrogen electrode (standard electrode potentials) are listed in Table 2.1. Metal elements such as Au, Pd, Hg, and Ag that have a small ionization tendency (large standard electrode potential) and are difficult to naturally oxidize are called "noble metals." Noble metal alloys or precious alloys, such as dental Au alloys, have high corrosion resistance because they contain noble metals as their main component. On the other hand, constituent elements in major metals for medical devices, such as Ti, Zr, and Ta, have a strong ionization tendency and are extremely easily passivated. Thus, the metals used for medical devices are noble alloys or passive alloys.

2.9 Corrosion Reaction

The dissolution or oxidation reaction of metals is as follows, assuming that the metal element is M as shown in Fig. 2.18.

$$M \rightarrow Mn+ + ne^- \quad (2.1)$$

It is expressed by the formula, and taking Fe as an example,

$$Fe \rightarrow Fe^{2+} + 2e^- \quad (2.2)$$

This reaction is called an anodic reaction. The anodic reaction cannot proceed unless a reaction occurs somewhere that consumes the electrons generated in the anodic reactions (2.1) and (2.2). In this case, on the same metal,

$$2H^+ + 2e^- \rightarrow H_2 \text{ (acidic aqueous solution)} \quad (2.3)$$

$$O_2 + H_2O + 4e^- \rightarrow 4OH^- \text{ (neutral/alkaline aqueous solution)} \quad (2.4)$$

Electrons are consumed by the above reactions. The reactions of formulas (2.3) and (2.4) are called cathodic reactions. What is important here is that an anodic

Table 2.1. Standard electrode potential versus standard hydrogen electrode (SHE) at 25°C.

Electrode reaction (oxidation-reduction reaction)	Standard electrode potential (V vs. SHE)		Order of practical corrosion resistance as bulk solid
$Au^{3+} + 3e^- \leftrightarrow Au$	1.498		Rh
$Pt^{2+} + 2e^- \leftrightarrow Pt$	1.18		Nb
$Ir^{3+} + 3e^- \leftrightarrow Ir$	1.156		Au
$Pd^{2+} + 2e^- \leftrightarrow Pd$	0.951		Ir
$Hg^{2+} + 2e^- \leftrightarrow Hg$	0.854		Pt
$Ag^+ + e^- \leftrightarrow Ag$	0.800		Ti
$Rh^{3+} + 3e^- \leftrightarrow Rh$	0.758		Pd
$Cu^+ + e^- \leftrightarrow Cu$	0.521		Ru
$Ru^{2+} + 2e^- \leftrightarrow Ru$	0.455		Hg
$2H^+ + 2e^- \leftrightarrow H_2$	0 (Standard)		
$Sn^{2+} + 2e^- \leftrightarrow Sn$	−0.138		Ga
$Mo^{2+} + 2e^- \leftrightarrow Mo$	−0.200		Zr
$Ni^{2+} + 2e^- \leftrightarrow Ni$	−0.257		Ag
$Co^{2+} + 2e^- \leftrightarrow Co$	−0.28		Sn
$In^{3+} + 3e^- \leftrightarrow In$	−0.338		Cu
$Fe^{2+} + 2e^- \leftrightarrow Fe$	−0.447		Be
$Ga^{3+} + 3e^- \leftrightarrow Ga$	−0.549		Hf
$Cr^{3+} + 3e^- \leftrightarrow Cr$	−0.744		Al
$Zn^{2+} + 2e^- \leftrightarrow Zn$	−0.762		In
$Nb^{3+} + 3e^- \leftrightarrow Nb$	−1.099		Cr
$V^{2+} + 2e^- \leftrightarrow V$	−1.175		Fe
$Mn^{2+} + 2e^- \leftrightarrow Mn$	−1.185		Ni
$Zr^{4+} + 4e^- \leftrightarrow Zr$	−1.45		Co
$Hf^{4+} + 4e^- \leftrightarrow Hf$	−1.55		Zn
$Al^{3+} + 3e^- \leftrightarrow Al$	−1.662		Mo
$Ti^{2+} + 2e^- \leftrightarrow Ti$	−1.630		V
$Be^{2+} + 2e^- \leftrightarrow Be$	−1.847		Mg
$Mg^{2+} + 2e^- \leftrightarrow Mg$	−2.372		Mn

reaction is always accompanied by a cathodic reaction. An electron conductor provided for the purpose of causing these reactions is called an electrode. The electrode where an anodic reaction occurs is called an anode; the electrode where a cathodic reaction occurs is called a cathode. Corrosion occurs when the reactions of formulas (2.1)–(2.4) proceed spontaneously without an excess or deficiency of electrons in the anodic and cathodic reactions. For example, in an acidic aqueous solution, Fe is calculated from the sum of formula (2.2) and formula (2.3):

$$Fe + 2H^+ \rightarrow Fe^{2+} + H_2 \text{ (generally } M + nH^+ \rightarrow Mn^+ + (n/2)H_2) \qquad (2.5)$$

However, whether or not the reaction in equation (2.5) proceeds spontaneously depends on the size of the Gibbs free energy, ΔG, of the reaction in equation (2.5). This energy, ΔG, is the energy (height) shown in Fig. 2.17. When a certain metal

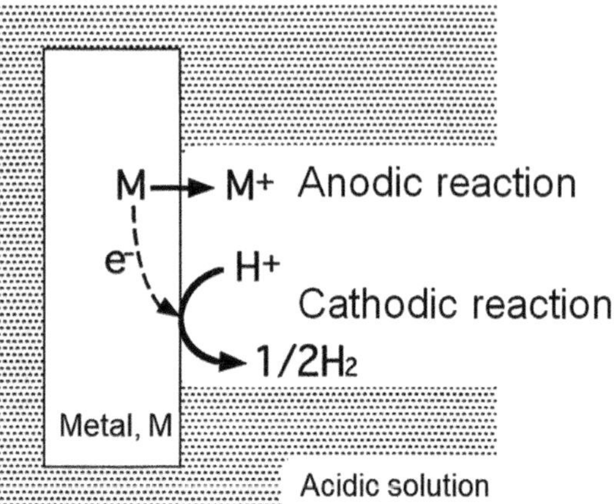

Fig. 2.18. Electrode reaction in an acidic solution. To corrode the metal, both anodic and cathodic reactions must occur simultaneously. If one of them is stooped, corrosion does not occur.

exists in an aqueous solution, the potential of the metal electrode when the oxidant, Ox, and the reductant, Red, are in equilibrium is called the equilibrium potential or redox potential E_{eq}, as shown in the following equation.

$$E_{eq} = E^0(\mathrm{Ox/Red}) + (RT/nF)\ln\{a(\mathrm{Ox})/a(\mathrm{Red})\} \quad (2.6)$$

where a is the activity (concentration), R is the gas constant, n is the valence of the oxidant, and F is the Faraday constant. Equation (2.6) is called the "Nernst equation". E^0 is the electrode potential when the standard electrode potential of hydrogen is set to 0 (based on the hydrogen electrode (natural hydrogen electrode: NHE or standard hydrogen electrode: SHE)) (Table 2.1). For example, in a Ti electrode, since Ti is a solid and its activity a(Ti) = 1, the equilibrium potential for the reaction $Ti \leftrightarrow Ti^{2+} + 2e^-$ is

$$E_{eq} = E^0(\mathrm{Ti^{2+}/Ti}) + (RT/4F)\ \ln a(\mathrm{Ti^{2+}}). \quad (2.7)$$

The larger E^0 is, the more negative ΔG is and the larger the absolute value, which means that metal dissolution or oxidation reactions are more likely to occur. E^0 corresponds to the ionization tendency of metals. In this way, the potential of a metal electrode is always expressed as a potential relative to a certain reference electrode.

2.10 Potential-pH Diagram

A potential-pH diagram is a phase diagram showing the potential-pH range in which metals, metal ions, and metal compounds can stably exist at a certain temperature. The potential-pH diagram is also called the Pourbaix diagram (Pourbaix 1966), named after its inventor. A potential-pH diagram is a diagram showing a stable region in an equilibrium state. Although it does not match the actual transient state, it is effective for predicting the state of a metal at a certain potential and pH.

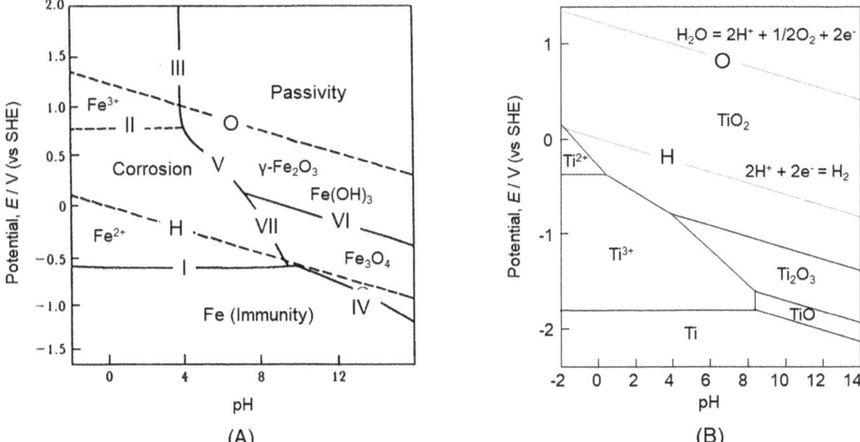

Fig. 2.19. Potential-pH diagram (Pourbaix diagram) of Fe-H_2O system (A) and Ti-H_2O system (B) at 298 K when titanium activity is 10^{-6} (Reproduced from the data of a reference (Pourbaix 1966)). In corrosion territory, corrosion progresses. In passivity territory, the material is passivated and covered by a passive oxide film. In immunity territory, bare metallic state is stable.

Figure 2.19A shows the potential-pH diagram of the Fe–H_2O system. The solid line (boundary line) in the figure shows the equilibrium potential determined by the equation (2.6) between the chemical species described on both sides of the solid line as a function of pH. Each region delimited by a boundary line can be classified into a stable region, a corroded region, and a passive region, depending on the state of existence of the corresponding chemical species. In the region marked "Fe" at the bottom of Fig. 2.19A, Fe is stable in a metallic state. Therefore, if the combination of Fe potential and solution pH is within the same range, no corrosion reaction of Fe can occur. This region is called the immunity zone. In the regions labeled "Fe^{2+}" and "Fe^{3+}", Fe becomes stable in the form of these soluble ions. In this potential-pH region, the Fe electrode continuously dissolves (corrodes) and becomes these ions, which is why it is called the corrosion zone. In addition, in the regions labeled "Fe_2O_3", "Fe_3O_4", and "$Fe(OH)_3$", rarely soluble metal compounds such as oxides and hydroxides are stable and become passive.

The dashed lines "H" and "O" in the figure respectively indicate the equilibrium potential of hydrogen evolution reaction of equation (2.8) and the equilibrium potential of oxygen evolution reaction of equation (2.9).

$$2H^+ + 2e^- \rightarrow H_2 \tag{2.8}$$

$$2H^+ + 1/2O_2 + 2e^- \rightarrow H_2O \tag{2.9}$$

In other words, at any given pH, if the immersion potential of Fe is lower than the dashed line "H", H_2 gas will be generated, and if it is higher than the dashed line "O", O_2 gas will be generated.

As shown in Fig. 2.19A, the boundary line "I" indicating the lower limit potential of the corrosion zone is located on the lower (base) potential side than the dashed line "H", regardless of pH. This means that the hydrogen evolution and

Fe dissolution occur at the same potential (on a single electrode). Moreover, the corrosion potential of Fe is between "H" and "I". Therefore, when Fe is immersed in an acidic aqueous solution, it dissolves while constantly generating hydrogen gas according to equations (2.2) and (2.8). Even in a neutral solution, if a certain concentration of oxygen is dissolved, the immersion potential of Fe will be higher than the dashed line "H", and the reduction reaction of dissolved oxygen (Equation (2.9)) will become a cathodic reaction without hydrogen evolution. Equation (2.2) becomes the anodic reaction, and the dissolution reaction of Fe proceeds as shown in equation (2.5), which is the sum of the reactions.

$$2Fe + O_2 + H_2O \rightarrow 2Fe^{2+} + 4OH^- \tag{2.10}$$

The boundary line in the figure merely indicates the equilibrium potential of one electrode reaction (single electrode reaction). The boundary line "I" in Fig. 2.19A only shows the equilibrium potential of equation (2.5), and at the same time the cathode potential of equation (2.3) or (2.4) that consumes electrons. If the reaction does not proceed, the Fe dissolution will not occur. The passive region in the potential-pH diagram merely indicates the range in which rarely soluble substances such as metal oxides and hydroxides exist stably from a thermodynamic perspective. In other words, there is no guarantee that these substances will actually act as a protective film. Even if it is made of a poorly soluble material, if the film is not dense and has good adhesion, the substrate metal will be corroded by repeated oxidation reactions and peeling through the defects.

Fig. 2.19B shows the potential-pH diagram of the Ti–H_2O system. Basically, it is the same as in the case of Fe–H_2O system, and corrosion reaction of Ti should not occur in the immunity region marked "Ti". However, it is difficult for Ti electrode to decrease real potential under this zone, because the hydrogen evolution occurs preferentially.

The potential-pH diagram used to evaluate corrosion is generally drawn with the ion activity (concentration) on the electrode surface as 10^{-6} mol L^{-1}. This is based on the idea that if the concentration of ions in equilibrium is less than 10^{-6} mol L^{-1} of activity, the electrode can be considered not corroded. The boundary lines in the potential-pH diagram are determined by calculation, so they can be calculated as freely as you like by changing the activity (concentration) of the ions.

2.11 Localized Corrosion

2.11.1 Outline

Uniform (overall) corrosion rarely occurs in metallic biomaterials; it is usually localized. This occurs because the surface oxide film is not repaired for some reason when it is damaged. When an anodic reaction and a cathodic reaction occur on the same electrode, if the locations where both reactions occur are separated and fixed for some reasons, corrosion progresses on the anodic side (Fig. 2.20). Causes of passive film destruction include pitting corrosion, crevice corrosion, grain boundary corrosion, and stress corrosion cracking. In galvanic corrosion, when metals with significantly different potentials come into contact with each other, the metal with

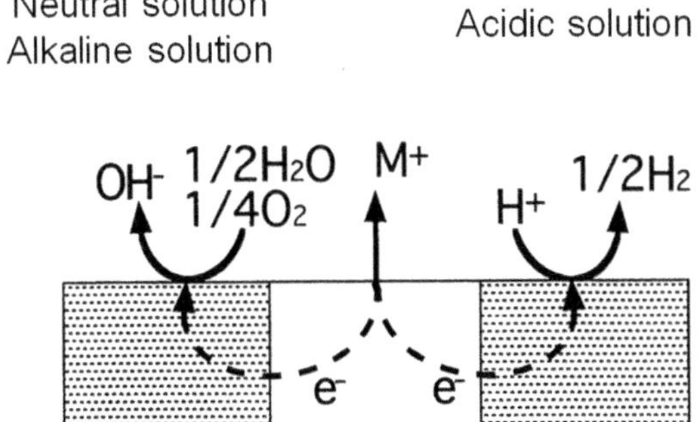

Fig. 2.20. Generation of local corrosion due to the formation of electrochemical cell in aqueous solutions due to the fixation of anodic site and cathodic site on a material.

a lower potential corrodes. The repassivation is hindered and a localized corrosion occasionally occurred along slip step (see the picture on Fig. 2.11) under cells and proteins.

2.11.2 Pitting Corrosion

The passive film is sometimes not repaired for some reason when it is damaged. Pitting occurs when passive metals such as Fe, Ni, and Al or their alloys are immersed in an aqueous chloride solution, as shown in Fig. 2.21A, where the passive film is locally destroyed and cannot be repaired. This is a localized corrosion that grows in the form of deep holes. Stainless steel suffers from pitting corrosion (see Section 5.6). In CP Ti, Ti alloys, and Co-based alloys, the passive film is chemically stable, so pitting corrosion does not normally occur on the free surface at room temperature. Pitting corrosion on the free surface increases the frequency of film destruction and repair when the electrode potential of the metal is high in a chloride solution, and eventually the film remains locally destroyed and cannot be repaired. This limiting potential is called the pitting potential. Pitting corrosion occurs in stainless steels and Ni–Ti alloys when chloride ions are present. Example of crevice corrosion is shown in Fig. 5.11.

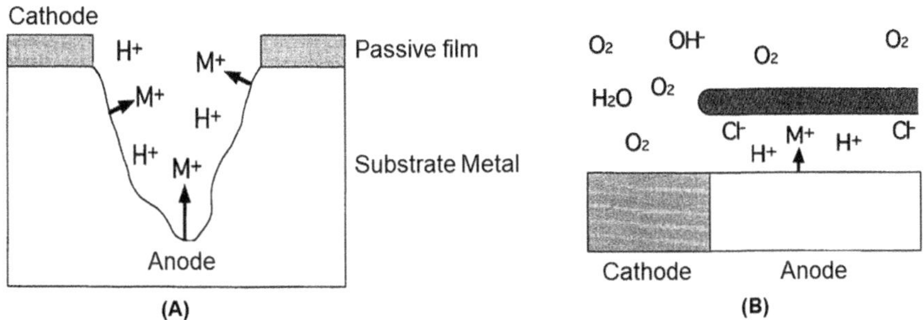

Fig. 2.21. Schematic illustrations of mechanisms of pitting corrosion (A) and crevice corrosion (B). Difference in concentration of proton and metal ions in the pore or crevice generates the electrochemical cell and accelerates the corrosion. These irreversible corrosion modes proceed with acceleration.

2.11.3 Crevice Corrosion

Crevice corrosion occurs when there is a locally high acidic chloride concentration in the solution in which mass transfer between inside crevice and outside open environment is prevented (Fig. 2.21B). In other words, crevice corrosion occurs when the solution side becomes locally high in acidic chloride concentration during a process in which mass transfer is hindered. At this time, the passive film becomes unstable and dissolves electrochemically. Locally high H^+ concentrations may occur near the fixation part of the bone plate and screw, or in the crevice between the plate and bone. Crevice corrosion can also occur on metal surfaces with attached cells. When cells adhere to a stainless steel surface, the area near the interface between the cells and the material is thought to become a site of crevice corrosion, as shown in Fig. 2.22. Example of crevice corrosion is shown in Fig. 5.10.

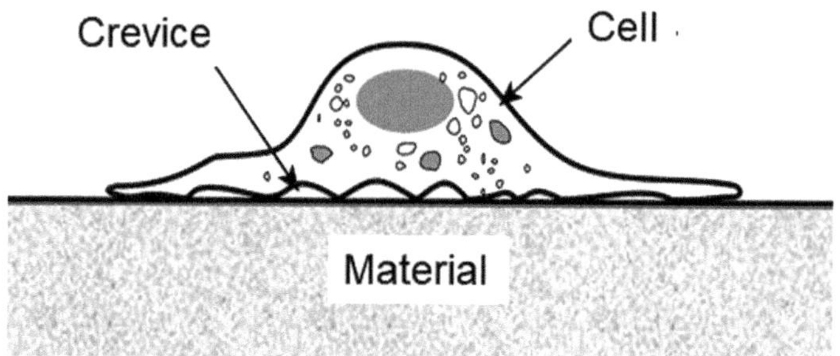

Fig. 2.22. Crevice formed between a cell and material surface.

2.11.4 Galvanic Corrosion

When different metals come into contact in an aqueous solution, the relatively noble metal becomes the cathode and the relatively base metal becomes the anode, forming a galvanic cell and allowing current (galvanic current) to generate. In medical implants, different metals sometimes come into contact, when different metals are used between the head and stem of an artificial hip joint or in spinal fixation in combinations of Co–Cr–Mo and Ti alloys. In addition, materials for dental crown restorations are often used with different metals in contact (Fig. 2.23). When dissimilar metals are present in the oral cavity, saliva and the internal tissues of the teeth become electrolytes, creating a potential difference between the dissimilar metals, generating an electromotive force, and when the two are short-circuited, a current flows (see Fig. 5.7). The difference in standard electrode potential in Table 2.1 is the potential difference. This current may corrode the base metals, which have relatively lower standard electrode potentials. Whether a combination of dissimilar metals accelerates corrosion can be determined by measuring galvanic current using a resistance-less ammeter. Galvanic corrosion of Ti–6Al–4V ELI alloy, Co–Cr–Mo alloy, and type 316L stainless steel, which are used in orthopedics, and a Zr1Mo alloy as a low-magnetic susceptibility material is evaluated in just saline (Manaka et al. 2023). No galvanic current is observed when the Ti–6Al–4V ELI and Co–Cr–Mo alloys are coupled. A slight galvanic current flows when type 316L stainless steel or the Zr1Mo alloy is coupled with the other alloys.

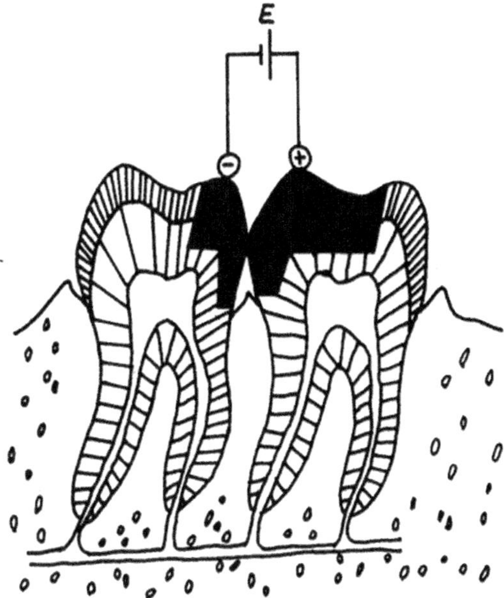

Fig. 2.23. Formation of a electrochemical cell by dissimilar metal contact in dental restorations (solid areas represent metal restoration) that generates Galvanic corrosion with a Galvanic potential of a value determined by the combination of metals (difference in the potential between metals shown in Table 2.1).

2.11.5 Intergranular Corrosion

Intergranular corrosion (grain boundary corrosion) occurs when there is non-uniformity in the structure of the material. When austenitic stainless steel such as type 316L is heated to a temperature range of 500 to 800°C, chromium carbide precipitates along the grain boundaries, and the Cr concentration decreases near the grain boundaries, resulting in poor corrosion resistance. Dental alloys formed by casting are prone to grain boundary segregation, which can lead to grain boundary corrosion.

2.11.6 Stress Corrosion Cracking

"Stress corrosion cracking" is a phenomenon in which the passive film is mechanically destroyed by the action of stress and corrosion occurs, or localized corrosion becomes the starting point for cracking. If dissolution is more dominant than repair of the passive film, pitting corrosion occurs, which initiates cracks from within the pitting site. In the former case, cracks that propagate through the grains grow; in the latter case, destruction occurs at grain boundaries.

2.11.7 Progress of Localized Corrosion

Once local corrosion occurs, a local electrochemical cell is formed with the passive film part becoming the cathode and the rupture part of the film becoming the anode, and corrosion progresses. In addition, in cases such as pitting corrosion, only OH^- of the H_2O in the solution is consumed inside the pit (pores created by pitting corrosion), and H^+ is accumulated in the pitting area, resulting in a decrease in pH (Fig. 2.21A). As a result, corrosion progresses even further. When a crack initiates due to fatigue fracture or fretting fatigue fracture, the crack initiation site can be thought of as the inside of a pit. The metal surface exposed by the propagation of the crack becomes an anode, and the surrounding area becomes a cathode, and corrosion progresses.

2.12 Biological Factors Affecting Corrosion Behavior

2.12.1 Outline

Specific *in vivo* factors affecting the corrosion of metals have been pointed out (Hanawa 2004, Jacobs et al. 1998, Pourbaix 1984, Virtanen et al. 2008). Here, the effects of body temperature, internal pH, calcium phosphate precipitation, dissolved oxygen concentration, proteins and amino acids, cells and cell matrices, body fluid circulation, material shape, and external stress on corrosion are explained.

2.12.2 Temperature and pH

Normally, the human body have homeostasis, so their internal body temperature is maintained at approximately 36–37°C, and the pH of their body fluids is maintained near neutrality due to the buffering effects of phosphoric acid, carbonic acid, protein, etc. However, immediately after the material is implanted into the body, the pH near the material surface drops to approximately 5.2 due to an inflammatory reaction (Hench and Ethridge 1975). Furthermore, in the oral environment, the temperature and pH fluctuate greatly depending on the intake of food and drink, and depending on the metabolism of oral bacteria, it takes more than 40 min for the pH to return to the original pH from below 5.0 (Stephan and Miller 1943a, b). Increased temperature and decreased pH are factors that accelerate corrosion, and can be a direct cause of destruction of the passive film and the associated release of large amounts of ions, especially in materials that are sensitive to localized corrosion such as stainless steel.

2.12.3 Calcium Phosphate Precipitation

Calcium phosphate precipitates on the surface of CP Ti and Ti alloys *in vivo* (see subsection 6.10.5). This calcium phosphate layer grows thicker over time and becomes an obstacle to mass transfer during corrosion reactions. Figure 2.24 shows the electrochemical impedance measurement (see section 3.9) results when CP Ti was immersed in a 0.9 mass% NaCl aqueous solution and Hanks' balanced salt solution for a long time. Impedance at 10 mHz, which corresponds to corrosion resistance, hardly changes in NaCl aqueous solution, while continues to increase in Hanks' solution. This indicates that the calcium phosphate layer formed on the CP Ti surface in Hanks' solution suppresses the corrosion reaction as it grows. On the other hand, in alloys that are highly sensitive to localized corrosion, such as stainless steel, corrosion may be accelerated due to the formation of crevices between the deposited calcium phosphate layer and the deposited calcium phosphate layer.

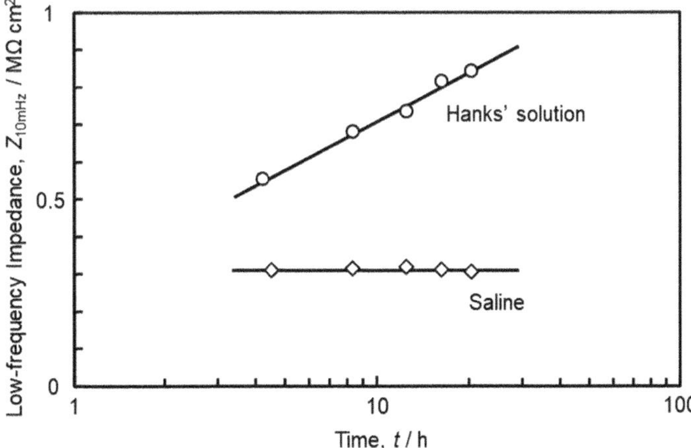

Fig. 2.24. Changes in low-frequency impedance (Z) of CP Ti immersed in Hanks' solution and saline at open-circuit potential (provided by Dr. Yusuke Tsutsumi, National Institute for Materials Science). The corrosion resistance in Hanks' solution increases with time, because calcium phosphate layer is formed that works as a barrier of corrosion.

2.12.4 Dissolved Oxygen Concentration

Dissolved oxygen in the solution is involved in cathode reactions and the formation, destruction, and repair of passive films. While the oxygen concentration in a solution exposed to the atmosphere is 7 ppm to 9 ppm, it drops to 1/4 of that in veins and 1/80 to 1/4 between cells (Black 1984). In an environment with a low dissolved oxygen concentration, while the cathodic reaction is suppressed, the repair of the passive film is also inhibited, so the corrosion behavior may be different, especially for passive alloys. Therefore, in order to properly reproduce the corrosive environment, the test solution must be adjusted to the desired dissolved oxygen concentration. Furthermore, when blowing gas into a test solution that has a carbonic acid buffering effect, such as Hanks' solution, it is necessary to consider not only the dissolved oxygen concentration but also changes in pH. If the pH changes significantly after degassing, it is possible to adjust the dissolved oxygen without causing pH fluctuations by changing the composition of the injected gas itself so that the partial pressure of carbon dioxide is in equilibrium with the carbonate ions in the test solution.

2.12.5 Proteins and Amino Acids

After inorganic ions, amino acids and proteins react first with the surface of metals implanted in living tissues. These organic species contain carboxyl groups, amino groups, and depending on the type, thiol groups, so they can affect the corrosion behavior of metals by adsorbing them to the surface or forming complexes with metal ions (Williams et al. 1988, Williams and Williams 1988). Whether these organic species promote or inhibit metal corrosion is thought to depend on the complex-forming and adsorption abilities of each organic species, while the details have not been clarified. During the repassivation of CP Ti in aqueous solutions, inorganic ions and proteins accelerate the repassivation of CP Ti, whereas certain amino acids slow it (Hanawa et al. 2004). Localized corrosion of Ti–6Al–4V alloy occurred after elongation when applied potential is nobler than some critical potential (Doi et al. 2013), which could not be determined with conventional electrochemical tests. In addition, proteins and cells adhered on Ti–6Al–4V alloy surface inhibit metal dissolution at newly created surface after rupture due to cyclic deformation to suppress crack initiation, whereas they accelerate crack propagation because dissolution at crack tip is accelerated in the occluded space formed under proteins and cells (Doi et al. 2016).

The type of protein that adsorbs to the surface of a metal immediately after implantation in a living body changes over time due to an exchange reaction from those with a smaller molecular weight to those with a larger molecular weight, as well known as "Vroman effect" (Vroman and Adams 1969). This effect must be taken into account when examining corrosion behavior in an environment where multiple proteins coexist.

2.12.6 Cells and Extracellular Matrix

The living body recognizes the implanted material as a foreign object, and macrophages, a type of immune cell, attach to it. If wear debris is released from the material even after long-term implantation, macrophages are induced to recognize the wear debris as a foreign object. Macrophages produce O^{2-}, a type of active oxygen, and O^{2-} reacts with water and immediately changes to H_2O_2. H_2O_2 forms peroxides ($Ti(OOH)(OH)_3$, $(Fe_{1-x}Cr_x)OOH$) with Fe, Cr, Ti, etc., in the passive film of stainless steel and Ti alloys (Pan et al. 1994, Hanawa 2003), it is thought that corrosion is accelerated by dissolving the passive film itself or reducing the protective properties of the film. As shown in Fig. 2.25, when macrophages are cultured with polyethylene wear particles on a CP Ti surface, the amount of Ti dissolution increases. However, when active oxygen dismutation enzyme is added, the amount of Ti dissolution decreases. This result shows that active oxygen, whose production increases due to the phagocytosis of wear particles, accelerates the corrosion of CP Ti (Mu et al. 2000). In this regard, in inflammatory condition, a destructive effect on the passive layer's resistance is triggered by H_2O_2, whereas in severe inflammatory condition, albumin, lactate, and H_2O_2 all have a synergistic effect towards decreasing the corrosion resistance of patterned Ti layers, while laser-assisted patterned Ti alloys surfaces have an improved corrosion resistance in simulated solutions compared to untreated Ti of the same composition (Bordbar-Khiabani and Gasik 2023).

When the inflammatory reaction at the initial stage of implantation subsides, cells adhere to the material surface via adhesive proteins and produce extracellular matrix. The types of cells that adhere to the material differ depending on the location where the material is implanted, and each type of extracellular matrix is produced. The main components of the extracellular matrix are fibrous proteins such as collagen, chondroitin sulfate, and polysaccharides. These molecules form a gel. When anodic polarization is performed while culturing fibroblasts on a stainless steel or CP Ti surface, an increase in the passivation current density and a drop in the pitting corrosion potential are observed on stainless steel, as shown in Fig. 2.26, while on

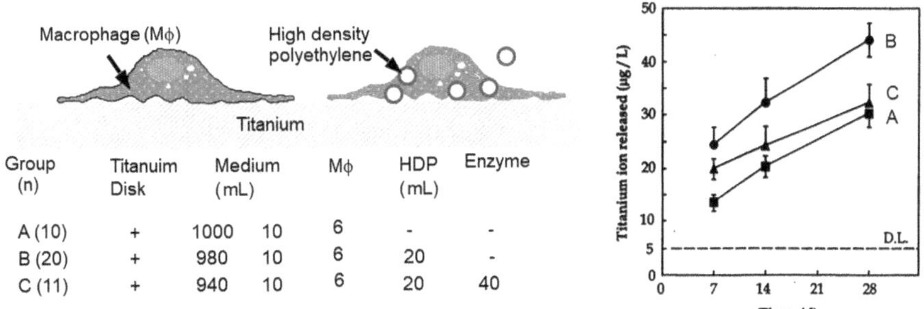

Fig. 2.25. Macrophages are incubated on CP Ti (A), that with high density polyethylene (HDP) powders (B), and that with enzyme (C). In the right figure, titanium ion release is observed by (A), the release amount increased with HDP powders (B), and the amount decreases in the addition of an active oxygen scavenging enzyme (C). Corrosion of CP Ti due to active oxygen generated by macrophage is shown (Reprinted with permission from Wiley et al. 2000. J. Biomed. Mater. Res. 49: 238–243.).

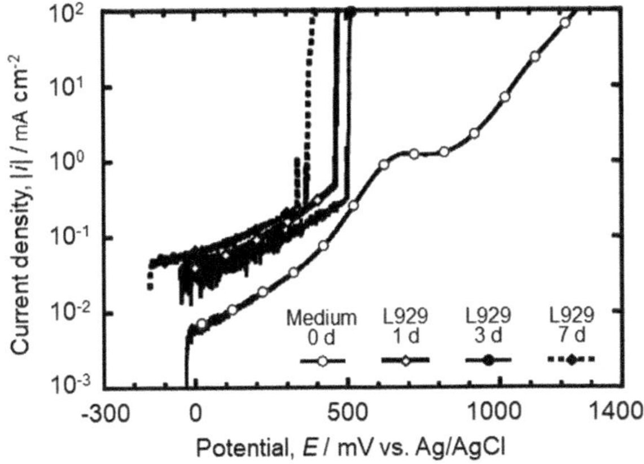

Fig. 2.26. Effect of culture days of mouse fibroblast L929 on the anodic polarization behavior of type 316L stainless steel (Reprinted with permission from Elsevier, Tang et al. 2006. Acta Biomater. 2: 709–715.). After 1 d incubation, extracellular matrix protect the surface against corrosion. After 3 d and 7 d incubation, pitting potential decreases, because crevice between cells and the material accelerate the corrosion.

CP Ti there is almost no effect (Tang et al. 2006, Hiromoto and Hanawa 2006a, b). When cathodic polarization was performed in a similar environment, a decrease in oxygen reduction current was observed in both stainless steel and CP Ti (Hiromoto et al. 2008a), as shown in Fig. 2.27. This indicates that the cells themselves and/or the extracellular matrix influence corrosion behavior as a diffusion barrier for dissolved oxygen and released metal ions.

2.12.7 Body Fluid Circulation

Blood circulates within blood vessels through forced convection caused by the cardiac beats. Body fluids circulate between cells through natural convection, transporting oxygen, and nutrients to cells. Therefore, the diffusion of released metal

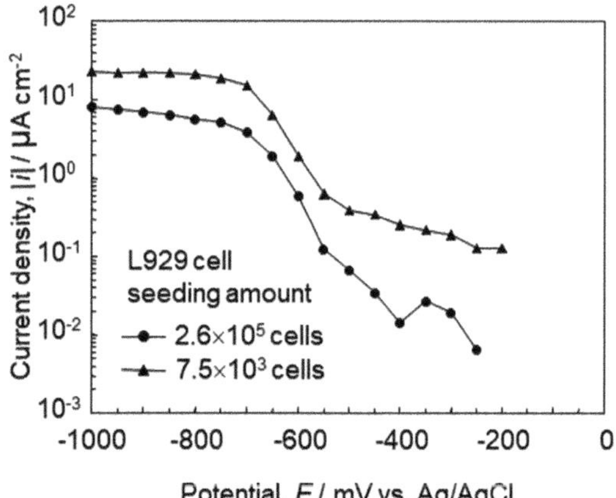

Fig. 2.27. Effect of seeding number of mouse fibroblast L929 on cathodic polarization behavior of CP Ti (culture time: 24 h) (Reprinted with permission from Japan Society of Corrosion Engineering, Hiromoto et al. 2008a. Zairyo-to-Kankyo. 57: 400–408). Seeded and incubated cells work as barrier against cathodic reaction.

ions and corrosion products offshore from the surface of materials implanted in the human body depends on the flow speed of blood, interstitial fluid, etc. The flow of solution not only increases the diffusion-limited current density but also inhibits the formation of a protective film, thereby promoting corrosion. In particular, for materials that require strict control of corrosion rate, such as bioabsorbable Mg alloys, it is necessary to evaluate the corrosion rate by considering body fluid circulation in the actual environment (Hiromoto et al. 2008b).

2.12.8 Geometric Structure of Material

Stainless steel is relatively sensitive to chloride ions, and the presence of crevices between materials can make this behavior more pronounced and crevice corrosion may occur. Because mass transfer is suppressed within the crevice, electrochemical cells are formed inside and outside the crevice, accelerating corrosion. The passive film of metals used for sliding parts of artificial joints and parts subject to fatigue loads is physically destroyed due to friction, wear, and deformation. When the new surface is exposed due to film destruction, repassivation occurs immediately, but some metal ions are released into the body fluid. In addition, repeated exposure and repassivation of new surfaces accelerates wear and fatigue associated with corrosion.

2.13 Safety

2.13.1 Concept of Toxicity

Metals themselves do not exhibit toxicity such as allergy or carcinogenesis, while metal ions or their derivatives such as oxides, hydroxides, salts, and complexes may exhibit toxicity when they combine with biomolecules and inhibit biological functions. Corrosion and wear are important when considering the toxicity of metals. There are several stages before metal ions and wear debris become toxic, and the

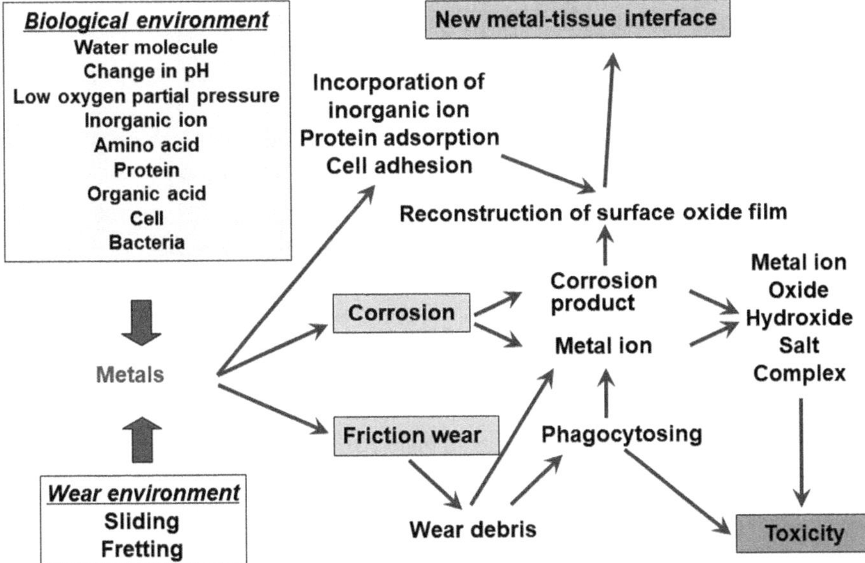

Fig. 2.28. Reactions occurred on metal surface in the human body and their effects. Corrosion and friction wear are origins of toxicity due to the generation of metal ions and wear debris. In actual reactions in the human body, biomolecules such as proteins influence these reactions.

reaction path of metals in the human body can be expressed as shown in Fig. 2.28. Metal ions and wear debris not only accumulate in the living tissue around the implanted material, but are also carried throughout the body by the circulation of body fluids. Some metal elements are dissolved in the urine and excreted. Toxic effects on the human body can be divided into local toxicity and systemic toxicity based on the extent of toxicity. It is also possible to classify toxicity into acute toxicity and chronic toxicity. Acute toxicity includes inflammation, local skin irritation, thrombus formation, necrosis, and allergy, while chronic toxicity includes canceration, ectopic calcification, granulation, immunotoxicity, and malformation.

Metal elements are released into the human body through corrosion and wear, and the reactivity of the released metal elements is also important. As shown in Fig. 2.29, metal ions immediately react with water molecules and anions, becoming stable as oxides, hydroxides, salts, etc. In another case, metal ions do not react with these or the reaction products are not stable. The probability of reaction with biomolecules is low in the former case, and high in the latter case. Examples of the former include Ti ions and Zr ions, and examples of the latter include Ni ions and Cu ions. In addition, each metal ion exhibits its own unique level of toxicity. To summarize the above, the toxicity of metal materials is

I. Ease of release of metal ions (corrosion resistance).
II. Activity of released metal ions or reactivity with surrounding molecules.
III. Toxicity of metal ions and their derivatives themselves.

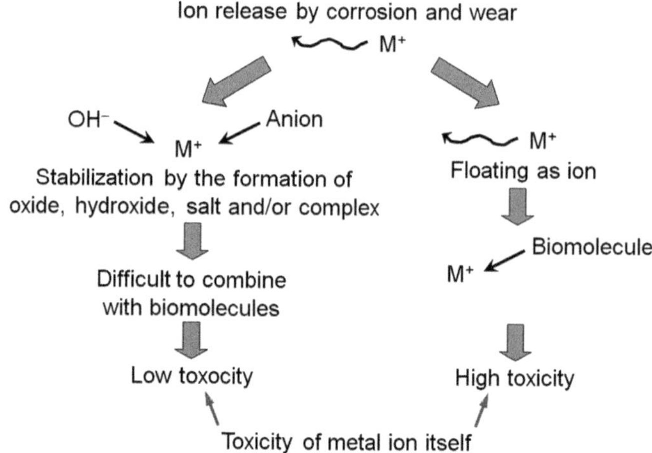

Fig. 2.29. Factors of toxicity in metals (Reprinted with permission from Corona Co., *Metallic Biomaterials* (Hanawa and Yoneyama: Corona Co., 2007), 77.). The toxicity of a metal is not determined only by direct toxicity of the metal ion that may release from the materials.

The toxicity of metals should be determined by integrating these factors. Considering all of the above factors, CP Ti and Ti alloys are highly safe materials.

2.13.2 Toxicity of Metal Elements

Among the metal elements, the "life elements" that exist in relatively large amounts in the human body are Na, Mg, K, Ca; those that exist in trace amounts (essential trace elements) include Cr, Mn, Fe, Co, Cu, Zn, Se, Mo; possibly essential elements include Li, Be, Al, V, Ni, Ge, As, Rb, Sr, Ag, Cd, Sn, Sb, Cs, Ba, W, Au, Hg, and Pb. Among these, As, Cd, Hg, and Pb are widely known as highly toxic metals. If a life element is deficient, it will cause a deficiency disease, and if it is taken in excess, a toxicity called excess disease will appear (Fig. 2.30). In other words, it is necessary to ingest appropriate amounts of life elements. On the other hand, elements that are not life elements, such as Ti and Zr, do not exhibit toxicity up to a certain threshold, but once that threshold is exceeded, the degree of toxicity increases as the amount increases. These threshold values vary depending on the element. In Fig. 2.30, the explanation was given using life elements and other elements as an example, and the above explanation also holds true even if these are replaced with chemical substances. In other words, the same holds true for *in vivo* substances and *in vivo* foreign substances (toxic substances); for example, the lethal dose (50%: LD_{50}) also holds true for the value when an *in vivo* foreign substance is ingested. Although Ti, Zr, Nb, Ta, and Hf used in new Ti alloys are not life elements, they are highly safe elements. The reason why these elements could not become life elements is thought to be because during the development and evolution of life, they were difficult to combine with biomolecules and could not be incorporated into living organisms. Even if these elements release from the material, they are not taken up by living organisms, so these elements are highly safe. Fig. 2.31 shows the correlation between the two types of cytotoxicity (Yamamoto et al. 1998). The smaller the IC_{50},

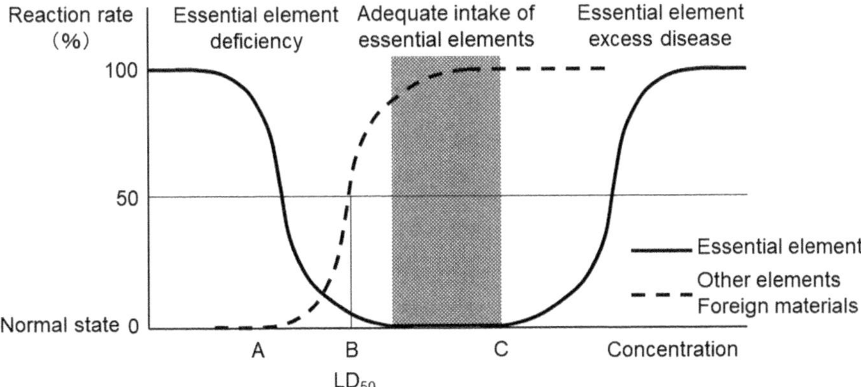

Fig. 2.30. Intake of essential biological elements and biological reactions. A: Minimum toxic dose of biologically non-essential elements, B: 50% reaction dose of biologically non-essential elements. Minimum toxic dose of biologically essential elements. LD_{50}: Half lethal dose (50% lethal dose at the time of fatal reaction) (Reprinted with permission from Corona Co., *Metallic Biomaterials* (Hanawa and Yoneyama: Corona Co., 2007), 78.).

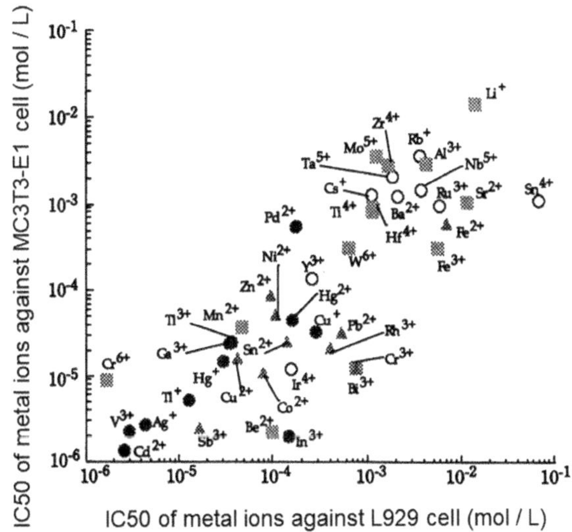

Fig. 2.31. Cytotoxicity (IC_{50}) of each metal ion to two types of cells and correlation between cells (Reprinted with permission from Wiley, Yamamoto et al. 1998. J. Biomed. Mater. Res. 39: 331–340.). Toxic tendency of a metal ion to one cell is almost same to another cell.

the stronger the cytotoxicity. The intensity of metal salts' cytotoxicity tends to be quite similar between MC3T3-E1 and L929 (the correlation coefficient of metal salts' IC50s is 0.82). The intensity of metal salts' cytotoxicity depends on the kinds of metal elements, their chemical states, and concentrations.

Although there are many studies on the carcinogenicity of compounds containing metal elements, little is known about the carcinogenicity of metals themselves. According to a monograph on carcinogens published by the World Health Organization (WHO) Cancer Research Center (IARC), there is no evidence that orthopedic metal implants are carcinogenic. There is inadequate evidence in humans for the carcinogenicity of metallic implants. There is limited evidence in experimental animals for the carcinogenicity of implants of metallic Cr, stainless steel, CP Ti, Ti-based alloys. However, pure Co, pure Ni, and Ni-13 ~ 16Cr-7Fe alloy "powders" have been found to be carcinogenic in animal experiments. Metals currently used for medicine require caution in environments where a lot of wear particles are generated, but otherwise they are not carcinogenic (IARC 1999).

2.14 Biocompatibility

2.14.1 Definition

Biocompatibility generally goes one step further than non-toxicity or safety, and refers to properties that have a favorable effect on living tissues. Recently, there has been a trend to indicate the target tissue, such as "hard tissue compatibility" and "blood compatibility", or to clearly describe the phenomenon itself, such as "tissue adhesion". Biocompatibility can be broadly divided into interfacial compatibility, which is mainly based on chemical reactions, and mechanical compatibility, which is based on mechanical effects. When a hard material is used in contact with soft tissue, the mechanical stress is repeated and the tissue is damaged. For example, dental implants and artificial joints apply non-physiological mechanical stimulation to bone tissue, which can lead to surrounding bone resorption. Conversely, when hard tissues such as bones are subjected to mechanical stimulation greater than normal, they may grow abnormally or become cancerous. When using metals for medical devices, several terms are used for the same meaning, such as hard tissue compatibility (osteoconductivity, osteocompatibility, osteogenic ability, and bioactivity in the field of bioceramics), depending on the situation to use, soft tissue compatibility (soft tissue adhesion), and blood compatibility (antithrombotic properties).

2.14.2 Bone Formation and Bone Bonding

Metallic devices that require hard tissue compatibility include dental implant fixtures and artificial hip joint stems and cups (Fig. 2.32). Among metals, Ti materials have particularly good hard tissue compatibility, and bone formation is rapid around CP Ti and Ti alloys among metals. Therefore, in orthopedics, bone screws and bone nails made of Ti alloys typically form calluses and assimilate into bone tissue after long-term implantation, causing the bone to refracture during retrieval (Sanderson et al. 1992). This is due to the fact that Ti alloys are compatible with hard tissues. Research and development of surface treatment techniques of CP Ti and Ti alloys for bone formation and mechanical anchoring are active (see Section 3.16 and Subsection 3.19.3).

2.14.3 Soft Tissue Adhesion

Adhesion between metals and soft tissue is important for dental implants, orthodontic implant anchors, percutaneous devices, and external fixator screws (Fig. 2.33). These components penetrate from inside the living tissue to the outside, and if soft tissue adhesion is incomplete, bacteria can invade and cause inflammation, leading to

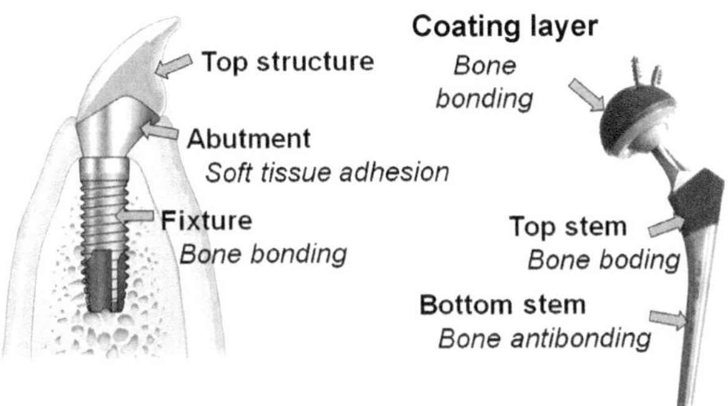

Fig. 2.32. Medical devices and locations that require hard tissue compatibility (bone formation and bone bonding), soft tissue adhesion.

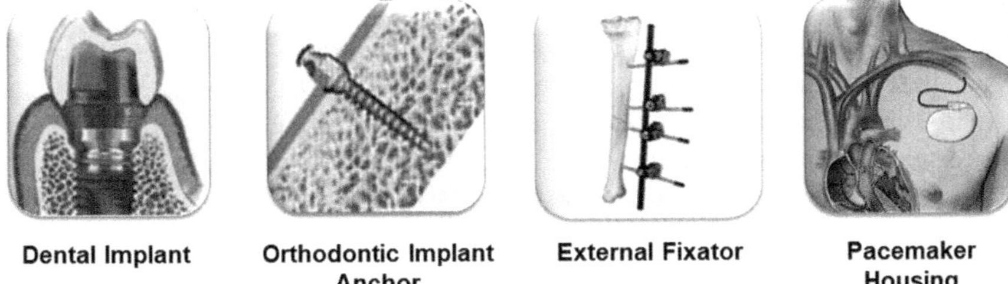

Fig. 2.33. Medical devices and locations that require soft tissue compatibility (soft tissue adhesion). In devices that are exposed from the inside of the body to the outside, if soft tissue does not sufficiently adhere to metal surface, bacteria invade from the crevice between them that induce infection.

loosening, shaking, and falling out. Even with other components that are completely implanted inside the body, if the soft tissue compatibility is not sufficient, fibrous tissue will cover the surrounding area. In particular, in dental implants, the bond between the connective epithelium and CP Ti is important, and although it is the main cause of periitis, it remains an unresolved problem. CP Ti is also known to have excellent soft tissue compatibility, but this only applies when it is completely implanted into the body. The chemical adhesion of soft tissue with CP Ti when penetrating through living tissue and the outside as described above has not been confirmed.

2.14.4 Blood Compatibility

Metals and several other metals are commonly used for devices for long-term intravascular use, such as heart valves, blood pumps, and pacemaker leads, as well as for temporary intravascular use, such as catheters and guide wires, because of their excellent mechanical properties. For metals to be used for intravascular devices, their blood compatibility is also important. However, our knowledge about the blood compatibility of these metals is little, even though these metals are commonly used for devices that are in direct contact with whole blood. Results of straightforward blood compatibility studies such as those proposed by the International Standardization Organization have not often been published. Also, comparisons between various metals and/or other materials have not been systemically performed, although more is known about the blood compatibility of variety of polymers. After sifting data from various *in vitro* studies, animal experiments and clinical reports, it is concluded that most metals seem to be less blood compatible than artificial polymers (Oeveren et al. 2000).

Protein adsorption and platelet adhesion to a material are important events for the formation of thrombus on the material and for the control of the blood compatibility of the material. The interaction of proteins with a metal surface occurs immediately after the metal contacts the blood, and then platelets attach to the surface. Since conventional metals are usually covered with surface oxide films (passive films), oxide films play an important role against protein adsorption and platelet adhesion to them. The compositions and chemical states of the surface oxide films on the above metals have been characterized. However, the relationship between those and the platelet-adhesion behavior on the metals remains unclear. The *in vitro* short term platelet adhesion accelerated by the addition of Ca^{2+} on various metals was evaluated. Metals used for medical devices, a type 316L stainless steel, a Co–Cr–Mo alloy, a Ti–6Al–4V alloy, a Ti–6Al–7Nb alloy, a Ni–Ti alloy, and a CP Ti, were immersed into platelet-rich plasma solution for 5 min and 20 min and the platelet adhesion and aggregation on the surfaces was observed by a scanning electron microscope as shown in Fig. 2.34 (Tanaka et al. 2009) (see Section 3.20). As a result, the platelet adhesion level on each metal after 5-min immersion into platelet-rich plasma solution was summarized in this order: stainless steel ≤ Co–Cr–Mo alloy < Ti–6Al–4V alloy < Ti–6Al–7Nb alloy < Ni–Ti alloy = CP Ti. This level in 5 min was almost remained after 20-min immersion. The platelet adhesion was inhibited on the stainless steel and Co–Cr–Mo alloy having Cr_2O_3-containing passive surface oxide film; that was accelerated on CP Ti and Ti alloys having TiO_2-contanining film. Cr_2O_3-containing

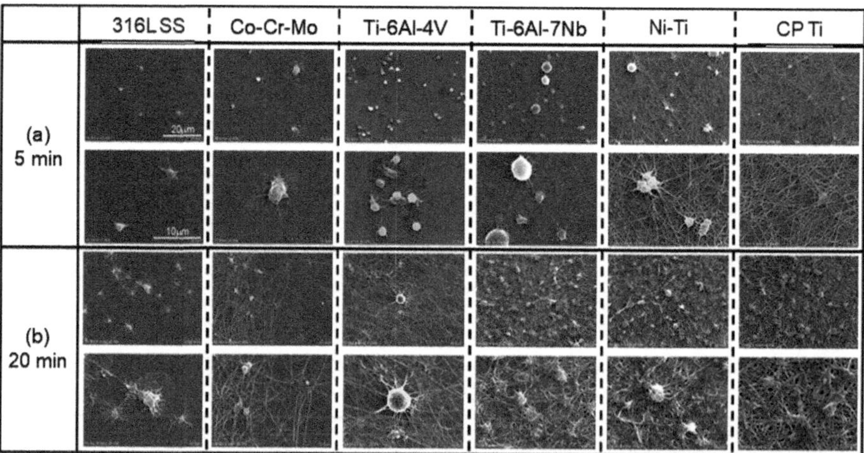

Fig. 2.34. Scanning electron micrographs of platelets spread on type 316L stainless steel, Co–Cr–Mo alloy, Ti–6Al–4V alloy, Ti–6Al–7Nb alloy, Ni–Ti alloy, and CP Ti at 5 min (a) and 20 min (b) (Reprinted with permission from Springer Nature, Tanaka et al. 2009. J. Artf. Org. 12: 182–186.). Adhesion of platelets and formation of fibrin network are prevented on type 316L stainless steel, while these are active on CP Ti and Ti alloys.

oxide film has larger permittivity than TiO_2-contanining film; the former has larger electrostatic force than the latter; the former adsorbs more albumins that worked as an inhibitory protein; the former inhibits the platelet aggregation. Therefore, the platelet adhesion and aggregation are controlled by the composition of surface oxide film on a metal due to the relative permittivity of the metal influencing the amount of adsorbed proteins.

References

Abrikosov, A.A. 2017. Fundamentals of the Theory of Metals. Dover, Mineola, NY, USA.

ASM Handbook Series, Vol. 1A-24A. 2023. ASM International, Materials Park, OH, USA.

ASM Handbook, Vol. 24. 2023. Additive Manufacturing Processes. ASM International, Materials Park, OH, USA.

ASM Handbook, Vol. 24A. 2023. Additive Manufacturing Design and Applications. ASM International, Materials Park, OH, USA.

Black, J. 1984. Biological Performance of Materials. Plenum, New York, USA.

Brandt, N.B. and S.M. Chudinov. 1975. Electronic Structure of Metals, Mir Publishers, Moscow, Russia.

Bordbar-Khiabani, A. and M. Gasik. 2023. Electrochemical behavior of additively manufactured patterned titanium alloys under simulated normal, inflammatory, and severe inflammatory conditions. J. Mater. Res. Technol. 26: 356–370.

Callister, W.D. and D.G. Rethwisch. 2015. Materials Science and Engineering, 9th ed. Wiley, Hoboken, NJ, USA.

Doi, k., S. Miyabe and S. Fujimoto. 2013. Breakdown of passive films and repassivation of Ti-6Al-4 V alloy with rapid elongation in simulated body fluid including osteoblast-like cells. J. Electrochem. Soc. 160: C576.

Doi, k., S. Miyabe, H. Tsuchiya and S. Fujimoto. 2016. Degradation of Ti–6Al–4V alloy under cyclic loading in a simulated body environment with cell culturing. J. Mech Behav. Biomed. Mater. 56: 6–13.

Hagihara, K. and T. Nakano. 2022. Control of anisotropic crystallographic texture in powder bed fusion additive manufacturing of metals and ceramics—A review. JOM 74: 1760–1773.

Hanawa, T. 2003. Reconstruction and regeneration of surface oxide film on metallic materials in biological environments. Corros. Rev. 21: 161–181.

Hanawa, T. 2004. Metal ion release from metal implants. Mater. Sci. Eng. C 24: 745–752.

Hanawa, T., Y. Kohyama, S. Hiromoto and A. Yamamoto. 2004. Effects of biological factors on the repassivation current of titanium. Mater. Trans. 45: 1635–1639.

Hiromoto, S. and T. Hanawa. 2006a. Electrochemical properties of 316L stainless steel with culturing L929 fibroblasts. J. Roy. Soc. Interface 3: 495–505.

Hiromoto, S. and T. Hanawa. 2006b. Corrosion of implant metals in the presence of cells. Corros. Rev. 24: 323–351.

Hiromoto, S., J. Ziegler and A. Yamamoto. 2008a. Morphological change of fibroblast cells on titanium and platinum cultured at anodic and cathodic potentials. Zairyo-to-Kankyo. 57: 400–408.

Hiromoto, S., A. Yamamoto, N. Maruyama, H. Somekawa and T. Mukai. 2008b. Polarization behavior of pure magnesium under a controlled flow in a NaCl solution. Mater. Trans. 49: 1456–1461.

Hench, L.L. and E.C. Ethridge. 1975. Biomaterials—The interfacial problem. Adv. Biomed. Eng. 5: 35–150.

IARC, WHO. 1999. IARC Monograph on the Evaluation of Carcinogenic Risks to Humans, Vol. 74, Surgical Implants and Other Foreign Bodies, International Agency for Research on Cancer, World Health Organization, Lyon, France.

Jacobs, J.J., J.L. Gilbert and R.M. Urban. 1998. Corrosion of metal orthopaedic implants. J. Bone Joint. Surg. 80A: 268–282.

Kelly, EJ. 1982. Electrochemical behavior of titanium. Mod. Aspect. Electrochem. 14: 319–424.

Ko, G., W. Kim, K. Kwon and T.K. Lee. 2021. The corrosion of stainless steel made by additive manufacturing: A review. Metals 11: 516.

Manaka, T., Y. Tsutsumi, Y. Takada, P. Chen, M. Ashida, K. Doi et al. 2023. Galvanic corrosion among Ti6Al4V ELI alloy, CoCrMo alloy, 316L-Type stainless steel, and Zr1Mo alloy for orthopedic implants. Mater. Tans. 64: 131–137.

McCafferty, E. 2010. Introduction to Corrosion Science. Springer, Berlin, Germany.

Mu, Y., T. Kobayashi, M. Sumita, A. Yamamoto and T. Hanawa. 2000. Metal ion release from titanium with active oxygen species generated by rat macrophages *in vitro*. J. Biomed. Mater. Res. 49: 238–243.

Oeveren, W.V., P. Schoen and C.A. Maijers. 2000. Blood compatibility of metals and alloys used in medical devices. pp. 211–214. Progress in Biomedical Research, IOP Science, Philadelphia, PA, USA.

Pan, J., D. Thierry and C. Leygraf. 1994. Electrochemical and XPS studies of titanium for biomaterial applications with respect to the effect of hydrogen peroxide. J. Biomed. Mater. Res. 28: 113–122.

Perez, N. 2016. Electrochemistry and Corrosion Science: Springer, Berlin, Germany.

Pourbaix, M. 1966. Atras of Electrochemical Equilibria. pp. 213–222. Pergamon, Oxford, UK.

Pourbaix, M. 1984. Electrochemical corrosion of metallic biomaterials. Biomaterials 5: 122–134.

Predeferri, P. 2018. Corrosion Science and Engineering: Springer, Berlin, Germany.

Revie, R.W. and H.H. Uhlig. 2008. Corrosion and Corrosion Control: An Introduction to Corrosion Science and Engineering: Wiley, Hoboken, NJ, USA.

Sander, G., J. Tan, P. Balan, O. Gharbi, D.R. Feenstra, L. Singer et al. 2018. Corrosion of additively manufactured alloys: A review. Corrosion 74: 1318–1350.

Sanderson, L., W. Ryan and P.G. Turner. 1992. Complications of metalwork removal injury. Injury 23: 29–30.

Stephan, R.M. and B.F. Miller. 1943a. A quantitative method for evaluating physical and chemical agents which modify production of acids in bacterial plaques on human teeth. J. Dent. Res. 22: 45–51.

Stephan, R.M. and B.F. Miller. 1943b. The effect of synthetic detergents on pH changes in dental plaques. J. Dent. Res. 22: 53–61.

Tanaka, Y., K. Kurashima, H. Saito, A. Nagai, Y. Tsutsumi, H. Doi et al. 2009. *In vitro* short term platelet adhesion on various metals. J. Artf. Org. 12: 182–186.

Tang, Y.C., S. Katsuma, S. Fujimoto and S. Hiromoto. 2006. Electrochemical study of Type 304 and 316L stainless steels in simulated body fluids and cell cultures. Acta Biomater. 2: 709–715.

Virtanen, S., I. Milošev, E. Gomez-Barrena, R. Trebše, J. Salo and Y.T. Konttinen. 2008. Special modes of corrosion under physiological and simulated physiological conditions. Acta Biomater. 4: 468–476.

Vroman, L. and A.L. Adams. 1969. Findings with the recording ellipsometer suggesting rapid exchange of specific plasma proteins at liquid/solid interfaces. Surf. Sci. 16: 438–446.

Williams, R.L., S.A. Brown and K. Merritt. 1988. Electrochemical studies on the influence of proteins on the corrosion of implant alloys. Biomaterials 9: 181–186.

Williams, R.L. and D.F. Williams. 1988. Albumin adsorption on metal surfaces. Biomaterials 9: 206–212.

Yamamoto, A., R. Honma and M. Sumita. 1998. Cytotoxicity evaluation of 43 metal salts using murine fibroblasts and osteoblastic cells. J. Biomed. Mater. Res. 39: 331–340.

CHAPTER 3

Evaluation Methods of Metallic Biomaterials

3.1 Introduction

Many textbooks have been published on how to evaluate metals, and this can be studied in universities' courses in the field of materials engineering. However, performance evaluations of metallic biomaterials for medical devices are often specially stipulated. In *in vitro* evaluation of mechanical property and corrosion resistance, an important issue is how to bring the environment closer to the actual *in vivo* environment. Although many of them are standardized by ISO and ASTM, evaluating materials in a biological environment requires a wide range of knowledge and experimental experience, and must be learned under the guidance of an experienced instructor. This chapter covers evaluation of mechanical property including strength and toughness, fatigue and fretting fatigue, and wear in simulated biological environments. Evaluation of corrosion resistance, adsorption of proteins, bone formation by simulated body fluids, and biological evaluation containing cell culture and animal experiment, are also explained. These are only overviews; refer to specialized books for details. In particular, biological evaluation using cells and animals requires a background in life science, so this book only provides an overview. Metals have advantages that cannot be obtained from other materials. However, in biological environment, the excellent property of metals may degrade and influence their safety and durability (see Chapter 5). Therefore, evaluation of metals in biological environments must be achieved. In this chapter, the minimum essentials for evaluation of metallic biomaterials are briefly explained, divided into mechanical property, surface property, and biological property.

3.2 Evaluation of Mechanical Property

Important mechanical properties for metallic biomaterials include strength, elongation to fracture, fracture toughness, Young's modulus, fatigue, fretting fatigue, and wear resistance. The fracture of materials and generation of wear debris in the living body cause directly significant damage to living tissue or indirect damage such as the release of cytokines through macrophages. In damaged areas where tissue replacement is required, even the tissue surrounding the implant is often made vulnerable. It is also important to have excellent mechanical compatibility to avoid major differences between the implant and living tissue.

Implants used in the human tissues (1) have significantly deteriorated mechanical properties compared to those in the air (or vacuum, inert gas), (2) even if the same material is used, the mechanical environment may vary depending on the purpose of use and location, and (3) the fact that many implant devices have complex shapes and movements. Therefore, there are various obstacles when evaluating the mechanical properties of medical materials. Currently, efforts are being made to establish a unified evaluation method for mechanical testing through ISO and ASTM specifications, but this is not necessarily fully developed. There are roughly three steps to evaluating the mechanical properties of medical materials.

In Vitro Material Test

As in the case of testing industrial materials, the test specimen is made into a simple shape (for example, a cylinder, a prism, etc.) that allows the shape characteristics to be excluded, and only the material characteristics are evaluated. The basic tests include tensile test, compression test, bending test, fatigue test, and wear test.

In Vitro Product Test

Tests on actual products or parts are essential to get approval for clinical application. However, because the product shape and usage environment differ, standardization is difficult and requires periodic review.

In Vivo Implantation Test

This is an *in vivo* implantation test that is mainly conducted in animal experiments, and it is possible to evaluate the interaction between materials and living tissues in a biological environment. However, there are large individual differences between animal species and even within the same species, data lacks universality and versatility, and complex reactions *in vivo* can make it difficult to extract and evaluate specific factors. Furthermore, from the perspective of animal welfare, compliance with the 3Rs (refinement; reduction; replacement) is essential under a legal document (Act on Welfare and Management of Animals 1973).

3.3 Strength and Toughness Test

The mechanical properties of a metallic biomaterial are usually first evaluated by tensile test (or compression test when the specimen size is small or for brittle materials). Fig. 3.1 shows typical stress-strain curve indicating specific values on the curve. In general, deformation of metals and ceramics can be classified into elastic strain and plastic strain, while in polymer materials, time-dependent viscoelastic behavior is added. “Elastic deformation” is a region governed by Hooke’s law, which corresponds to the deformation of a spring, and returns to its original shape when the load is removed. On the other hand, when the load exceeds a certain level, the material shape remains deformed even after the load is removed. This permanent deformation is called "plastic deformation". In metals and ceramics, stress increases linearly due to elastic deformation in the low strain region. In the case of metals, after reaching a constant stress, the slope decreases, and as work hardens, plastic deformation progresses. This transition stress from elastic deformation to plastic deformation is called "yield strength", or "elastic limit", and is an important index that reflects the strength of the material. Furthermore, the maximum stress until fracture is called "ultimate tensile strength (UTS)", the strain at fracture is called "elongation to fracture" (fracture strain in compression tests), and the energy absorption (corresponding to the area under the stress-strain curve or integration of stress-strain curve) until fracture is called "facture toughness". Tensile tests are usually performed by applying a fixed amount of crosshead displacement in a uniaxial direction at a constant rate, and display the stress-strain curve. Because there is a difference between the crosshead displacement and the practical material strain due to the rigidity of the equipment and jig used for mechanical test, it is in fact desirable to calculate the strain from the direct displacement of the material being evaluated. A number of methods are used for direct displacement, including methods that evaluate strain gauges directly contacted with the specimen, methods that measure displacement through image processing using laser beams, etc. The calculated stress and strain are "nominal stress" and "nominal strain", respectively, which are analyzed using the initial cross-sectional area and initial length of the specimen. On the other hand, "true stress" and "true strain" are also used, which takes into account the cross-sectional area and length of specimen during deformation. When the amount of strain is small, nominal stress and nominal strain may be used, while when deformation progresses relatively uniformly up to a large strain under constant volume conditions, it is better to evaluate using true stress and true strain. Figure 1.6 shows the stress-strain curves of typical medical materials and cortical bone determined by tensile and compression tests. The inset shows an enlarged view of the region indicated by the dashed line, that is, the vicinity of the elastic deformation region. These stress-strain curves represent the mechanical characteristics of metals, ceramics, and polymers.

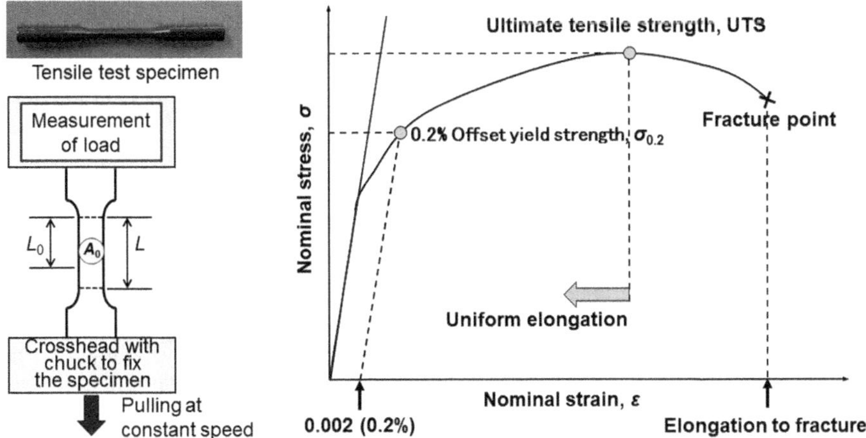

Fig. 3.1. Picture of a tensile test specimen, schematic diagram of tensile test method, and explanation of a model stress strain curve.

The slope of the stress-strain curve during elastic deformation is Young's modulus, which reflects the elastic properties of the material. Generally, when applying metals to implants, etc., they are used within their elastic limits. Therefore, when implanting into bone, the difference in elastic modulus with the bone is important. As is clear from the inset in Fig. 1.6, Young's modulus is relatively high for ceramics such as alumina (Al_2O_3) and zirconia (ZrO_2), moderate for metals, and lower for polymers than cortical bone. Even among metals, the Young's modulus differs depending on the interatomic potential. For example, the value is significantly lower in a β-type Ti alloy than in a Co–Cr alloy. Furthermore, ceramics do not undergo plastic deformation at room temperature and have low fracture toughness, whereas metals exhibit moderate strength (yield strength and UTS) and elongation to fracture, making them highly tough and suitable for use as implants under load.

3.4 Fatigue and Fretting Fatigue Test

"Fatigue" is involved in most of the causes of *in vivo* failure of metallic biomaterials. Fatigue basically progresses through the initiation and propagation of a crack due to to-and-fro motion of dislocation. Since dislocation motion occurs even below the yield strength, fracture may occur under extremely low repeated stress of less than half the yield strength. *In vivo*, the effects of corrosion and fretting wear are added, and the life time due to fatigue *in vivo* is sometimes much lower than that *in vitro*.

"Fretting" refers to wear and sometimes corrosion damage of loaded surfaces in contact while they encounter small oscillatory movements tangential to the surface. Fretting is caused by adhesion of contact surface asperities, which are subsequently fractured by the small movement. This fracture generates wear debris. The area where such fretting wear occurs may become the starting point of fatigue fracture, and this type of fracture is called "fretting fatigue" fracture. A schematic diagram of the fretting fatigue test is shown in Fig. 3.2 (JSME S015 2002). A uniaxial repeated load is applied to the test specimen, and at the same time, a constant compression force (variation within ±5%) is applied through the contact piece using a pressing jig. Real fretting fatigue conditions vary depending on the product and the part in which it is used. According to a specification (ASTM E2789-10 2021), it is possible to evaluate the fretting fatigue characteristics of materials. *In vivo*, the addition of corrosion to fretting fatigue has a greater effect on crack propagation than on crack initiation.

Durability test methods for implant products themselves are specified by ISO, ASTM, etc. (ISO 7206-4 2010, ASTM F-1612-95 1995). Figure 3.3 shows the design of test specimen of artificial hip joints. Fig. 3.4 shows the specimen orientation during the test of an implant without anteversion. The test should be conducted under the following conditions: (1) the elastic modulus of the embedding medium is within the range of 3 to 5 GPa, (2) the load is applied as a sine wave, and the deflection is stopped when the deflection exceeds a predetermined value, and the number of repetitions or elapsed time of operation are recorded, (3) the minimum load to be applied to the specimen is 200 to 300 N, and (4) the frequency during loading should be 1 to 30 Hz, and the recommended frequency is 1 Hz for non-metallic materials and 4–30 Hz for metallic materials.

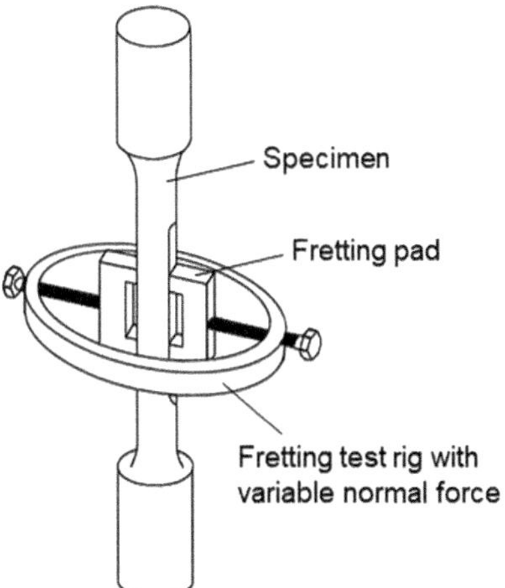

Fig. 3.2. Schematic diagram of fretting fatigue test specimen (Reproduced with permission from The Japan Society of Mechanical Engineers, *JSME Standard Fretting Fatigue Test Configuration*, JSME S 015-2002.).

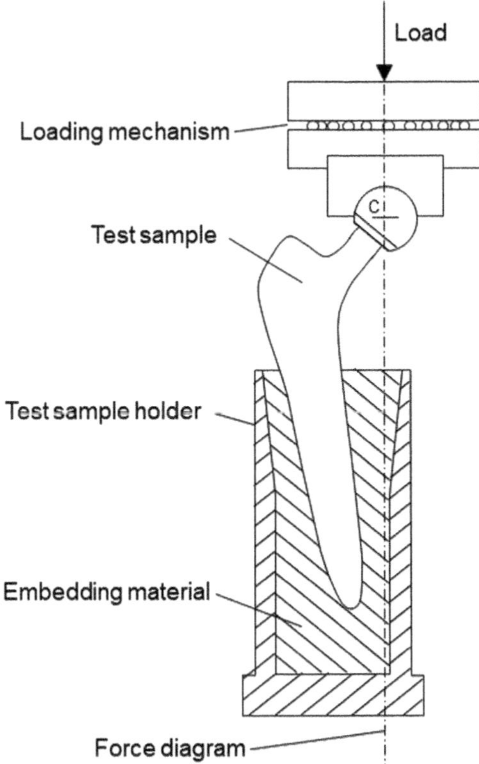

Fig. 3.3. Schematic diagram of the general arrangement of hip implant test samples (Reprinted with permission from International Organization for Standardization, ISO 7206-4:2010 2020.).

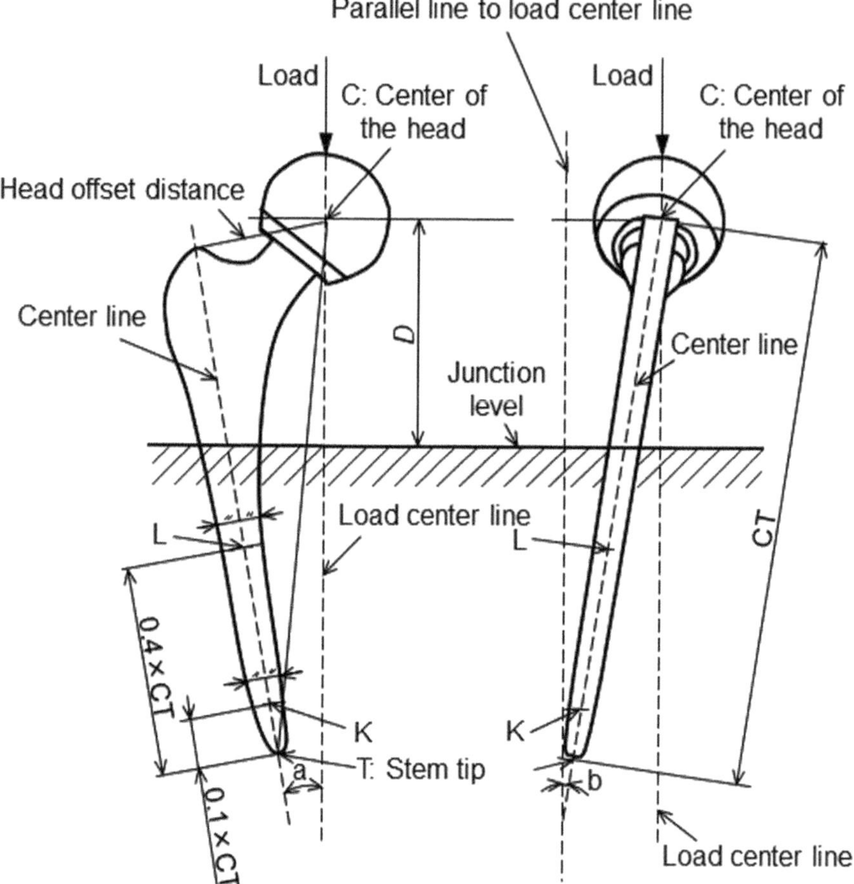

Fig. 3.4. Sample orientation during testing with an artificial hip stem without anteversion (Reprinted with permission from International Organization for Standardization, ISO 7206-4:2010 2020.).

Similarly, the fatigue test method for artificial knee joints is specified by ASTM, etc., and a test method that simulates the *in vivo* stress state between the tibia and knee joint is specified (ASTM F1800-04 2017).

3.5 Wear Test

Wear is defined as a phenomenon in which material gradually separates from its surface due to mechanical action caused by friction with solids, powder, etc. Wear analysis items include wear loss, scratches and deterioration of the friction surface, size of wear particles, and the formation of a metal transfer film on the mating worn surface. Wear of sliding parts in artificial joints *in vivo* involves a complex interplay of plastic deformation, fatigue, creep, etc., and is strongly influenced by surface conditions, friction speed, load conditions, lubricants, atmosphere, etc., so it is difficult to standardize wear evaluation. The development of artificial joints ultimately requires joint simulator testing, and material selection at the test piece level

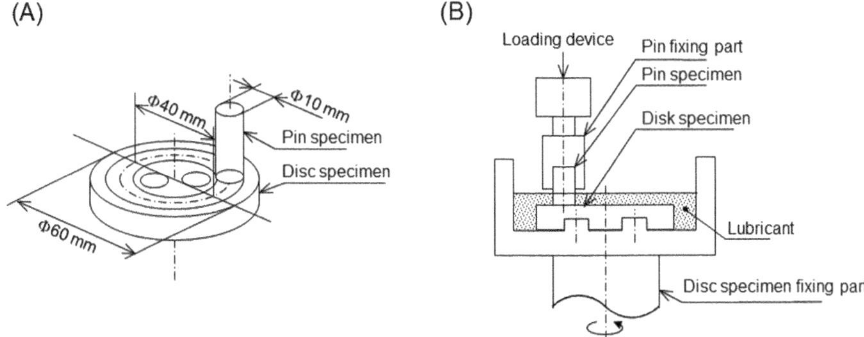

Fig. 3.5. An example of the shape of a test piece in the pin-on-disk method of wear testing (A) and a schematic diagram of the test equipment (B) (Reprinted with permission from Japan Industrial Standards Committee, JIS T0303. 2000. Figures 1 and 2.).

has been standardized (ASTM F732 1991, ISO 6474 1994). The pin-on-disc method is a test method in which a pin test piece is pressed against a sliding disk under a constant load. An example of the test piece dimension and a schematic diagram of the test equipment are shown in Fig. 3.5 (JIS T0303 2000). A soft material is used as the pin test piece to prevent wear due to digging. Only the disk side is rotated and load is applied from the pin side. To keep the concentration of lubricant constant, evaporated water volume must be considered. The specific wear amount of the test piece is calculated using the following equation. The worn volume is the mass of the test piece when the sliding distance is 2×10^6 mm and the amount of decrease in the mass of the test piece at the end of the test (sliding distance of about 10^8 mm).

$$w = (W_1 - W_2)/P \cdot L \cdot \rho \quad (3.1)$$

where w is specific wear amount of the test piece (mm^2/N), W_1 is mass (g) when sliding distance is 2×10^6 mm, W_2 is mass (g) at the end of test (sliding distance approximately 10^8 mm), P is Load = $p \cdot S$ (N), p is friction surface pressure (MPa), S is friction surface area (mm^2), L is sliding distance (mm) = Total sliding distance (mm) $- 2 \times 10^6$ mm, ρ is the density of the test piece (g/mm^3). The friction surface pressure during the test must be 2.5 MPa or more and the sliding speed is approximately 20 mm/s. The candidates of lubricant are a saline, a phosphate buffered physiological salt solution (PBS), an aqueous solution containing about 30 vol% serum, etc., and the temperature must be 37 ± 2°C.

3.6 Joint Simulators

To ultimately evaluate an artificial joint, it is necessary to use an artificial joint simulator that simulates the movement of an artificial joint in a simulated body fluid. Fig. 3.6 shows the appearance of the knee joint simulator. The knee joint simulator is a device that simulates normal human walking by applying periodic variations in the flexion/extension angle and contact force to the interface between the femoral component and the tibia component. The tibia component is free to move relative to the femur

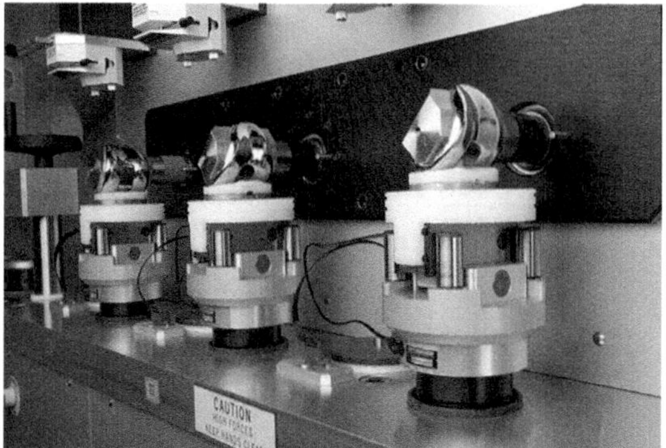
Fig. 3.6. Appearance of knee joint simulator (fatigue wear tester) test (Provided by AMTI Force & Motion.).

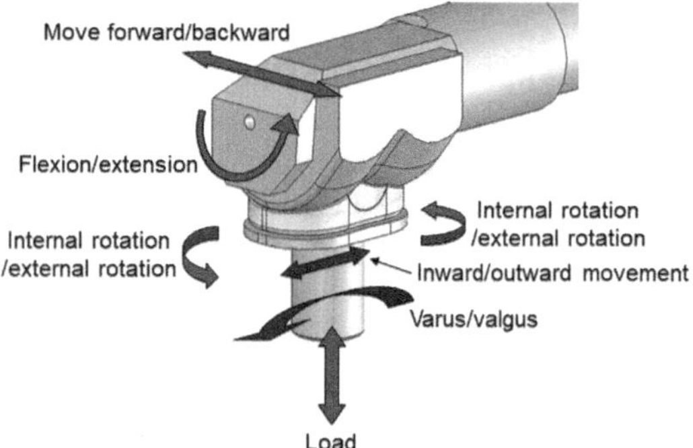

Fig. 3.7. Example of control axis of knee joint simulator.

under the influence of the applied contact force. This movement has all degrees of freedom except the flexion/extension angle, which follows a specific cyclic variation. The operation of such a knee joint simulator is specified by ISO (ISO 14243-1:2009 2020). It specifies the relative angular motion between connected components to be used in wear tests, the pattern of applied loads, test speed and duration, sample composition, and test environment. The simulator performs displacement control, and as shown in Fig. 3.7: (i) flexion/extension, (ii) internal rotation/external rotation (external rotation), (iii) axial load, (iv) varus/valgus, and (v) the two axes of medial/ lateral translation. Anterior-posterior motion is restricted by the standard. This is actually a force controlled axes that takes into account the ligaments that act while the femoral component is moving relative to the tibial component. For the knee joint, the reference position is equivalent to 0° of flexion (full extension) *in vivo*. The test solution used was bovine serum (25 ± 2%) diluted with deionized water, and with appropriate treatment and exchange, the temperature was maintained at 37 ± 2°C and at 1 ± 0.1 Hz to simulate human walking. Furthermore, an evaluation method for the wear of tibia components using a gravimetric method is specified. The testing is a combination of load and displacement controlled axes.

Figure 3.8 shows the appearance of the hip joint simulator. Regulations regarding simulator operation, wear amount, etc., are established (ISO 14242-1 2018, ISO

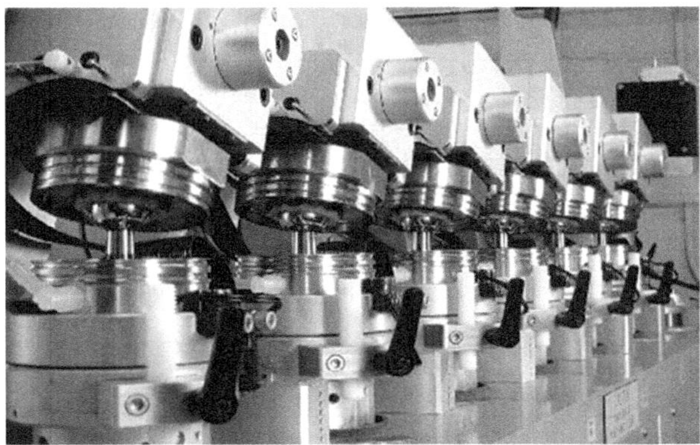

Fig. 3.8. Exterior view of the hip joint simulator test (Provided by AMTI Force & Motion.).

14242-2 2016). Four axes of the hip joint are controlled: (1) flexion/extension, (2) internal rotation/external rotation, (3) adduction/abduction, and (4) load. The test is conducted using the center of the femoral head as the reference point. In recent years, implants whose surfaces are coated with hydroxyapatite, etc., have also been widely used. Shear and tensile tests at the interface between metal substrate and coated ceramics are specified (ASTM F1044-05 2018, ASTM F1147-05 2022).

3.7 Test Solution of Corrosion Resistance

Metallic biomaterials come in a wide variety of types and applications, such as orthopedics cardiology, and dentistry, and the required properties vary widely. Therefore, it is necessary to carefully consider conditions such as the type of material and the environment in which it will be used, and select an evaluation method according to the purpose. The *in vivo* environment is an extremely complex corrosion environment in which there are many factors that affect the corrosion behavior of materials. A simulated body fluid (SBF) is generally used as a test solution, and there are many types of it, as summarized in Table 3.1. Each solution has its own characteristics. The more complex the composition of the SBF, the better the ability to simulate the biological environment in which the material is used, but it becomes more difficult to prepare, store, and handle. On the other hand, since it is impossible to completely reproduce the environment in which a material is used, it is necessary to consider in advance the factors that have a large effect on corrosion behavior in the environment where the material is exposed. Carrying out corrosion evaluations under reproduced conditions is the key to obtaining the most efficient results that are close to the practical situation.

3.8 Polarization Test

3.8.1 Anodic Polarization Test

Corrosion of metallic biomaterials is caused by two reactions: a reaction in which the metal releases electrons and is oxidized to metal ions (anodic reaction), and a reaction in which the released electrons are received to reduce dissolved oxygen,

Table 3.1. Typical test solutions (simulated body fluid) used in corrosion tests.

Solution	Characteristics
Saline	The simplest composition (0.9mass% NaCl). Isotonic with extracellular solution.
Ringer's solution	Physiological saline solution with approximately the same osmotic pressure as serum containing Na^+, K^+, Ca^{2+}, and Cl^-. A physiological saline solution that is a substitute for body fluids is generally called Ringer's solution, and various compositions are used.
Phosphate Buffered Saline: PBS	The pH is buffered by phosphate ions. Concentration of phosphate ion is relatively high.
Hanks' solution: HBSS	The pH is buffered by phosphate ions and carbonate ions. Simulating extracellular fluid.
Kokubo's simulated body fluid; SBF in the field of bioceramics	Simulating plasma components. There are several compositions. Containing supersaturated Ca^{2+} and is used to evaluate calcium phosphate or HA formation.
Minimum Essential Medium: MEM	Containing organic species such as amino acids in addition to inorganic salts. Mainly used as a cell culture medium.
Serum	Solution removed blood cells and some blood clotting factors from blood. Containing about 7% proteins, inorganic salts, and amino acids.
Cell culture medium	Main components are inorganic species such as Na, K, Ca, Mg, P, Cl, etc., proteins, amino acids, vitamins, hormone, etc. A semi-synthetic culture medium containing MEM and serum is often used.

hydrogen ions, and water molecules in the solution (cathodic reaction) (see Section 2.9). These electrochemical reactions occur in pairs. Therefore, corrosion resistance can be evaluated by electrochemical measurement. Applying an external potential or current to a corrosion system is called "polarization," and polarization test is a method to obtain various information from the response. Potentiodynamic polarization test or linear sweep voltammetry is the most common, applying an overpotential with a constant potential gradient. Polarization test methods are specified (ASTM F2129-19a 2019). The electrochemical cell contains three types of electrodes: a working electrode (specimen), a counter electrode, and a reference electrode, as shown in Fig. 3.9. The tip of the reference electrode is placed close to the working electrode to minimize the effect of voltage drop (IR drop) due to solution resistance. In a polarization test, a "potentiostat" measures the current response between the working and counter electrodes in response to changes in the potential difference between the working and reference electrodes. Typically, a saturated calomel electrode (SCE) or standard silver-silver chloride electrode (SSE; Ag/AgCl) is used as the reference electrode, and Pt is used as the counter electrode. The main test solutions used for corrosion and electrochemical evaluation of metallic biomaterials are listed in Table 3.1, taking into consideration the environment in which the material is used and the special characteristics of the biological environment. The solution temperature is maintained at 310 K (37°C), which is close to body

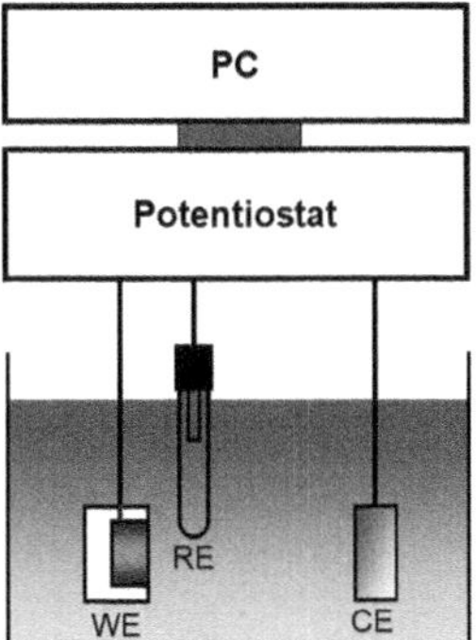

Fig. 3.9. Example of electrochemical cell for polarization test. WE: working electrode. RE: reference electrode. CE: counter electrode.

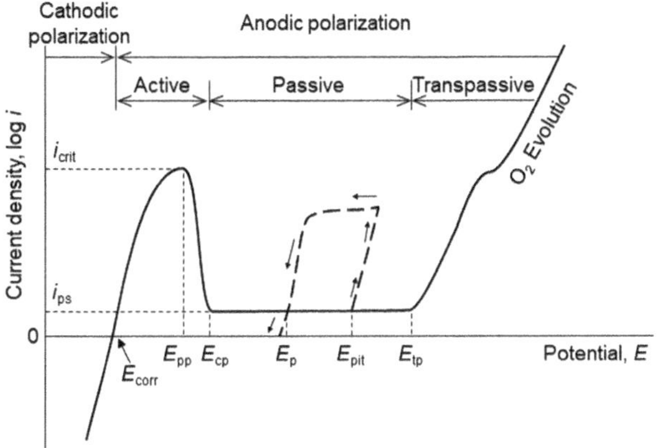

Fig. 3.10. Polarization curve of alloy showing passivation phenomenon. E_{corr}: corrosion potential, E_{pp}: passivation potential, E_{cp}: passivation completion potential, E_p: protection potential, E_{pit}: pitting potential, E_{tp}: transpassivation potential, i_{crit}: critical passivation current density, and i_{ps}: passivation current density.

temperature, and the dissolved oxygen concentration is adjusted according to the usage environment and test purpose.

A schematic diagram of the anodic polarization curve of an alloy exhibiting the passivation with the parameters on the curve are shown in Fig. 3.10. When a metal is polarized from corrosion potential (E_{corr}), the current shows an active region, and when it reaches a certain critical passivation current density (i_{crit}), the current density becomes very small on the order of μA cm^{-2}. The current density in this region is called current density in passive state (i_{ps}), indicating the protection of the passive film against general corrosion of the substrate metal. At even higher potentials, the current increases again due to pitting corrosion, crevice corrosion, transpassivation, or oxygen evolution. To determine the cause of the current increase, it is necessary to confirm corrosion pits on the specimen surface after the test. Note that most passive alloys such as Ti alloys, Co-based alloys, and stainless steels are already passivated in the atmosphere or immediately after immersion in a solution, so active regions rarely appear on the anode polarization curve.

Pitting potential (E_{pit}) indicates the resistance to local destruction of the passive film by chloride ions, etc., or the low stability of the passive film itself. The initiation of pitting corrosion has an incubation period because unstable pitting corrosion repeatedly occurs and repassivates, and then one of pit grows stably. In addition, factors such as the shape and distribution of defects such as inclusions exposed on the material surface are stochastically involved in the possibility of unstable pitting corrosion and repassivation, resulting in variations in the pitting corrosion potential. For this reason, it is necessary to measure the pitting potential at least three times and evaluate it statistically. Measuring protection potential (E_p) is effective in predicting the risk of pitting corrosion. The protection potential is determined as the potential at which the anodic current intersects the passive region by reversing the potential sweep direction after sufficient pitting has grown through anodic polarization.

3.8.2 Tafel Extrapolation Method and Polarization Resistance Method

The natural potential (corrosion potential) of a metal immersed in an aqueous solution is the potential at which the magnitudes of the anodic and cathodic reactions occurring on the surface are balanced. As shown in Fig. 3.11, when the specimen is polarized from the corrosion potential in both anode and cathode directions, in the region where the overvoltage (η) is sufficiently large, theoretically, the following "Tafel equation" is expressed.

$$\eta = a + b \log i \tag{3.2}$$

A Tafel region in which the logarithm of potential and current shows a linear relationship is obtained. Here, the slopes of the straight lines on the anodic and cathodic sides are called anodic and cathodic Tafel coefficients (b_a and b_c), respectively, with expressed in a unit of V. The method of determining the corrosion current density (i_{corr}), which corresponds to the corrosion rate, from the intersection points of the extrapolated lines, is called the "Tafel extrapolation method." On the other hand, in an environment such as a neutral solution where the oxygen reduction is the main cathodic reaction and a critical current density (dashed line in the figure) appears, the intersection point of the extrapolated diffusion limited current line and the anodic Tafel line is the corrosion current. However, in the case of alloys or solutions containing oxygen acids, multiple redox reactions occur in parallel, so a clear Tafel region often does not appear. This results in a serious reading error, so careful analysis is required.

On the other hand, when a slight overvoltage of approximately ±5 mV is applied, which is close to the corrosion potential, the potential and current show a linear relationship as shown in Fig. 3.12. The slope of this straight line is polarization resistance (R_p). This value is correlated to the reciprocal of the corrosion current, and can be converted to the corrosion current using the following formula with the values of the Tafel coefficients b_a and b_c for the anode and cathode.

$$R_p = \frac{b_a b_c}{i_{corr}(b_a + b_c)} \tag{3.3}$$

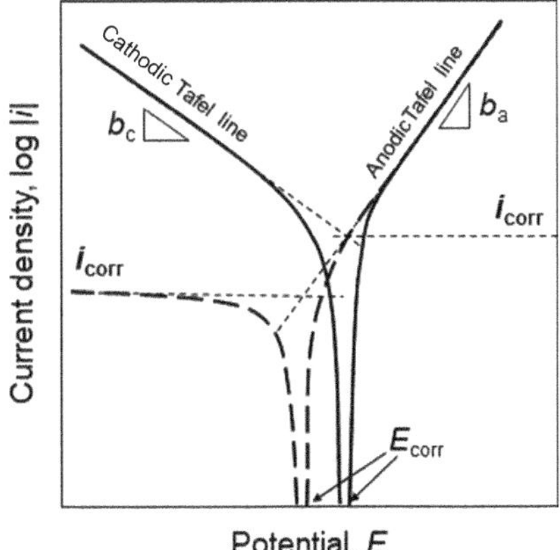

Fig. 3.11. How to determine corrosion current density using Tafel extrapolation method. E_{corr}: corrosion potential, i_{corr}: corrosion current density, b_c: cathodic Tafel coefficient, b_a: anodic Tafel coefficient. Solid line: when Tafel straight line is obtained for both cathode and anode polarization. Dashed line: when the cathode reaction is involved in the spread of oxygen.

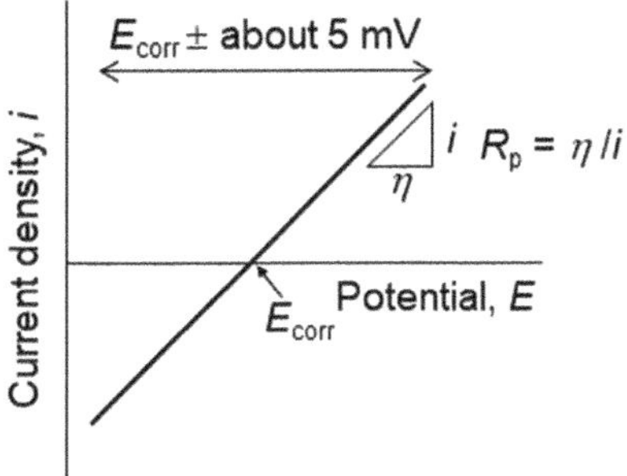

Fig. 3.12. How to find polarization resistance. R_p: polarization resistance, E_{corr}: corrosion potential, η: overvoltage, and i: current density.

3.9 Electrochemical Impedance Method

Electrochemical impedance spectroscopy (EIS) is a test method that evaluates the current response of an electrode at each frequency to the application of a minute sinusoidal AC potential of several mV to 20 mV. It is used to analyze electrode reaction mechanisms and measure corrosion rates. The feature is that continuous *in situ* measurements are possible without adding any disturbance to the system. The electrochemical characteristics near the surface of a metal corroding in an aqueous solution are simulated by an equivalent circuit as shown in Fig. 3.13, which includes circuit components such as charge transfer resistance, solution resistance, and electric double layer capacitance. By measuring the frequency characteristics of the impedance in the range of about 1 mHz to 1 MHz, the value of the circuit component is obtained, when the simulated curve of the assumed equivalent circuit most closely matches the measured data. The equivalent circuit becomes complicated due to an increase in circuit components with various factors such as the roughness of the specimen surface, the presence of a film, and the adsorption of

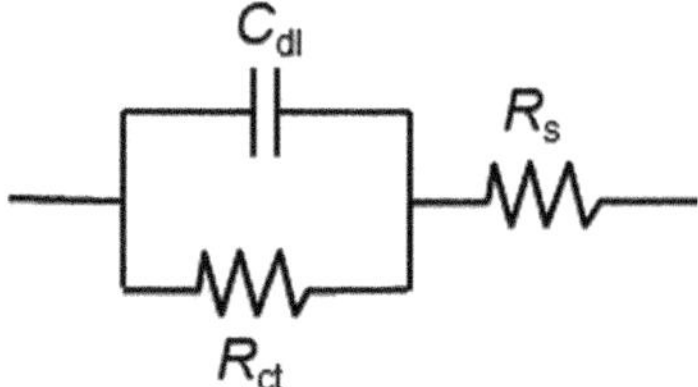

Fig. 3.13. Equivalent circuit near corroded metal surface. R_s: solution resistance, R_{ct}: charge transfer resistance, and C_{dl}: electric double layer capacitance.

solution components. Equation (3-4) is an impedance equation that corresponds to the simplest circuit, the equivalent circuit in Fig. 3.13, where j is an imaginary unit and ω is the angular velocity. In a reaction system simulated by such a simple circuit, impedance corresponding to solution resistance and corrosion resistance (charge transfer resistance on the circuit) is measured on the high frequency side and low frequency side, respectively.

$$Z(j\omega) = R_s + \frac{1}{j\omega C_{dl} + \frac{1}{R_{ct}}} = R_s + \frac{R_{ct}}{1 + \omega^2 C_{dl}^2 R_{ct}^2} - j\frac{\omega C_{dl} R_{ct}^2}{1 + \omega^2 C_{dl}^2 R_{ct}^2} \tag{3.4}$$

Changes in impedances (Z) of CP Ti in saline and Hanks' solution are shown in Fig. 2.24. The impedance in Hanks' solution increases with time that indicates corrosion resistance increases with time, while in saline it is almost constant. Calcium phosphate formation on CP Ti in Hanks' solution works as a resistance, resulting in the apparent corrosion resistance increases.

3.10 Dissolution Test

The main corrosion resistance evaluation method other than the electrochemical method introduced in the above is the dissolution test. This is a test method that determines the corrosion rate by immersion of the material in a test solution for a certain period and then measuring the concentration of released metal ions. Although it is more time-consuming and labor-intensive compared to electrochemical methods, it has the advantage of being easy to interpret the results, providing results that are highly similar to the real environment, and being able to measure each element individually. The main procedures for medical materials are specified (ISO 10271 2020). In addition to the simulated body fluids shown in Table 3.1, the test solutions include aqueous solutions containing lactic acid, hydrochloric acid, amino acid, and mixed aqueous solutions of sodium chloride. Lactic acid is used for corrosion-accelerated tests. A test vessel that has high chemical resistance can be sealed tightly, and has a shape that minimizes contact between the specimen and the vessel. After removing the specimen, the metal ion concentration in the solution is measured using inductively coupled plasma (ICP) analysis or atomic adsorption (AA) analysis. The weight of released metal ion is determined by the following formula.

$$W = V(C - C_0)/S \tag{3.5}$$

where W is the dissolution amount per unit area, V is the volume of test solution, C is the concentration in the solution in which the specimen is immersed, C_0 is the concentration of the blank solution, and S is the contact area between the specimen and the solution.

3.11 Tarnish Test

Surface observation to evaluate corrosion is the simplest qualitative evaluation method. In a corrosive environment, the color tone changes as corrosion products and precipitates form or accumulate on the surface of metals, or as the surface roughness changes. In particular, dental Au and Ag alloys react with trace amounts of soluble sulfides contained in saliva, producing metal sulfides and causing tarnish. Discoloration of dental materials not only indicates signs of deterioration due to corrosion, but also poses a problem from an esthetics perspective. In the color change test for dental materials, the specimen is immersed in an aqueous sodium sulfide solution, and the color change is determined visually or with a color difference meter or colorimeter (ISO 10271 2020). Using a testing machine with a power unit, there are two types of tests: dynamic tests in which the specimen is repeatedly immersed into and withdrawn from the test solution at room temperature, and static tests in which the specimen is continuously immersed.

3.12 Corrosion Potential Measurement

The natural potential (open-circuit potential) obtained when the material is in an open circuit state without being connected to an external power source can also be an important indicator in evaluating corrosion behavior. The natural potential in a corrosion system is called the "corrosion potential." As shown in Figs. 3.10 and 3.11, the corrosion potential is a potential in a non-equilibrium state, determined from the balance of anode and cathode reactions. Generally, an increase in corrosion potential indicates passivation and stabilization of the passive film, i.e. an increase in corrosion resistance, and a decrease in corrosion potential indicates a decrease in corrosion resistance. Fluctuations in the corrosion potential mean that changes are occurring in the reactions at the electrode surface. The value of corrosion potential itself is often misused as a value that indicates high corrosion resistance. However, corrosion potential varies depending on not only the material but also the environmental conditions. It should be noted that corrosion potential does not simply indicate superiority or inferiority of corrosion resistance, because it is also affected by standard electrode potential of component element of the alloy. Figure 3.14 shows change in the open circuit potential of CP Ti in saline and Hanks' solution.

The advantages of corrosion potential measurement are that it can be measured with a simple device and that it can be measured continuously over a long term without adding any disturbance to the corrosion system. Especially for passivated metals, it

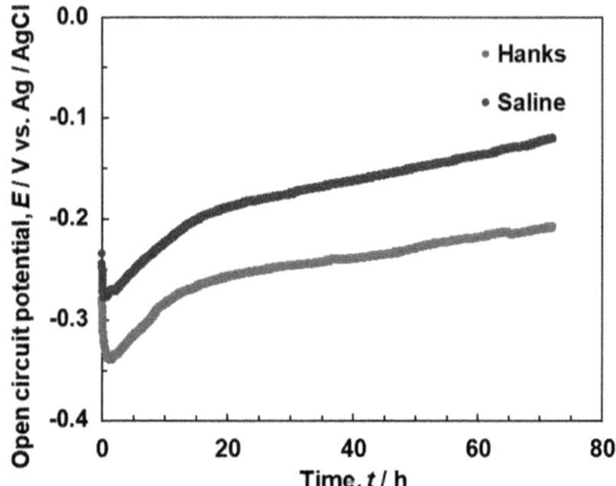

Fig. 3.14. Change in open circuit potentials or corrosion potential of CP Ti in Hanks' solution and saline for 72 h (Reprinted with permission from Taylor & Francis, Kim et al. 2022. Sci. Technol. Adv. Mater. 23: 322–331.).

is useful to compare the effects of changes in alloy composition, surface treatment conditions, and environments, or to investigate changes in corrosion behavior over long time, from several days to several months (ISO16429 2004). In situations where the passive film is unstable and does not provide sufficient protection, resulting in repeated destruction and repassivation, rapid fluctuations in the corrosion potential can be observed. However, since corrosion potential measurement is a qualitative evaluation, it is desirable to use it in conjunction with other electrochemical measurement methods. In addition to simulated body fluids, aqueous solutions with adjusted concentrations, pH, and deaeration condition are used.

3.13 Tribocorrosion Tests

"Tribocorrosion" is a material degradation phenomenon resulting from interactive effects between wear and corrosion. It is commonly found in engineering applications (e.g., biomedical implants and marine equipment) which involve relative motion of contacting metals in a corrosive environment. In other words, tribocorrosion deals with the wear and friction that occurred due to the implants pieces rubbing against one another like hip joint and spine implant, while corrosion is an electrochemical process taking place due to the presence of corrosive species—existing in the body around the implant—leading to the implant's surface degradation. Models describing tribocorrosion of passive metals in sliding contacts are reviewed (Cao and Mischler 2018). Different categories of models (two-body or three-body contact models, lubricated tribocorrosion model, empirical models, multi-degradation models) are found in the literature. Through the identification of relevant chemo-mechanical degradation mechanisms, robust analytical expressions accurately predicting the overall material loss in tribocorrosion have been developed. A critical appraisal of the main electrochemical techniques and evaluation methods used in tribocorrosion research with special emphasis on sliding and fretting situations involving passive metals is performed (Mischler 2008). Tribocorrosion model and the effect of bovine serum albumin (BSA) on wear and friction is explained by the consideration of physical factors such as changes in viscosity and double layer structure, because in the present results no tribofilm formation is observed (Yoneyama et al. 2020). Also, numerical methods have been used to describe time dependent transitions in tribocorrosion. Various investigations have outlined its influential role in the medical devices and disparate routes have been introduced to address this problem (Shahini et al. 2022). The use of several types of alloys, the application of various types of coatings, and the production of porous layers are some of these efforts made till now. The commonly used tribochemical methods adopted in the analysis of tribocorrosion and putting forward some of the models and environmental factors affecting the tribocorrosive behavior of Co–Cr–Mo alloys, a widely-used class of biomaterial for orthopedic implants, are reviewed (Toh et al. 2017). In addition, a theoretical approach to predict currents and voltages over time utilizing the concepts of heredity integrals, area-dependent surface impedance, contact mechanics and the high field physics of oxide repassivation is investigated (Gilbert and Zhu 2020). The coupled integrals were shown to predict the overall current–potential–time behavior for Co–Cr–Mo alloy surfaces under several controlled fretting corrosion conditions (loads, sliding speeds, etc.) with a high degree of similarity. These models can be adapted to numerical analyses of tribocorrosion to predict performance.

3.14 Points to Note in Corrosion Tests

Corrosion of metals is a complex phenomenon that exhibits a wide variety of behaviors depending on the combination of the material and the environment. Corrosion of metallic biomaterials in particular is an environment in which various factors have a complex effect, so the corrosion behavior that should be evaluated will differ depending on the type of material and the purpose of use. Therefore, in corrosion evaluation, it is necessary to predict the corrosion behavior that may occur based on the characteristics of the target device and the corresponding environment, and to select an evaluation method based on these situations. To exactly achieve this evaluation, sufficient knowledge of corrosion and electrochemistry is required. Relying on measurements and interpretation of results by instructions, or simply relying on the analysis results of the software included with the equipment, may lead to serious misjudgments. When handling metallic biomaterials for the human body, the risk of unexpected corrosion must be reduced to a minimum. The international standard for corrosion testing of orthopedic materials (ISO 10271) states that "measurement results should be interpreted based on electrochemical experience and professional skills."

3.15 Characterization of Passive Film

Elements that are important for medical metallic materials, such as Ti, Zr, and Ta, are extremely easily oxidized, and as explained in the Section 2.9, they become passivated by being covered with a passive film (surface oxide film). The passive film is extremely thin (1 to 5 nm) and transparent, so it cannot be seen with the naked eye. Generally, the rate of formation of a passive film is extremely fast, so the film tends to become amorphous (non-crystalline). Amorphous films have no grain boundaries and have few other structural defects, so they have excellent corrosion resistance.

A feature of metallic biomaterials such as CP Ti, Ti alloys, Co-based alloys, and stainless steels, are that their surfaces are covered with a passive film in normal living tissues, and even if they are ruptured for some reason, they can immediately self-repair. In addition, Ta and Pt group alloys exhibit corrosion resistance through passive films.

X-ray photoelectron spectroscopy (XPS) is effective for evaluating the composition and thickness of passive films. Since the passive film is extremely thin, the entire film and the substrate metal can be detected. Figure 3.15A shows an XPS spectrum in the Ti 2p electron binding energy region from Ti sputter-deposited on a glass substrate. It can be decomposed into a total of eight spectra derived from zero-valent (metallic state), divalent, trivalent, and quadrivalent (oxide states) 2 $p_{3/2}$ orbital electrons and 2 $p_{1/2}$ orbital electrons (Asami et al. 1993, Hanawa et al. 1998). The passive film on CP Ti contains not only Ti^{4+} but also Ti^{3+} and Ti^{2+}. Simultaneously, the underlying metallic state (zero valence) is detected through the surface film, indicating that the film is extremely thin. Figure 3.15B shows a spectrum in the O 1s binding energy region from the same sample as Fig. 3.15A. There is a shoulder on the high energy side and it can be separated into at least three spectra. These are caused by oxides, hydroxides, hydroxyl groups, bound water, or adsorbed water (Asami and Hashimoto 1977), and the ratio of the integrated intensities of each spectrum directly indicates the existence property of each chemical state. In other words, the binding energy increases as the oxide becomes OH^- in its reduced state and H_2O in its further reduced state. Passive oxide films usually contain hydroxide and bound water, and passive films on CP Ti in particular are stabilized by containing H_2O.

In addition, in the case of a film that is thin enough to be detected in its entirety by XPS, by using the angular resolution method (Fig. 3.16), which changes the detection angle of photoelectrons, it is possible to detect the film in the depth direction non-destructively without using argon ion sputtering. It is possible to analyze state changes along depth of the film. Since the distance that photoelectrons can travel through a solid is fixed, the lower the angle, the more photoelectrons will be detected near the surface, and by changing the detection angle, it is possible to analyze the composition and state that change in the depth direction (Akiyama et al. 1997). Since this method is non-destructive, there is no change in the chemical state. Figure 3.17 shows the depth variations of the $[OH^-]/[O^{2-}]$ ratio and Ti^{4+} fraction in the passive

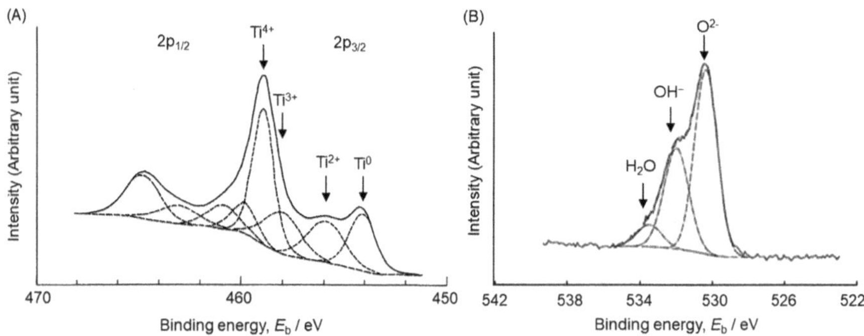

Fig. 3.15. XPS spectra in the Ti 2p electron binding energy region (A) and in the O 1s electron binding energy region (B) from CP Ti sputter-deposited on a glass substrate.

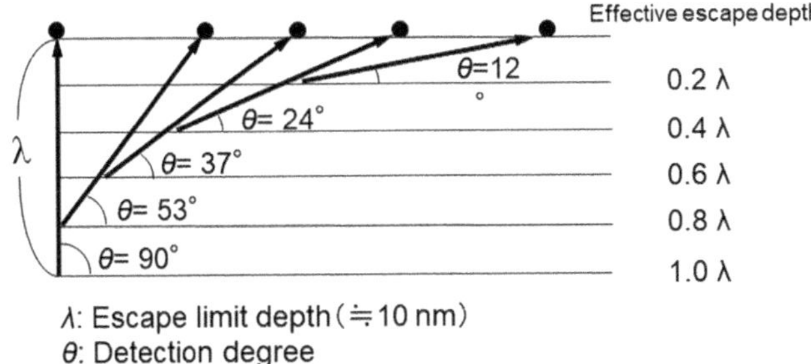

Fig. 3.16. Change in effective escape depth of photoelectron according to the detection angles of the photoelectron.

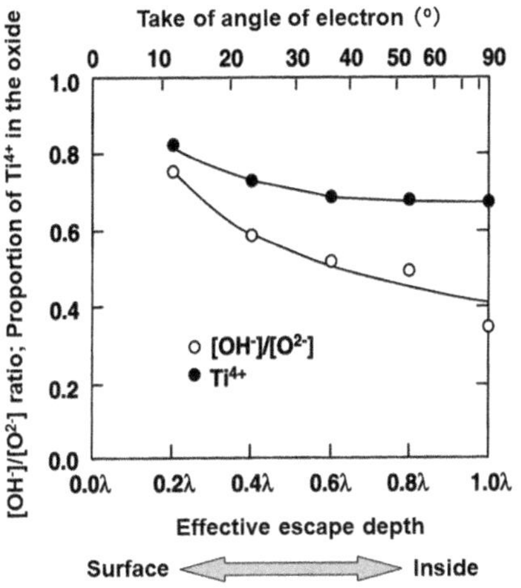

Fig. 3.17. Changes in depth direction of $[OH^-]/[O^{2-}]$ ratio and Ti^{4+} ratio of CP Ti surface oxide film by XPS angle resolution method shown in Fig. 3.16.

oxide film on CP Ti determined by the angle resolution method. The smaller the photoelectron escape angle, the more information near the surface can be obtained. It can be seen that the closer to the surface there are, the more hydroxyl groups or hydroxides there are, and the more Ti^{4+} there is.

3.16 Adsorption of Proteins

When the material comes into contact with biological tissue, protein adsorption begins immediately. Protein adsorption affects subsequent cell adhesion, corrosion of metals, etc. It is also possible that biological functions may be affected by denaturation of the adsorbed proteins. Protein adsorption on metal and oxide surfaces has been analyzed by many methods (Ivarsson and Lundström 1986). The conformation of proteins plays an important role in exerting their functions, and it is important to understand the changes in conformation (Fig. 3.18) when adsorbed onto material surfaces. Since proteins are charged substances, their conformational changes during adsorption depend on the electrostatic force on the surface of the metal. The strength

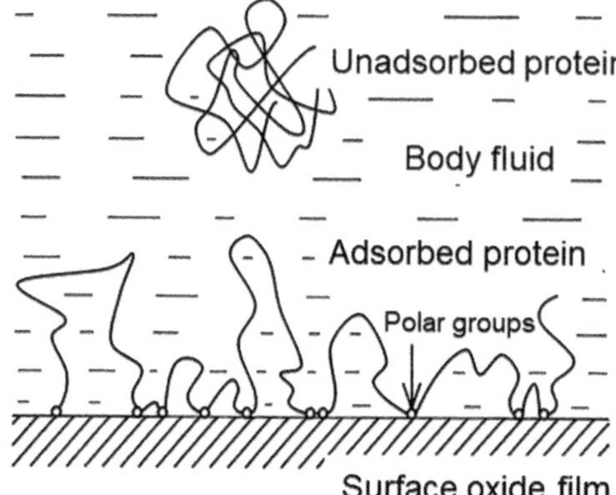

Fig. 3.18. Conformational change of a protein adsorbed on a solid surface.

of the electrostatic attraction of adsorption is determined by the dielectric constant, and the larger the dielectric constant, the smaller the electrostatic attraction. Table 3.2 lists the relative permittivity of water and oxides, and the relative permittivity of Co–Cr–Mo alloy and stainless steel calculated from the oxide values and surface oxide composition (Lide 2006). The dielectric constant of TiO_2 is large compared to others and is close to that of water, so it is expected that the change in conformation during protein adsorption will be small. When fibrinogen is adsorbed onto the surfaces of pure Au and CP Ti in Hanks' solution, it is adsorbed more thickly on the CP Ti surface than on the Au surface, even though it adsorbs more on pure Au than on CP Ti (Sundgren et al. 1986). This is because the Ti surface has a large dielectric constant because it is covered with TiO_2, whereas the dielectric constant of Au is much low because there is no oxide film on the surface. The change in fibrinogen conformation is smaller on the Ti surface where it is adsorbed thicker. In this way, the adsorption amount can be evaluated using an ellipsometer based on the difference in relative thickness of the protein adsorption layer. In addition, when the amount of adsorption is small, the relative size of adsorption can be compared using the C/Ti ratio of the XPS peak for CP Ti and Ti alloys. Other methods include adsorbing proteins labeled with fluorescent substances and observing them using a fluorescence microscope, and methods of desorbing and quantifying the adsorbed proteins.

3.17 Evaluation of Bone Formation Ability by Simulated Body Fluids

Evaluation of bone formation ability is evaluated by immersion in simulated body fluid and characterization using scanning electron microscopy (SEM), energy dispersive X-ray spectroscopy (EDS), X-ray diffractometry (XRD), XPS, etc. Therefore, it cannot be used to evaluate materials whose bone formation ability is promoted by the action of biomolecules such as bone morphogenetic factors such as BMP or cell adhesion peptides. In addition, the surface roughness of the substrate strongly influences the formation of calcium phosphate by immersion in SBFs. Calcium phosphate is easily formed on polishing scratches, grooves, and gaps, and the rougher the surface of the material, the faster the calcium phosphate is formed. Therefore, caution must be required when comparing materials whose surface

Table 3.2. Relative dielectric constant of water and oxide (Data from Lide, D.R. [Ed.]. 2006. CRC Handbook of Chemistry and Physics, 87th ed. RC Press, Boca Raton, FL, USA).

Water/Oxide	Relative dielectric constant	Temperature (°C)	Frequency (Hz)
H_2O	80.1	20	-
TiO_2	85.8-170	25	10^6
Ta_2O_3 (α)	30-65	−196	10^3
Ta_2O_3 (β)	24	19	10^3
CuO	18.1	Ambient	2×10^6
CoO	12.9	25	$10^2 \sim 10^3$
ZrO_2	12.5	Ambient	2×10^6
Cr_2O_3	12.0	Ambient	2×10^6
Al_2O_3	9.3-11.5	25	$10^2 \sim 8 \times 10^9$
SiO_2	4.5-4.6	Ambient	10^5
Fe_2O_3	4.5	Ambient	$10^5 \sim 10^7$
Co–Cr–Mo alloy ASTM F799-95	13.1	-	-
Type 316L stainless steel	4.5	-	-

roughness and morphology have changed due to surface treatment with materials before the treatment. A commonly used SBF to evaluate bone formation ability is so-called "Kokubo's solution,"[1] which is relatively prone to calcium phosphate formation. During immersion in the solution, HA-like precipitates are observed with SEM and XRD to determine bone formation ability (ISO 23317 2007, Kokubo and Takadama 2006). SBF is a term that broadly encompasses solutions shown in Table 3.1, and does not refer only to Kokubo's solution. It cannot be used for materials that dissolve rapidly in the Kokubo's solution, such as biodegradable materials like tricalcium phosphate (TCP).

Similar evaluations can be made by immersion in Hanks' solution, which does not contain glucose, although apatite precipitation does not occur as markedly as in the Kokubo's solution. The advantage of Hanks' solution is that electrochemical treatment and electrochemical measurements can be performed in the solution. Extra components can be easily applied, such as proteins to evaluate the effects of proteins. Calcium phosphate formation is reduced in the presence of protein (Serro et al. 1997).

3.18 Outline of Biological Evaluation

Cells are the smallest unit of life, and cell culture tests are one of the important items in evaluating the properties of medical materials in the biological environment. In cell culture tests, the cells used must be selected according to the purpose. In order to make a final evaluation of the developed biomaterial, the necessary conditions such

[1] In the field of bioceramics, only Kokubo's solution is called SBF, but SBF is a term that refers to a wider range of simulated body fluids as shown in Table 3.1.

as biosafety (non-toxicity), functionality, biocompatibility, and durability must be evaluated using animal experiments. Since animal experiments involve sacrificing the animal's life for human health, it goes without saying that the basis for using animals and the purpose of the experiment are essential. Institutions that conduct animal experiments are required to establish an "animal experiment committee" to conduct appropriate animal experiments, such as reviewing experimental plans submitted by experimenters and deciding whether to approve them. Applicants must submit an animal experiment plan to the animal experiment committee of their institution and obtain approval for the details of the animal experiment plan. It is necessary to attend a designated seminar on animal experimentation, learn about the principles behind animal experimentation standards, and obtain animal experimentation qualifications. The 3Rs are a philosophy regarding standards for animal experiments, and represent the three elements of replacement, reduction, and refinement, and were proposed by British researchers (Russell and Burch 1959). Replacement refers to lower animal species without consciousness or sensation, substitution to *in vitro*, and elimination of duplicate experiments. Reduction refers to reduction in the number of animals used, and use of the minimum number of animals scientifically necessary. Refinement refers to things such as reducing suffering, euthanasia measures, and improving the breeding environment.

However, this book does not cover specific methods of biological evaluation of medical devices using cell culture or animal experiments, or molecular biological evaluation. These biological assessments require skill with appropriate equipment and supervised training, and should be directed directly in the appropriate laboratory. Biological evaluation methods for medical devices are detailed in ISO (ISO 10993-1 2018, ISO 10993-2 2022, ISO 10993-3 2014, ISO 10993-4 2017, ISO 10993-5 2009, ISO 10993-6 2016, ISO 10993-7 2008, ISO 10993-9 2019, ISO 10993-11 2017, ISO 10993-15 2019, ISO 10993-17 2023, ISO 10993-18 2020, ISO 10993-19 2020).

3.19 Toxicity Evaluation

When a new material is developed, it undergoes two types of evaluations: *in vitro* evaluations such as cytotoxicity tests, and *in vivo* evaluations such as animal experiments, before clinical examination of implantation into the human body. The problem with animal experiments is difference in species. There is an unbridgeable gap between humans and animals, and when conducting animal tests, various corrections have been made in an effort to apply experimental results to humans. This extrapolation to humans is still a major challenge in animal experiments. Furthermore, a new issue that has emerged since the 1970s is the need to consider animal welfare. This is widely recognized worldwide, and the current situation is that unnecessary animal experiments are completely prohibited. It is essential that animal experiments that must be carried out be kept to the minimum necessary, and that treatment should be done in a way that does not cause suffering to the animals. A series of these measures has already been enacted into law in developed countries in the name of animal welfare.

Cytotoxicity tests should be performed first to confirm the safety of biomaterials. Although the importance of cytotoxicity testing has increased due to restrictions on animal testing, it cannot completely replace animal testing. The cells used are cell lines or primary cells extracted from tissues extracted from animals or humans, depending on the purpose. In relative proliferation rate tests for colony formation of cell types, 50% inhibitory concentration (IC_{50}) is an indicator of toxicity (Fig. 3.19). The lower the IC_{50} concentration, the less metal is required to cause toxicity, and the toxicity is stronger. The cytotoxic effects of most chemicals can be compared by comparing IC_{50} values. IC_{50} is the LD_{50} in Fig. 2.30 applied to cell proliferation. It is known that IC_{50} is almost independent of cell type. Figure 2.31 shows the correlation between the two types of cytotoxicity with IC_{50}.

In contrast to such cytotoxicity tests in static environments, materials used under wear condition require cytotoxicity tests using dynamic extraction. As shown in Fig. 3.20, this is done by applying abrasion to the metal in the cell culture solution, and adding the culture solution (extract solution) containing metal wear debris and metal ions to a culture solution in which cells are actually cultured. This is a method to examine the relationship between an increase in the proportion of extract and a decrease in cell proliferation rate. If you examine only the effects of released metal ions, filter the extract and add it to the cell culture medium. In addition, depending on the intended use, it is necessary to conduct sensitization tests, mutagenicity tests, irritation tests, etc.

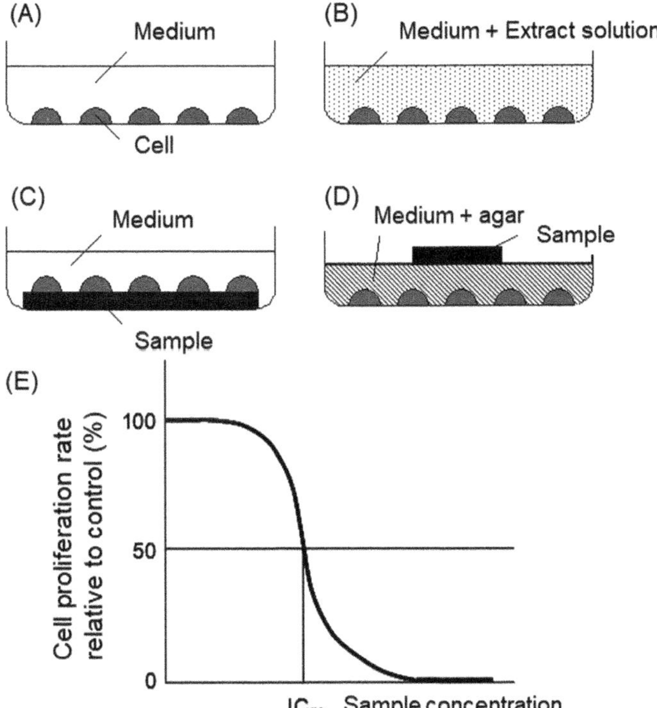

Fig. 3.19. Cell culture test method, evaluation of cell proliferation in the presence of controls and specimens, and determination of IC_{50}. (A) control, (B) extractable test, (C) direct contact test, (D) indirect contact test (agar overlay method), and (E) schematic diagram of how to determine LC_{50} (Reprinted with permission from Corona Co., *Metallic Biomaterials* (Hanawa and Yoneyama: Corona Co., 2007), 80.).

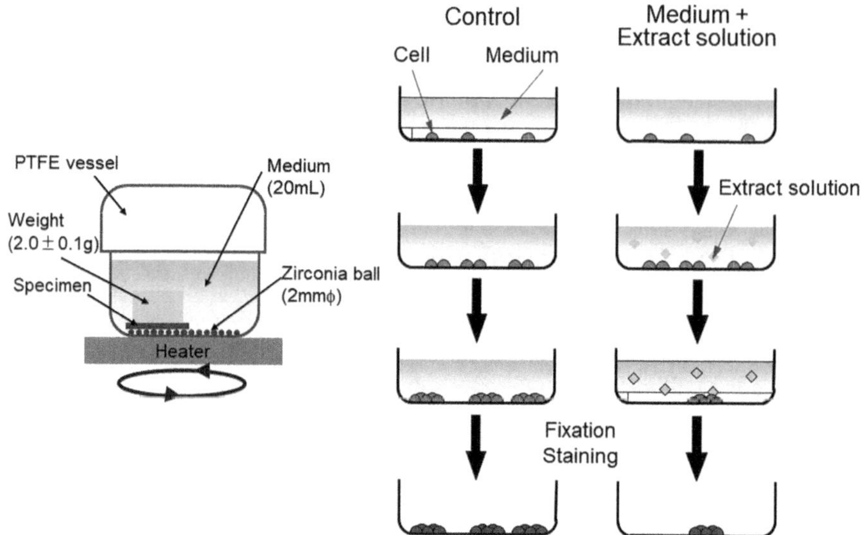

Fig. 3.20. Cytotoxicity evaluation method using dynamic extraction (Reprinted with permission from Corona Co., *Metallic Biomaterials* (Hanawa and Yoneyama: Corona Co., 2007), 81.).

3.20 Cell Compatibility/Functionality Evaluation

3.20.1 Selection of Cell Types

A cell is the smallest unit of life, and cell culture tests are one of the important items in evaluating the properties of medical materials in the biological environment. Biological tissues can be broadly divided into soft tissue and hard tissue, and this section provides an overview of the cytocompatibility and functionality evaluation.

In cell culture tests, the cells used must be selected according to the purpose. Cells used in cell culture tests can be divided into two types: cell lines and primary cultured cells. Established cell lines can be purchased or distributed from cell banks such as ATCC in the United States, and information such as culture methods can be obtained from the place of purchase or distribution. Furthermore, since information can be collected from other researchers who have used the same cell line, it is relatively easy to plan experiments using established cell lines. However, many established cell lines have undergone repeated subcultures since their establishment, and the various properties of the cells have changed to a greater or lesser degree. Furthermore, although cell lines derived from various tissues have been established, there are limits to their types, so it may not be possible to obtain a cell line that perfectly matches the purpose. These problems can be solved by using primary cultured cells. Primary cultured cells are cells that are separated from a living body and cultured outside the body until the first passage. Because primary cultured cells are separated from living tissue, cells that meet the purpose can be obtained. Furthermore, primary cultured cells and cells that have been passaged from primary culture with a small number of passages have fewer mutations compared to established cell lines. However, these cells require higher technology and cost than established cell lines, and are also complicated in many ways, such as the difficulty of obtaining a single cell population. The decision as to whether to use established cell lines or primary cultured cells is largely left to the discretion of each researcher.

3.20.2 Outline of Cell Culture Evaluation

In cell culture tests, tissue compatibility is evaluated by observing and comparing conditions such as adhesion, extension, and proliferation of cells in the material. If the culture equipment is transparent, cells in culture can be directly observed while still alive using a phase contrast microscope (Fig. 3.21). However, when cells are cultured on opaque materials such as metals, they cannot be observed using a phase-contrast optical microscope, so SEM or fluorescence microscope must be used. Observation of cells using these microscopes requires step-by-step processing as shown in Fig. 3.22, and it is impossible to observe living cells with the exception of some techniques.

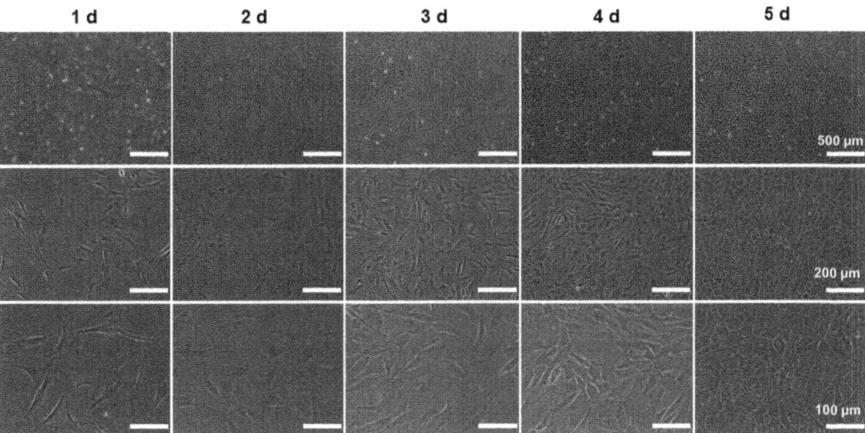

Fig. 3.21. Time transient of osteoblast-like cells (MC3T3-E1) cultured on a sputter deposited Ti thin film observed using a phase contrast optical microscope (provided by Dr. Peng Chen, Tohoku University.).

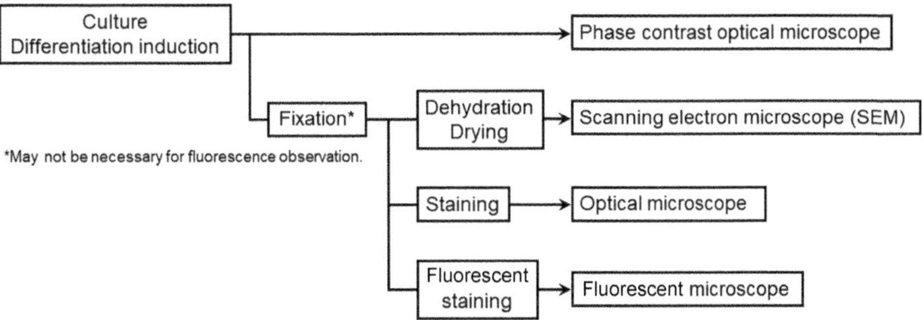

Fig. 3.22. Flow of cell sample processing up to observation with various microscopes.

Cell Fixation

Cell fixation is performed for the purpose of preserving the state of cells during culture. Fixation can render cells and their organs inactive and stabilize their structure. As cell fixatives, aldehyde-based fixatives such as formaldehyde (formaldehyde; formalin) or glutaraldehyde (glutaraldehyde) are generally used. Formaldehyde penetrates into tissues quickly and has excellent preservation properties such as enzyme activity, but glutaraldehyde has better fixative power. Karnovsky's fixative solution (Karnovsky 1965), which is a mixture of formaldehyde and glutaraldehyde, is also used to take advantage of the strengths of each other. In addition, for SEM observation, it is necessary to impart electrical conductivity to the sample, so after pre-fixing with Karnovsky's fixative, etc., post-fixing is sometimes done using osmium tetroxide (osmic acid). Osmium tetroxide is excellent at fixing phospholipids, which are components of biological membranes.

Observation of Cells Using Scanning Electron Microscopy (SEM)

SEM allows observation at extremely high magnifications of 100,000 to 100,000 times or more. Furthermore, because it has an extremely deep focus, it is possible to obtain three-dimensional images. These features have made SEM an indispensable method for observing cells on materials. Figure 3.23 is an SEM image of cells adhering and spreading on the material. It can be seen that the state of cell adhesion and spreading can be observed in great detail. Since SEM observation is performed in a vacuum, it is necessary to perform the following steps before observation: (I) fixation, (II) dehydration, and (III) drying, as shown in Fig. 3.22. In order to observe cell adhesion and spreading in detail, it is desirable to perform pre-fixation with an aldehyde-based fixative followed by post-fixation with osmium tetroxide. In addition, if you want to observe cells without damaging them as much as possible, it is better to perform critical point drying after dehydration. *t*-butyl alcohol freeze-drying is also an effective drying method.

Observation of Cells by Staining

Because the cells are extremely thin and almost colorless and transparent, they cannot be recognized at the optical microscope level. Therefore, in order to observe cells on opaque equipment using an optical microscope, it is necessary to stain the cells with a dye to emphasize differences in absorption. However, if a staining solution is added directly to cells in culture, the state of the cells will change immediately, so fixation must be performed before staining. Giemsa's staining is often applied to observe the adhesion and spread of cells in materials. This method stains cells blue-purple, and stains cell nuclei particularly strongly. Figure 3.24 shows Giemsa staining of cells cultured on CP Ti. The original photograph is in color and stained purple. There are a wide variety of staining solutions depending on the purpose of use, such as hematoxylin (stains cell nuclei), eosin (stains cytoplasm), and Janus green (stains mitochondria).

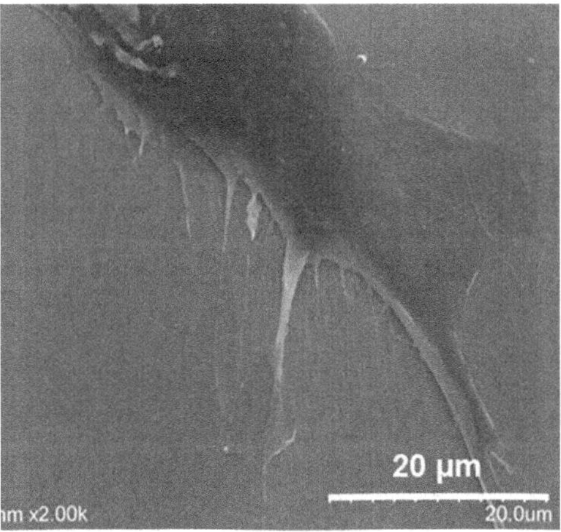

Fig. 3.23. Scanning electron microscopy (SEM) observation of the spread of osteoblast-like cells (MC3T3-E1) adhering to the Zr surface.

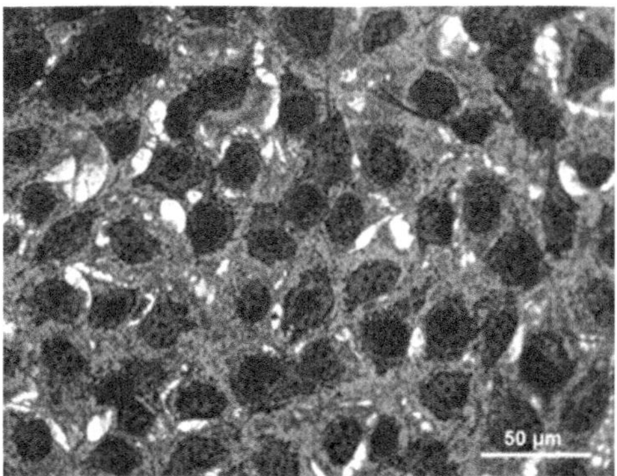

Fig. 3.24. Giemsa-stained osteoblast-like cells (MC3T3-E1) adhered on CP Ti.

Fluorescence Observation of Cells

Fluorescence observation using a fluorescence microscope is also an effective method for observing cells on a sample. Fluorescence observation has high detection sensitivity because it allows observation of only the target object against a dark background. In addition, a wide variety of fluorescent substances can be selected depending on the purpose, and multiple targets can be detected and observed simultaneously by utilizing differences in fluorescence wavelength. Figure 3.25 shows the actin, vinculin, and cell nucleus of cells on a sample that were each fluorescently stained and observed using a fluorescence microscope. The original photograph is in color, with actin emitting red fluorescence, vinculin emitting green fluorescence, and the cell nucleus emitting blue fluorescence. The figure on the far right is a composite of each image. Staining methods for fluorescence observation include methods that directly bind fluorescent dyes to specific molecular structures

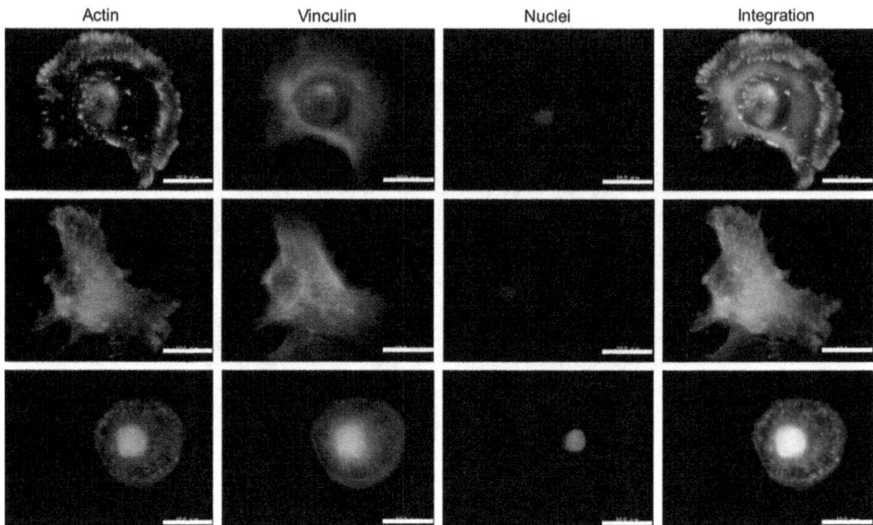

Fig. 3.25. Appearance of cells on the material surface by fluorescence observation (scale bar: 50 μm) (Provided by Dr. Peng Chen, Tohoku University.).

or intracellular organelles (fluorescent staining), and methods that use antibodies labeled with fluorescent substances (fluorescent antibodies). Another method is to introduce fluorescent proteins such as GFP (green fluorescent protein) into cells and observe living cells in real time.

Cell Migration

Cell migration is important for tissue reconstruction such as morphogenesis and wound healing. Cells actively migrate on equipment with excellent cell compatibility. There are several methods to measure cell migration: the wound healing method and the Boyden chamber method. The evaluation of cell migration using the wound healing method can be observed that cells migrate to fill the gaps over time.

Cell Count

On a material that does not have excellent cell compatibility, cells will proliferate slowly or die. Therefore, evaluating cell proliferation is also an important indicator as a method for evaluating cell compatibility and functionality. The most common method for measuring the number of adherent cells on equipment is to collect cells from culture equipment by enzyme treatment, etc., and count the number of cells using a hemocytometer. To measure the number of living cells, trypan blue staining solution is used, which selectively stains only dead cells. This method is inexpensive, but requires experience and skill. In recent years, methods for measuring living cells that utilize intracellular enzyme activity, such as the MTT method, WST-1 method, and WST-8 method, are often used. Recently, software has been developed that uses computer image processing to recognize and count cells within a unit area.

3.20.3 Hard Tissue Compatibility Evaluation

Hard tissue compatibility evaluation in cell culture tests is performed by measuring and observing the differentiation status of osteoblasts that have undergone bone differentiation induction on the material. Once osteoblasts differentiate, they eventually embed themselves in the bone matrix they secrete and become osteocytes. The phenomenon in which cells form bone matrix around themselves is called calcification, and evaluating the timing and amount of calcification is an important indicator in hard tissue compatibility evaluation. Famous osteoblast cell lines include mouse-derived MC3T3-E1, human-derived MG-63, and Saos-2. Furthermore, as mentioned above, since various properties of established cell lines change with passage, they are sometimes referred to as osteoblast-like cells.

In hard tissue compatibility evaluation, it is also important to detect and evaluate various proteins that are expressed in stages until osteoblasts differentiate into bone cells. Typical proteins include type I collagen and alkaline phosphatase (ALP) in the early stages of differentiation, and bone sialoprotein, osteonectin, osteopontin, and other proteins in the middle to late stages of differentiation. Osteocalcin and other substances are expressed (Setzer et al. 2009). When evaluating ALP as an indicator, the following must be noted. The activity of ALP increases immediately after osteoblast differentiation begins, and reaches its maximum level at the beginning of mineralization. Thereafter, the activity decreases once and then increases again (Kuboki et al. 1992). This shows that ALP is deeply involved in mineralization, and the time when ALP activity reaches its peak is an important indicator of osteogenic differentiation. It is believed that the amount of ALP activity is an indicator of differentiation, but there is a report that there is no correlation between the amount of ALP activity and mineralization, and the relationship between the amount of ALP activity and the state of bone differentiation needs to be carefully discussed (Beck Jr. et al. 1998).

Protein evaluation methods include direct qualitative and quantitative determination of proteins produced by cells, and gene expression analysis by extracting messenger RNA (mRNA), which carries the genetic information of proteins, from cells. Osteoblasts undergo osteogenic differentiation after adhering to and spreading on culture equipment, so the evaluation of cell adhesion is also an important item in the initial evaluation of hard tissue compatibility.

Measurement of Calcification Amount

In the evaluation of osteoblast calcification, methods are widely used to stain and observe calcified sites using alizarin red S staining or von Kossa staining. Figure 3.26 shows the evaluation of calcification of osteoblast-like cells (MC3T3-E1 cells) that were induced to differentiate into bone on a CP Ti surface using alizarin red S staining. The original photo is in color, with dark black areas dyed red. In addition, to quantify the amount of calcification, there are two methods: after staining the calcified site, the dye is eluted into a solvent, and the amount of dye in the solvent is quantified using ICP, etc. Methods such as calculating the area of calcified parts using image analysis software are used.

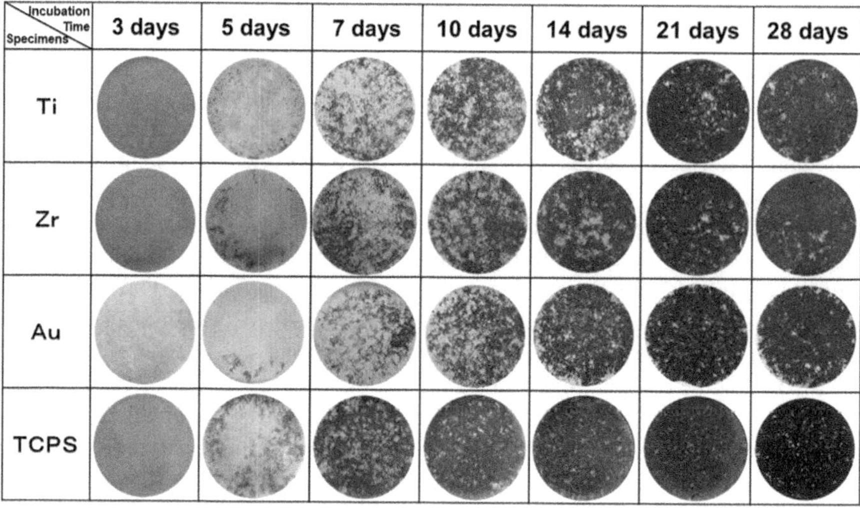

Fig. 3.26. Calcification of osteoblast-like cells (MC3T3-E1) on sputtered Ti, Zr, Au thin film and a tissue culture polystyrene dish (TCPS) (Provided by Dr. Peng Chen, Tohoku University.).

Protein Measurement

Enzyme-linked immunosorbent assay (ELISA) and Western blotting are often used to identify and quantify proteins. These methods detect and quantify target proteins using antibodies that specifically bind to proteins, and are capable of measuring a wide variety of proteins. Compared to Western blotting, ELISA has higher quantitative sensitivity and is a simpler method. On the other hand, Western blotting detects the target protein after separating it by electrophoresis, so it has higher detection accuracy than ELISA. In addition, kits for qualitative or quantitative determination of the amount of specific proteins are also commercially available. The most commonly used kit for hard tissue compatibility evaluation is the ALP activity evaluation kit.

Gene Expression Analysis

For gene expression analysis, reverse transcription polymerase chain reaction (RT-PCR) and DNA microarray are commonly used. Other methods include northern blotting, which detects RNA, and southern blotting, which detects DNA fragments. PCR is a method that selectively amplifies a DNA fragment of interest. RT-PCR is a method in which complementary DNA (cDNA) is created by performing reverse transcription using the target RNA as a template, and PCR is performed based on this cDNA. RT-PCR can detect even minute amounts of RNA and is relatively easy to operate, making it one of the most widely used methods for gene expression analysis. In addition, methods for quantifying the amount of amplified genes include real-time RT-PCR, in which the PCR amplification product is monitored in real time using a fluorescent reagent and quantified in the exponential amplification region, and the amplified product after PCR is subjected to agarose gel electrophoresis. A method of quantifying the density of the obtained band by quantifying it using image analysis software is being used. Because the latter lacks quantitative properties, it is also called semi-quantitative PCR.

A DNA microarray is also called a DNA chip, and uses fluorescently labeled DNA or RNA in a specimen (target) to detect hundreds to tens of thousands of types of cDNA or oligo DNA (probes) arranged and immobilized on a substrate. This method qualitatively and quantitatively evaluates the target genes corresponding to each probe on the substrate by hybridizing the probes. By using mRNA as a target, gene expression in a sample can be analyzed. With DNA microarrays, the expression of hundreds to tens of thousands of genes can be measured at once, and gene expression patterns can be analyzed by clustering. However, since DNA microarrays are basically a method for measuring the expression of a large number of genes at once, the obtained data may contain outliers that appear to be far from the true values. Therefore, when performing gene expression analysis using DNA microarrays, it is desirable to select genes based on the obtained data and examine expression values using quantitative PCR.

3.21 Antithrombotic Evaluation

All metallic biomaterials used in devices placed in blood contact such as stents, heart valves, pacemakers and temporary blood contact devices such as guidewires and catheters are demanded to have blood compatibility. For example, stent restenosis is thought to occur due to thrombus formation on the stent surface, neointimal growth due to increased migration and proliferation of smooth muscle cells, and accumulation of extracellular matrix. One way to prevent this is to select materials and design surfaces that prevent blood clots from occurring on the surface of metal stents.

Thrombus formation occurs by adhesion and aggregation of platelets (primary aggregation). Adherent platelets are activated and undergo secondary aggregation (crosslinking) via fibrinogen in plasma. In addition, plasma proteins such as fibrinogen are initially adsorbed on the surface of metallic materials and influence platelet activation and subsequent thrombus formation.

In order to evaluate the blood compatibility of a material, it is appropriate to implant the material into the blood vessels of an animal such as a dog for a certain period of time, then remove the entire blood vessel and observe the condition of the material's surface. Since animal experiments are limited, a platelet adhesion test is performed as a preliminary evaluation. The general platelet adhesion test procedure is shown in Fig. 3.27. When using human whole blood, each institution uses human cells, so notification and permission are required in accordance with the regulations of each institution, as well as explanation and consent from the blood sample and de-identification of the material. Human whole blood collected from a healthy volunteer is added with 3.8% sodium citrate at a ratio of 1:9 to the blood to inhibit coagulation, and then centrifuged (293 K, 140 G, 15 min). The blood cell components were separated into two layers, and the supernatant, platelet rich plasma (PRP), was extracted. The remaining plasma is further centrifuged (293 K, 1400 G, 30 min) to obtain platelet poor plasma (PPP), a supernatant that is separated into two layers. After measuring the number of platelets in PRP and PPP using a hemocytometer,

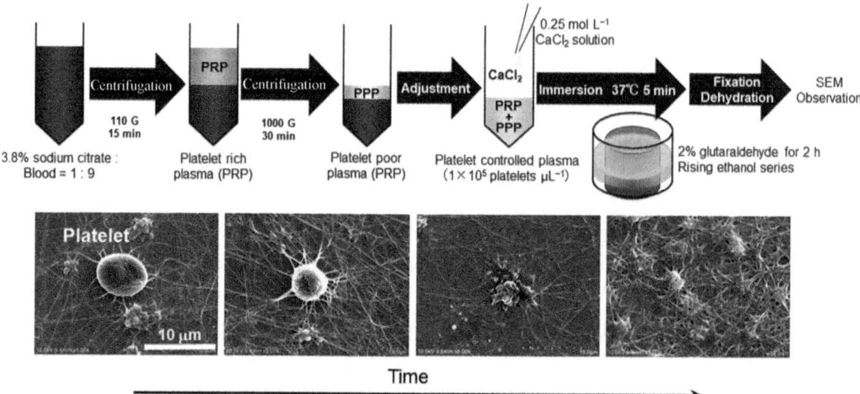

Fig. 3.27. Platelet adhesion test method using human whole blood (top) and morphological changes and fibrin network formation due to activation of platelets adhered to Au (bottom).

mix and prepare the platelet count to 1.0×10^5 μL^{-1}. Ca^{2+} is an important factor that causes platelet aggregation and activation (morphological change). To activate adhered platelets early, add 0.25 mol L^{-1} $CaCl_2$ to the prepared platelet plasma solution to increase the coagulation rate. Each substrate (placed in a 310 K incubator for 30 min before immersion) was immersed in the accelerated solution for 5 min and 20 min (310 K). After soaking, wash with PBS(-) and fix with 2% glutaraldehyde (for at least 2 h). After that, dehydration was performed in an ascending series (15 min each) with 30%, 50%, 70%, 90%, and 100 vol% ethanol, and observed with SEM. Bottom pictures in Fig. 3.27 shows the process of platelet adhesion, platelet activation (aggregation), and fibrin network formation on Au using this method. A platelet adhesion test shown in Fig. 2.34 is performed by this method.

3.22 Bacterial Adhesion/Biofilm Formation Evaluation

Bacteria attached to materials do not simply multiply and form colonies, but also form a biofilm that even includes nutrient supply channels. Aggregates of attached bacteria produce quorum sensing (QS) signals to increase their density, and the bacteria proliferate to form a mature biofilm. The formed biofilm creates channels that take in nutrients. In dentistry, plaque and tartar are a type of biofilm, and it is well known that they cause caries and periodontal disease. In addition, it is known that bacterial invasion of dental implants at the bone-implant interface can cause problems such as loosening. In recent years, in orthopedics, the majority of cases in which implanted parts have to be removed during treatment are due to infections, and these infections are caused by biofilms that form on the surfaces of implanted parts. No method has been established to evaluate biofilm formation in medical materials. It is necessary to develop a contrast method that can directly observe the ease with which biofilms form, the ease with which biofilms come off, and the formation of biofilms within the human body. Regarding oral bacteria, biofilm formation is being performed using artificial oral cavity devices (Ono et al. 2007). Currently, there is no

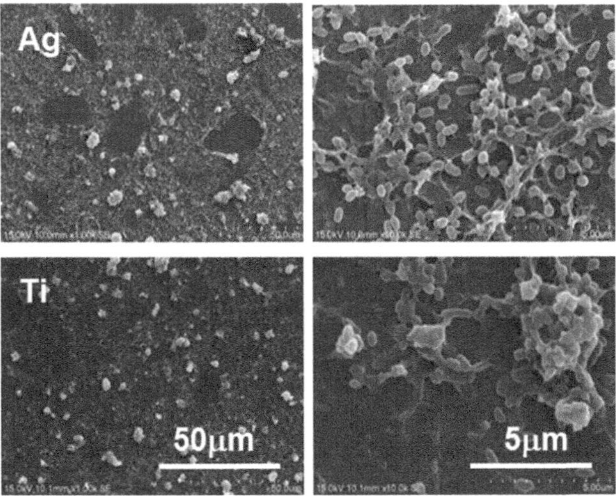

Fig. 3.28. Adhesion of *S. mutans* MT8148 to Ag and CP Ti surfaces.

standard protocol for evaluating biofilm formation, and it is difficult to compare the results of individual studies. Figure 3.28 shows the adhesion and biofilm formation of *S. mutans* on each material surface observed using this method.

3.23 Animal Experiment

In order to make a final evaluation of the developed biomaterial, the necessary conditions such as biosafety (non-toxicity), functionality, biocompatibility, and durability must be evaluated using animal experiments. Since animal experiments involve sacrificing the animal's life for human health, it goes without saying that the basis for using animals and the purpose of the experiment are essential. When biomaterials are implanted, local reactions and systemic reactions occur, both acute and chronic. On the implant material side, material deterioration and elution are thought to occur. Of course, before conducting animal experiments, it is necessary to conduct material property tests and cell experiments to test the rate of deterioration, cytotoxicity, irritability, etc. This is true even if a new device is developed using the same material with improved durability or functional properties; unlike *in vitro*, the *in vivo* environment is quite dynamic, because unpredictable bio-material interactions may occur. By conducting these preliminary tests, an appropriate plan for animal experiments can be made.

Outline of the experimental procedures for animal experiments that require general anesthesia, assuming small animals, is summarized in Fig. 3.29. Animal experiments should not be conducted unless the rationale for using animals and the purpose of the experiment are clear. Animal experiments should be carefully planned and conducted after learning the techniques under experienced experts.

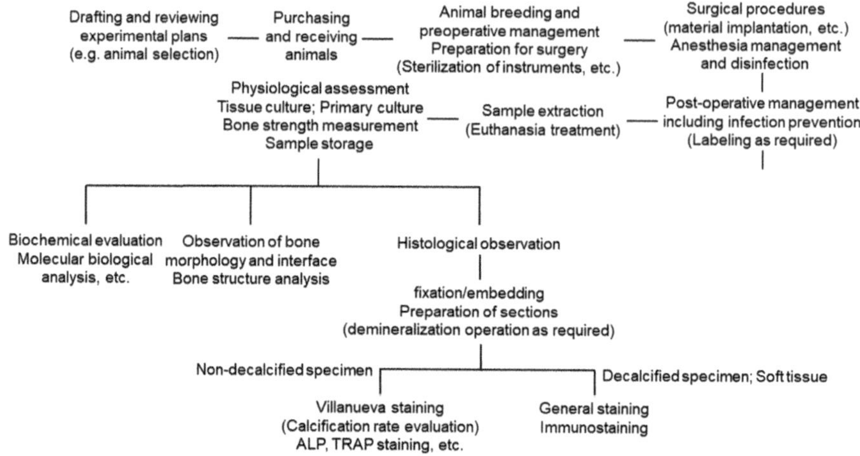

Fig. 3.29. Animal implant evaluation process.

References

Act on Welfare and Management of Animals. 1973. Food and Agriculture Organization of the United Nations, Roma, Italy.

Akiyama, E., A. Kawashima, K. Asami and K. Hashimoto. 1997. An angle-resolved XPS study of the in-depth structure of passivated amorphous aluminum alloys. Corros. Sci. 39: 1351–1364.

Asami, K. and K. Hashimoto. 1977. The X-ray photo-electron spectra of several oxides of ion and chromium. Corros. Sci. 17: 559–570.

Asami, K., S.C. Chen, H. Habasaki and K. Hashimoto. 1993. The surface characterization of titanium and titanium-nickel alloys in sulfuric acid. Corros. Sci. 35: 43–49.

ASM Handbook, Vol. 1A-24A. 2023. ASM International, Materials Park, OH, USA.

ASTM E2789-10. 2021. Standard Guide for Fretting Fatigue Testing. American Society for Testing and Materials, West Conshohocken, PA, USA.

ASTM F1044-05(2017)e1. 2018. Standard Test Method for Shear Testing of Calcium Phosphate Coating and Metallic Coatings. American Society for Testing and Materials, West Conshohocken, PA, USA.

ASTM F1147-05(2017)e1. 2022. Standard Test Method for Tension Testing of Calcium Phosphate and Metallic Coatings. American Society for Testing and Materials, West Conshohocken, PA, USA.

ASTM F1612-95. 1995. Standard Practice for Cyclic Fatigue Testing of Metallic Stemmed Hip Arthroplasty Femoral Components with Torsion Tibial Tray Components of Total Knee Joint Replacements. American Society for Testing and Materials, West Conshohocken, PA, USA.

ASTM F1800-04. 2004. Standard Test for Cyclic Fatigue Testing of Metal Tibial Tray Components of Total Knee Joint Replacements. American Society for Testing and Materials, West Conshohocken, PA, USA.

ASTM F2129-19a. 2019. Standard Test Method for Conducting Cyclic Potentiodynamic Polarization Measurements to Determine the Corrosion Susceptibility of Small Implant Devices. American Society for Testing and Materials, West Conshohocken, PA, USA.

ASTM F732. 1991. Standard Practice For Reciprocating Pin-on-Flat Evaluation of Friction and Wear Properties of Polymeric Materials for Use in Total Joint Prostheses. American Society for Testing and Materials, West Conshohocken, PA, USA, 1991.

Beck, Jr., G.R., E.C. Sullivan, E. Moran and B. Zerler. 1998. Relationship between alkaline phosphatase levels, osteopontin expression, and mineralization in differentiating MC3T3-E1 osteoblasts. J. Cell Biochem. 68: 269–280.

Callister, W.D. and D.G. Rethwisch. 2011. Materials Science and Engineering, 9th ed. Wiley, Hoboken, NJ, USA.

Cao, S. and S. Mischler. 2018. Modeling tribocorrosion of passive metals—A review. Curr. Opin. Solid State Mater. Sci. 22: 127–141.

Gilbert, J.L. and D. Zhu. 2020. A metallic biomaterial tribocorrosion model linking fretting mechanics, currents, and potentials: Model development and experimental comparison. J. Biomed. Mater. Res. Appl. Biomater. 108B: 3174–3189.

Hanawa, T., K. Asami and K. Asaoka. 1998. Repassivation of titanium and surface oxide film regenerated in simulated bioliquid. J. Biomed. Mater. Res. 40: 530–538.

Hanawa, T. and T. Yoneyama. 2007. Metallic Biomaterials, Corona Co., Tokyo, Japan.

ISO 10271:2020. 2020. Dental metallic materials–Corrosion test methods for metallic materials, International Organization for Standardization, Geneva, Switzerland.

ISO 10993-1:2018. 2018. Biological evaluation of medical devices. Part 1: Evaluation and testing within a risk management process. International Organization for Standardization, Geneva, Switzerland.

ISO 10993-2:2022. 2022. Biological evaluation of medical devices. Part 2: Animal welfare requirements. International Organization for Standardization, Geneva, Switzerland.

ISO 10993-3:2014. 2014. Biological evaluation of medical devices. Part 3: Tests for genotoxicity, carcinogenicity and reproductive toxicity. International Organization for Standardization, Geneva, Switzerland.

ISO 10993-4:2017. 2017. Biological evaluation of medical devices. Part 4: Selection of tests for interactions with blood. International Organization for Standardization, Geneva, Switzerland.

ISO 10993-5:2009. 2009. Biological evaluation of medical devices. Part 5: Tests for in vitro cytotoxicity. International Organization for Standardization, Geneva, Switzerland.

ISO 10993-6:2016. 2016. Biological evaluation of medical devices. Part 6: Tests for local effects after implantation. International Organization for Standardization, Geneva, Switzerland.

ISO 10993-7:2008. 2008. Biological evaluation of medical devices. Part 7: Ethylene oxide sterilization residuals. International Organization for Standardization, Geneva, Switzerland.

ISO 10993-9:2019. 2019. Biological evaluation of medical devices. Part 9: Framework for identification and quantification of potential degradation products. International Organization for Standardization, Geneva, Switzerland.

ISO 10993-11:2017. 2017. Biological evaluation of medical devices. Part 11: Tests for systemic toxicity. International Organization for Standardization, Geneva, Switzerland.

ISO 10993-15:2019. 2019. Biological evaluation of medical devices. Part 15: Identification and quantification of degradation products from metals and alloys. International Organization for Standardization, Geneva, Switzerland.

ISO 10993-17:2023. 2023. Biological evaluation of medical devices. Part 17: Toxicological risk assessment of medical device constituents. International Organization for Standardization, Geneva, Switzerland.

ISO 10993-18:2020. 2020. Biological evaluation of medical devices. Part 18: Chemical characterization of medical device materials within a risk management process. International Organization for Standardization, Geneva, Switzerland.

ISO 10993-19:2020. 2020. Biological evaluation of medical devices. Part 19: Physico-chemical, morphological and topographical characterization of materials. International Organization for Standardization, Geneva, Switzerland.

ISO 14242-1:2014/Amd 1:2018. 2018. Implants for surgery, Wear of total hip-joint prostheses, Part 1: Loading and displacement parameters for wear-testing machines and corresponding environmental conditions for test. International Organization for Standardization, Geneva, Switzerland.

ISO 14242-2:2016. 2016. Implants for surgery, Wear of total hip-joint prostheses, Part 2: Methods of measurement. International Organization for Standardization, Geneva, Switzerland.

ISO 14243-1:2009/Amd 1:2020. 2020. Implants for surgery, Wear of total knee-joint prostheses, Part 1: Loading and displacement parameters for wear-testing machines with load control and corresponding environmental conditions for test. International Organization for Standardization, Geneva, Switzerland.

ISO 16429:2004(en). 2004. Implants for surgery – Measurements of open-circuit potential to assess corrosion behavior of metallic implantable materials and medical devices over extended time periods. International Organization for Standardization, Geneva, Switzerland.

ISO 23317. 2007. Implants for surgery. In vitro evaluation for apatite-forming ability of implant materials. International Organization for Standardization, Geneva, Switzerland.
ISO 6474. 1994. Implant for surgery - Ceramic materials based on high purity alumina second edition. International Organization for Standardization, Geneva, Switzerland.
ISO 7206-4:2010. 2020. Implants for surgery - Partial and total hip joint prostheses - Part 4: Determination of endurance properties of stemmed femoral components with application of torsion. International Organization for Standardization, Geneva, Switzerland.
Ivarsson, B. and I. Lundström. 1986. Physical characterization of protein adsorption on metal and metal oxide surfaces. CRC Critic. Rev. Biocompatibility 2: 1–96.
JIS T 0303:2000. 2000. Testing method for wear resistance of materials for artificial joints by pin-on-disk method. Japanese Standard Association Group, Tokyo, Japan.
JSME S 015-2002. 2002. JSME standard fretting fatigue test configuration. The Japanese Society of Mechanical Engineering, Tokyo, Japan.
Karnovsky, M.J. 1965. A formaldehyde-glutaraldehyde fixative of high osmolality for use in electron-microscopy. J. Cell Biol. 27: 137-138A.
Kim, S.C., T. Hanawa, T. Manaka, H. Tsuchiya and S. Fujimoto. 2022. Band structures of passive films on titanium in simulated bioliquids determined by photoelectrochemical response: principle governing the biocompatibility. Sci. Technol. Adv. Mater. 23: 322–331.
Kokubo, T. and H. Takadama. 2006. How useful is SBF in predicting in vivo bone bioactivity? Biomaterials 27: 2907–2915.
Kuboki, Y., A. Kudo, M. Mizuno and M. Kawamura. 1992. Time-dependent changes of collagen cross-links and their precursors in the culture of osteogenic cells. Calcif. Tissue Int. 50: 473–480.
Lide, D.R. [Ed.]. 2006. CRC Handbook of Chemistry and Physics, 87th ed. RC Press, Boca Raton, FL, USA.
Mischler, S. 2008. Triboelectrochemical techniques and interpretation methods in tribocorrosion: A comparative evaluation. Tribol. Int. 41: 573–583.
Russell, W.M.S. and R.L. Burch. 1959. The Principles of Humane Experimental Technique, Methuen, London, UK.
Serro, A.P., A.C. Fernandes, B. Saramago, J. Lima and M.A. Barbosa. 1997. Apatite deposition on titanium surfaces—the role of albumin adsorption. Biomaterials 18: 963–968.
Setzer, B., M. Bächle, M.C. Metzger and R.J. Kohal. 2009. The geneexpression and phenotypic response of hFOB 1.19 osteoblasts to surface-modified titanium and zirconia. Biomaterials 30: 979–990.
Shahini, M.H., H.E. Mohammadloo and B. Ramezanzadeh. 2024. Recent approaches to limit the tribocorrosion of biomaterials: A review. Biomass Convers. Biorefin. 14: 4369–4389.
Sundgren, J.E., P. Bodö, B. Ivarsson and I. Lundström. 1986. Adsorption of fibrinogen on titanium and gold surfaces studied by ESCA and ellipsometry. J. Colloid Interface Sci. 113: 530–543.
Wei Quan Toh, W.Q., X. Tan, A. Bhowmik, E. Liu and S.B. Tor. 2017. Tribochemical characterization and tribocorrosive behavior of CoCrMo alloys: A review. Materials 11: 30.
Yoneyama, C., S. Cao, A.I. Anna Igual Munoz and S. Mischler. 2020. Influence of bovine serum albumin (BSA) on the tribocorrosion behaviour of a low carbon CoCrMo alloy in simulated body fluids. Lubricants 8: 61.

CHAPTER 4

Medical Use of Metals

4.1 Introduction

The advantages of metals compared to ceramic and polymeric materials are that they have greater strength and plasticity, and therefore greater fracture toughness. In other words, it is difficult to be fractured. Therefore, it is used in fractured bone fixators, artificial joints, and screwing devices, that are applied heavy loads. In addition, since the amount of deformation from the start of plastic deformation to fracture (elongation to fracture) is large, it is used for components such as spinal rods, maxillofacial plates, and mini plates that must be plastically deformed in the operating room according to the shape of bones and skeleton. Another important property of metals is that they can be elastically deformed, and stents, embolic coils, guide wires, etc., take advantage of this property. Stents are folded metal mesh tubes that are transported to the affected area through blood vessel using a catheter and placed in narrowed regions. Stents are also used to dilate bile ducts and esophagus. For this purpose, elasticity that expands from the folded state and rigidity that can resist the contraction force of the blood vessel are required. Furthermore, since stent treatment is performed while performing X-ray contrast, good X-ray contrast performance is required, so the use of metals is essential. Attempts to manufacture orthodontic wires from polymers have been going on for half a century, but polymers tend to creep at body temperature and gradually lose their elasticity, so the use of metal is essential. The clasps of partial dentures must also be made of metals for the same reason. In these medical components, metals cannot be replaced with other materials mainly due to mechanical reliability. Metals are also essential for surgical instruments. Comprehensive handbook on metals for medical devices should be referred (ASM Handbook Vol. 23, Vol. 23A 2023).

4.2 Use of Metals for Medical Devices

Table 4.1 shows medical devices that consist of metals and the types of metals used. Metals that come into contact with living tissues run the risk of exhibiting toxicity if they are dissolved as metal ions due to corrosion or become wear debris due to friction wear. Therefore, high corrosion resistance is absolutely necessary for metals

Table 4.1. Metals used for medical devices.

Clinical division	Medical device	Material
Orthopedics	Spinal fixation	CP Ti; Ti–6Al–4V; Ti–6Al–7Nb; 316L SS
	Bone fixation (bone plate, screw, wire, bone nail, mini-plate, etc.)	CP Ti; Ti–6Al–4V; Ti–6Al–7Nb; Co–Cr–W–Ni; 316L SS
	Artificial joint; Bone head	Ti–6Al–4V; Ti–6Al–7Nb; Ti–15Mo–5Zr–3A; Ti–6Al–2Nb–1Ta–0.8Mo; Co–Cr–Mo; Zr–Nb; 316L SS; Fe–Cr–Ni–Co
	Spinal spacer	Ti–6Al–4V; Ti–6Al–7Nb; 316L SS
Cardiology	Implant-type artificial heart (housing)	CP Ti
	Pace maker (case) (electric wire) (electrode) (terminal)	CP Ti; Ti–6Al–4V Co–Cr–Ni–Mo–Fe; Ni–Co CP Ti; Pt–Ir CP Ti; 316L SS; Pt
	Artificial valve (frame)	Ti–6Al–4V
	Stent	Co–Cr–Ni–Mo; Co–Cr–Ni–W–Fe; Co–Cr–Fe–Ni; 316L SS; Ni–Ti; Ta
	Catheter	304 SS; 316L SS; Co–Cr; Ni–Ti; Au; Pt–In
	Guide-wire	316L SS; Co–Ni–Cr–Mo; Ni–Ti
	Embolization wire	Pt
	Aneurysm clip	CP Ti; Ti–6Al–4V; Co–Cr–Ta–Ni; Co–Cr–Ni–Mo–Fe; 630 SS
Otolaryngology	Artificial inner year (electrode)	Pt
	Artificial eardrum	316L SS
Dentistry	Filling	Au foil; Ag–Sn(–Cu) amalgam
	Inlay; Crown; Bridge; Clasp; Post; Denture base	Au–Cu–Ag; Au–Cu–Ag–Pt–Pd; Ag–Pd–Cu–Au; Co–Cr–Mo; Co–Cr–Ni; Co–Cr–Ni–Cu; CP Ti; Ti–6Al–7Nb; 304 SS; 316L SS
	Thermosetting resin facing crown; Metal-ceramic restoration	Au–Pt–Pd; Ni–Cr
	Solder	Au–Cu–Ag; Au–Pt–Pd; Au–Cu; Ag–Pd–Cu–Zn
	Dental implant	CP Ti; Ti–6Al–4V; Ti–6Al–7Nb; Au
	Orthodontic wire	Ni–Ti; Ti–Mo; Co–Ni–Cr–Mo; 316L SS
	Magnetic attachment	Sm–Co; Nd–Fe–B; Pt–Fe–Nb; 444 SS; 447J1 SS; XM27 SS; 316L SS
	Treatment device (bar, scaler, periodontal probe, dental tweezers, raspatory, etc.)	304 SS
General surgery; Diagnostics	Needle of syringe	304 SS
	Scalpel	420J1 SS
	Suture stapler	630 SS; 304 SS
	Surgical robot	SS
	CT; MRI; PET	SS
	Endoscope	SS

SS: Stainless steel

used for medical implant devices, so noble metals and corrosion-resistant metals (mainly passive metals and alloys) are used.

In orthopedics, it is used in artificial hip and knee joints, bone fixators, spinal fixators, and spinal spacers that bear heavy loads. The use of metals is essential in reconstructing the motor and skeletal functions of locations that are subject to such heavy loads. Another important property of metals is that they can be elastically deformed, and stents and guide wires that require flexible deformation along blood vessels utilize this property. In dentistry, when the shape or function of a tooth is partially impaired due to caries or trauma, restoration is performed using artificial materials. These medical devices can be broadly classified into three types.

I. Devices that are completely implanted within the patient's body and remain in the body for a long term or semi-permanently.

II. Devices that are inserted into the patient's body or come into contact with human tissue but are removed after a short term.

III. Devices used without implantation or insertion into patient's body.

Artificial joints, bone fixators, spinal fixation devices, stents, artificial valves, cerebral aneurysm clips, and dental implants fall under category I. Since they are in contact with living tissue for a long term, they are required to have not only long-term safety but also long-term durability, bone formation ability, soft tissue adhesion, and sterilizability. Therefore, CP Ti, Ti alloys, Co-based alloys, stainless steels, Pt, etc., are used. Stents, stent grafts, cerebral aneurysm clips, and embolic coils are medical devices that have made minimally invasive medical treatment possible. A cardiac pacemaker is also a medical device that is left in the body for a long term.

Guide wires, catheters, endoscopes, scalpels, injection needles, staples, dental endodontic files, probes, scalers, etc., fall under category II. Orthodontic wires also fall into this category. Short-term safety, short-term durability, lubricity within blood vessels and organs, flexibility, balance between rigidity and flexibility, antibacterial properties, and sterilization are required. This is also a medical device that usually uses metals due to the requirements for strength and rigidity. In particular, scalpels, endodontic files, probes, scalers, etc., need to be as hard as tools. Mainly stainless steel and Co-based alloys are used.

Metals used for parts of surgical robots that do not come into contact with the human body and for the bodies of diagnostic equipment such as X-ray computed tomography (CT), and magnetic resonance imaging (MRI) fall under category III, while these materials are used as structural materials for the bodies of devices. Electromagnetic properties are important depending on the device. Usually stainless steel, steel materials, etc., are used.

4.3 Orthopedics

4.3.1 Metals in Orthopedics

As the elderly population increases, the number of age-related degenerative diseases such as osteoarthritis and musculoskeletal diseases like osteoporosis will increase, and the importance of treatment for locomotive syndrome will become increasingly important so that the elderly can maintain self-reliance in life. Since the decline in motor function is often directly linked to bedridden status, the reconstruction of these functions and the regeneration of bone tissue are extremely important issues. Many metallic biomaterials are used for artificial joints, bone fixators, spinal fixators, vertebral spacer, and intervertebral spacer. Metals which exhibit stable functionality over long term even under mechanically severe environments are the mainstay of current orthopedic treatment. There are reviews and books on orthopedic implant materials (Rony et al. 2018, Szczesny et al. 2022, Tapscott and Wottowa 2023).

4.3.2 Artificial Joints

Cases in which artificial joints are applicable include rheumatoid arthritis, osteoarthritis, fractures around joints, and tumorous diseases, and are used to restore joint function that has been destroyed due to disease or trauma. In the treatment of musculoskeletal diseases, artificial joints as shown in Fig. 4.1 are essential. Artificial joints used in clinical practice include artificial hip joints, knee joints, shoulder joints, elbow joints, ankle joints, and finger joints. The market for artificial joints continues to expand as the aging population increases (Fig. 4.2) (Predence Research 2023).

Total hip arthroplasty (THA), developed by Charnley in the 1960s, is still the model most commonly used in clinical practice, although various models have since appeared (Charnley 1961). The artificial hip joint consists of a femoral component on the femoral side and an acetabular component on the pelvic side (Fig. 4.3). The acetabular component consists of an acetabular preparation cup and liner. The Charnley hip prosthesis and femoral component consist of a femoral stem consisting of type 316L stainless steel, Co-Cr-Mo alloys, or Ti alloys and a sliding

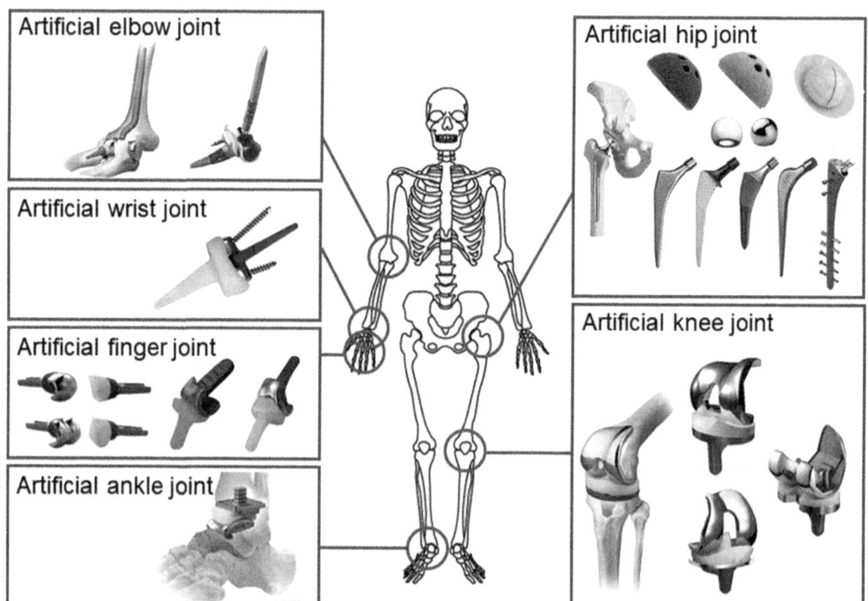

Fig. 4.1. Examples of artificial joints (Provided by Teijin Nakashima Medical Co., Ltd.).

head consisting of Co-Cr-Mo alloys. The acetabular component forms the joint with ultra high molecular weight polyethylene (UHMWPE) socket, which is fixed to the acetabulum using poly(methyl methacrylate) (PMMA) bone cement. The sliding parts that play a role in the joint function are basically made of a combination of metals and polymers, so over many years of use, the polymer UHMWRE wears out and wear debris is generated. Wear debris invades the interface of the artificial joint, causing osteolysis around the stem, and the repeated mechanical stress on the artificial joint during daily life activities generates loosening of the artificial joint. The survival rate with the end point of revision surgery for loosening 25 years after Charnley THA is approximately 90% for the femoral component and approximately 75% for the acetabular component. The amount of wear on the femoral head and socket varies depending on the combination of materials (Fig. 4.4). To reduce this wear, artificial hip joints made of ceramics-on-ceramics or metal-on-metal are attracting attention. However, ceramics have low fracture toughness values, and they may be at risk of fracture due to mechanical loads in daily life. With metal-on-metal combinations, the generation of wear debris is seen as a clinical problem, but acetabular components made from a combination of highly wear-resistant Co-Cr-Mo alloys have been growing in Europe and other regions. In addition, irradiation of gamma ray followed by heat treatment (Oonishi et al. 1992), the addition of vitamin D to UHMWPE (Lan et al. 2021), and the coating of 2-methacryloyloxyethyl phosphorylcholine (MPC) polymer (Kyomoto et al. 2009, Ishihara 2015) have been utilized to improve the wear resistance of UHMWPE. However, it is necessary to wait for clinical results in long-term cases.

There are two types of stem fixation to the femoral cortical bone: a cement fixation type with PMMA bone cement and a cement-less type that does not use bone cement. In the case of cement fixation, the polymerization heat of the cement and the toxicity of residual monomers may have harmful effects on the patient. Artificial joint systems that do not use bone cement at all are called cement-less systems; systems that only partially use bone cement are called hybrid systems. In the case of cement-less stems, the roughened surface created by plasma spraying of CP Ti on the top of the stem generates mechanical anchoring and increase bonding force with the bone (Fig. 4.3B). Furthermore, research is continuing to improve the surface of metals to integrate them with bone (see Chapter 10). Completely removing bone cement once

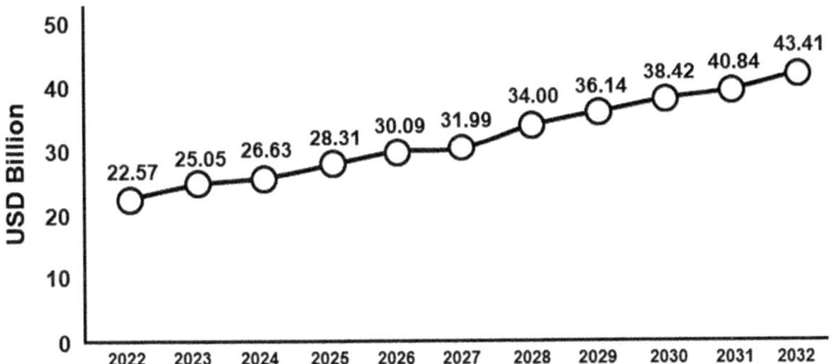

Fig. 4.2. Artificial market size. Reproduced from data by Precedence Research (Reproduced from the data of a reference (Predence Research 2023).

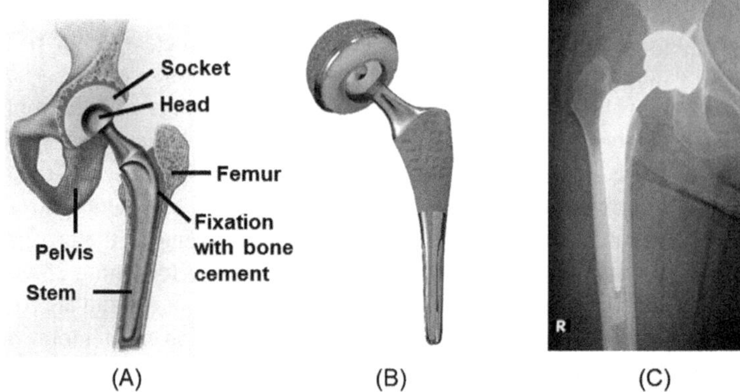

Fig. 4.3. Examples of Charnley's artificial hip joints bone cement type (A), cement-less type (B) (provided by Striker Japan), and X-ray image (C) (Provided by Dr Takuya Konno, National Hospital Organization.).

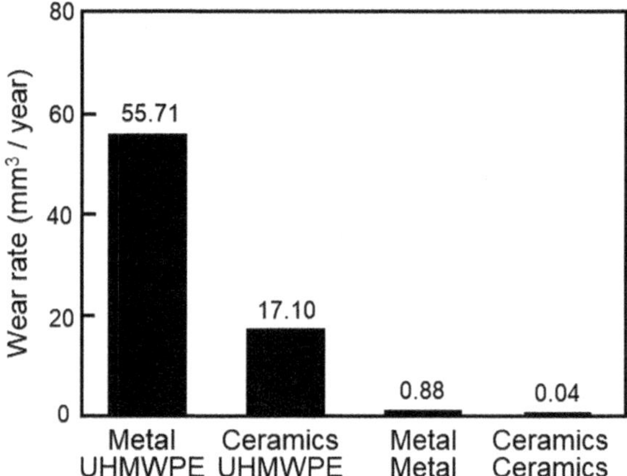

Fig. 4.4. Differences in the amount of wear due to the combination of sliding parts of artificial hip joints (Reproduced from Research report: Development and evaluation technology for artificial joints, Research and Development of Medical Welfare Equipment Technology, NEDO, Japan (2000).).

injected during reoperation is cumbersome and time-consuming, so going cement-less has the advantage of reducing the burden on patients and surgeons.

Since the 1890s, when artificial knee joints were created using ivory, attempts were made in the 1940s to create artificial knee joints in which only the femoral side was covered with metals and in which only the tibia side was covered with metals. Later, based on the success of bone cement and polyethylene for artificial hip joints, a similar combination was introduced for artificial knee joints. In the 1970s, total knee joint prosthesis was developed with a design that is now the prototype. Afterward, further improvements have been made to improve the fixation with the bone, improve the durability of the material, and expand the range of motion (angle of bending and straightening) up till the present. An example of an artificial knee joint is shown in Fig. 4.5. Most of the sliding parts of artificial knee joints are a combination of Co-Cr-Mo alloy and UHMWPE. Although it depends on the

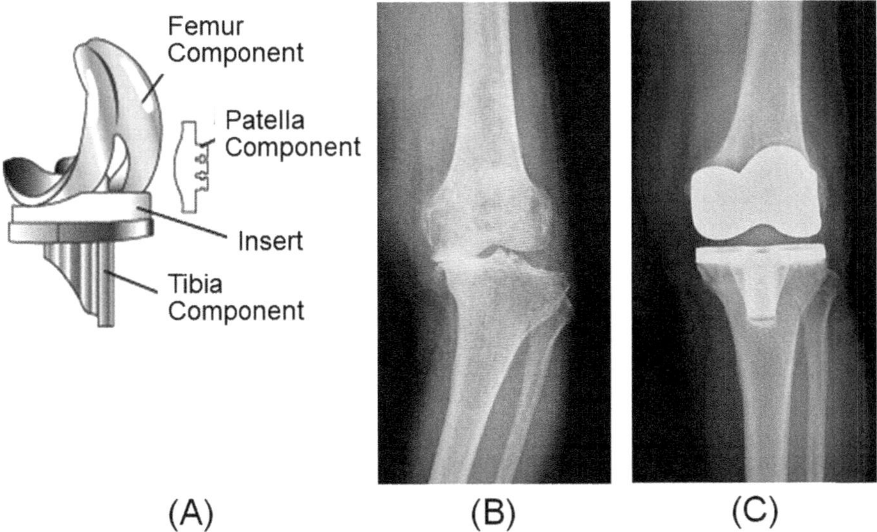

Fig. 4.5. (A) Schematic diagram of an artificial knee joint (provided by Stryker Japan Co., Ltd.), (B) X-ray image before artificial joint replacement. The articular cartilage on the medial side of the knee joint has worn away, and the joint space has disappeared, and (C) X-ray image after joint replacement surgery (Provided by Dr. Takuya Konno, National Hospital Organization.).

preoperative condition, most patients will be able to bend their knees to about 100° to 140° after discharge from the hospital.

Due to recent advances in surgical instruments and technology, minimally invasive surgery (MIS), which performs artificial joint replacement with small incisions, is rapidly gaining popularity. Minimally invasive surgery will shorten the hospital stay and allow patients to return to society sooner, so the application of MIS to artificial hip joints and knee joints will progress further in the future, and specialized equipment is currently being actively developed.

The global joint reconstruction devices' market size was valued at USD 26.06 billion in 2022 and is anticipated to grow at a compound annual growth rate (CAGR) of 4.4% from 2023 to 2030. Based on the joint type, the market for joint reconstruction devices is segmented into knee, hip, shoulder, and ankle. The knee segment is expected to have a significant revenue share in 2022 and is anticipated to grow at a significant rate over the forecast period. With the population getting older, the occurrence of conditions such as osteoarthritis that frequently necessitate knee surgeries is also rising. Progress in surgical methods, implants, and artificial joints enhances the success and availability of knee surgeries, motivating individuals to consider treatment—these are the factors driving the growth of the segment (Grand View Research 2023).

4.3.3 Bone Fixators

For fractured bone fixation, usually a plate and screws in which a plate is placed on the outside of the cortical bone and fixed with screws (Fig. 4.6A), a bone nail

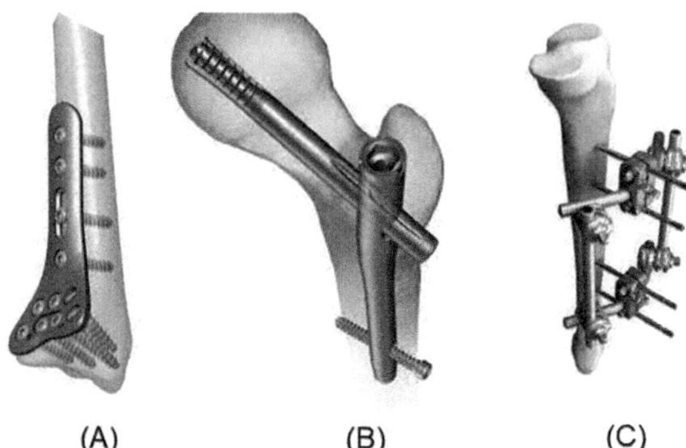

Fig. 4.6. Bone fracture fixation material. (A) Locking plate and screw, (B) intramedullary nail, and (C) external fixation device (Provided by Striker Japan Co. Ltd.).

in which a rod is inserted into the bone marrow and fixed from within the bone (Fig. 4.6B), and an external fixator from outside the human body (Fig. 4.6C), are used. In order to heal the fractured bone, it is necessary to provide a certain level of stability to the fractured site for several months. In other words, it is necessary to maintain the mechanical stability of the affected area using a highly rigid material such as metals. During the bone healing process at the fracture site, the fracture site is initially filled with immature or soft bone, and is gradually remodeled into strong, mature bone with collagen fibers running in an orderly manner. Appropriate mechanical stimulation is essential to form this strongly matured bone. The Young's modulus of the metals used for bone fixation is much higher than that of cortical bone, so the metal absorbs most of the mechanical load applied to the fractured region. Therefore, if internal fixation metal is left in place for a long term, bone maturation may be delayed. This may induce bone resorption, leading to bone fragility (device related osteoporosis or osteopenia). This mechanical load blocking of the bone by internal fixation metal is called "stress shielding" (McAfee et al. 1989) (see Section 5.10 and Fig. 5.19).

Most conventional bone fixation materials were made of stainless steel, while in recent years Ti alloys and Co–Cr–Mo alloy have been increasingly used. Because Ti alloy has high biocompatibility, when using Ti alloy screws or bone nails implanted into the bone marrow, callus may form around the material during the fixation period, making removal difficult (Schmalzried et al. 1991). Stainless steel ones are used if they need to be removed after healing.

We meet the needs of clinical practice by color-coding using the anodic oxidation method (anodizing) to make it easier to distinguish between left and right, body part, and size.

4.3.4 Spinal Fixators and Spacers

Metal implants in spine surgery are used to correct and fix spinal deformities such as vertebral fractures and scoliosis (Figs. 4.7A and 4.7B). It is also used in surgeries to stabilize severe spinal instability caused by tumors or degenerative diseases, and to maintain corrected position until bone union is complete. The purpose of spinal

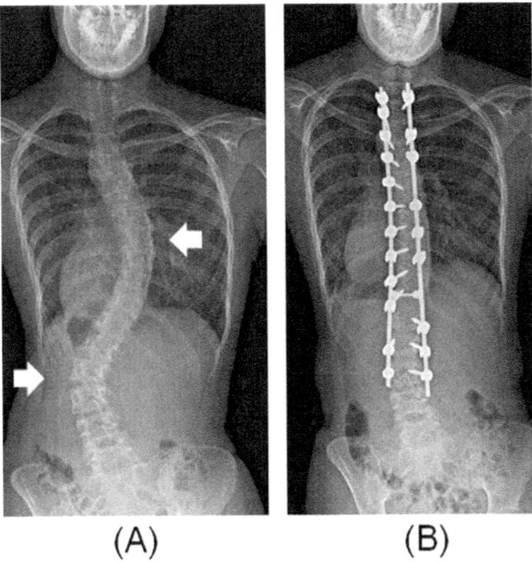

Fig. 4.7. Corrective surgery using pedicle screw and rod system for scoliosis. (A) Preoperative X-ray image. Allows for scoliotic curves around 60 degrees. (B) Postoperative X-ray image. Scoliosis has been corrected to about 20°, and thoracic deformity has also been corrected. (Provided by Dr. Manabu Ito, National Hospital Organization).

implants is exposed to the mechanical load until the surgical site has osseointegrated and stabilized. Therefore, spinal implants are used until the complete bone healing. Spinal fixation devices are always used as a system, as shown in Fig. 4.8. The components are plate fixation with screws, rod fixation with screws, wire fixation, cage fixation, and transforaminal lumbar interbody fusion (TLIF) or plif lumbar interbody fusion (PLIF) with intervertebral spacers (Fig. 4.8B). Variety of shapes and sizes are available depending on the purpose. For spinal fixation devices, Ti alloy is usually used in Japan, but stainless steel is also often used in Europe and the United States (Sin et al. 2009).

The first attempt to fix the spine using a metallic biomaterial was conducted in 1891 using silver wire (Hadra 1891). Thereafter, stainless steel internal fixation materials appeared in the 1930s, then spinal instrumentation surgery rapidly developed after the publication of the Harrington method (Harrington 1962). In the 1960s, when spinal implants had not yet been developed, patients were forced to lie down in order to keep the treated area at rest for several months while bone healing was completed. However, with the improved fixation of spinal implants in recent years, a few days after the surgery, the patient is able to get out of bed and walk, which plays a major role in improving the patient's QOL. However, if bone alliance is not completed in the implanted region, repeated mechanical stress on the implant over a long term will cause fatigue and fracture, so it is important to complete bone alliance in the implanted region. Remarkable technologies in recent years are artificial intervertebral discs and artificial facet joints, which reconstruct the spinal column while preserving mobility rather than fixing the spinal column and sacrificing mobility. Artificial intervertebral discs have been widely used mainly in Europe and the United States. In terms of mid- to long-term clinical results, there have been occasional cases of failure of artificial discs in the lumbar vertebrae, and it

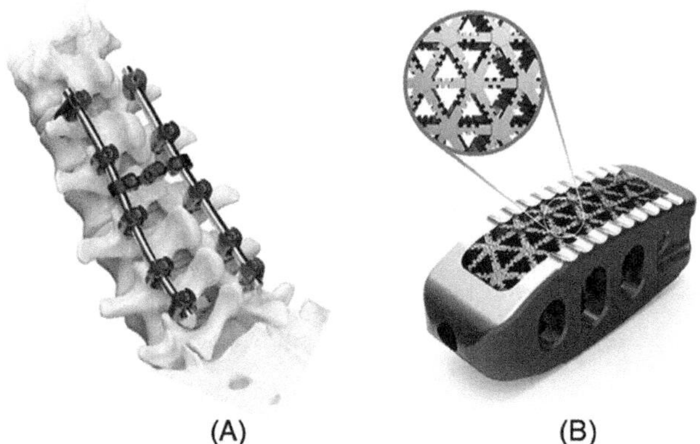

Fig. 4.8. Spinal fixation rod and pedicle screws (A) and spinal fusion spacer (B) (Provided by Teijin Nakashima Medical Co., Ltd.).

is difficult to surpass conventional reconstructive surgery in terms of clinical results. It is necessary to accumulate long-term clinical results in the future.

The biomechanically strongest fixation required among spinal implant is the pedicle screw system (Figs. 4.7 and 4.8A), in which screws are implanted in the left and right pedicles of each vertebrae and connected with rods or plates. Surgery to correct and fix the lumbosacral vertebrae using this technique is increasing. The morphology of each individual vertebra is slightly different, and the morphology of the surgical site also differs depending on the level of the spine, so rods and plates are bent during surgery depending on the circumstances of the surgical site. Spinal rods require plastic deformation in the surgical field, and plastic deformability and spring back after deformation are important properties. It is also necessary to consider the elongation to fracture and embrittlement due to work hardening after deformation (see Subsection 5.9.6 and Fig. 5.18). It is necessary to fully understand the superiority and inferiority of Ti–6Al–4V ELI alloy and Co–Cr–Mo alloy are being debated. Currently, internal fixation devices made of Ti alloy with a variety of designs are on the market, and are highly biocompatible and allow for post-surgical MRI evaluation. This is because artifacts around stainless steel implants occur during MRI imaging, making it impossible to evaluate the disease state.

In addition to screws and rods, many vertebral spacers and intervertebral spacers are used to replace the defective part after removing a vertebral body due to a tumor or fracture. Traditionally, autologous bone was harvested from the pelvis and lower limb bones to fill in the defect, but in order to alleviate pain at the bone harvest site, cages (cage-like) made of HA, CP Ti, carbon fiber, and absorbable materials are now being used. This method is used to fill in excess autologous bone produced during surgery. Poly(ether ether ketone) (PEEK) is used as a spinal spacer, but infections frequently occur because it does not adhere to living tissue, so it is now coated with CP Ti to make it adhesive to tissue. Recently, spinal spacers with novel designs that take bone orientation into consideration have been developed and commercially available as UNIOS® (Fig. 4.8B). This spacer promotes bone formation and excellent bone quality without bone grafting, and its principle has been clarified (Ishimoto et al. 2022, Matsugaki et al. 2023).

The global spinal implants and devices' market size was worth USD 12.8 billion in 2022 and is expected to grow at a compound annual growth rate (CAGR) of 5.2% from 2023 to 2030. The market growth is driven by the rise in spinal cord injuries (SCIs) globally. The compression of the spinal nerve or damage results in injury to the external side of the vertebral column. The main causes of this compression include spine degeneration, bone fractures, or abnormalities like hematomas or herniated discs (Global Market Insights 2023a).

4.4 Cardiology

4.4.1 Catheter and Guidewire

In recent years, intravascular treatment using stents and embolic wires has attracted attention as a minimally invasive treatment for cardiovascular disease and brain disease. Both treatments were made possible only when it became possible to diagnose vascular occlusion or malformation through catheter examination. This involves inserting a thin tube (called a catheter) with a diameter of about 2 mm into the heart or brain from an artery in the groin, wrist, elbow, etc., and injecting a contrast agent from the tip to see the detailed structure of the artery. This is a visual inspection (Fig. 4.9).

A technology is required to deliver the catheter to the affected area without getting lost through the complex blood vessels within the body. Catheters need to be pressure resistant because contrast media and other substances must be injected against blood flow. If the polymer is used alone, the tube will have a thick wall, so a tube with a metal mesh is used. In order to further reduce the wall thickness, it is necessary to realize high elasticity and high strength of the metal as the core material. Superelastic tubes are being developed for this purpose. Type 304 stainless steel,

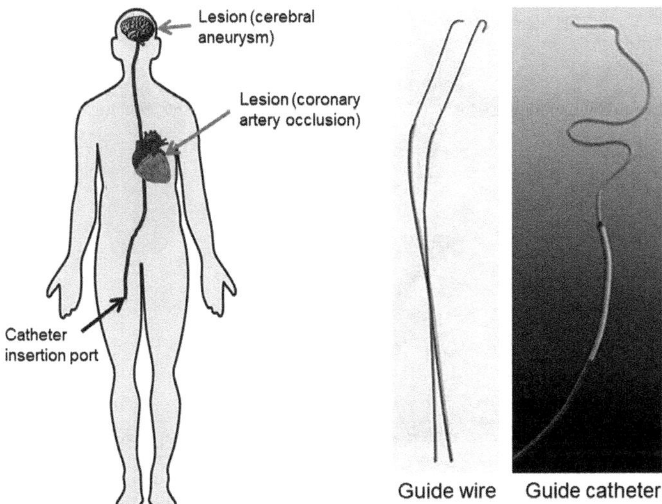

Fig. 4.9. Diagram of catheter insertion route, guide wire, and guide catheter (Provided by Dr. Akio Kishida, Tokyo Medical and Dental University.).

type 316L stainless steel, Co-based alloy, Ni–Ti alloy, Au, and Pt–In alloy are used for catheters.

The guidewire is inserted into the lumen of the catheter and used with its tip exposed (Fig. 4.9). In the operating room, the tip is bent by the surgeon, inserted into a blood vessel under X-ray vision, and pushed out to the affected area. At the blood vessel bifurcation, the wire is rotated and the bending of the tip is used to select an appropriate branch, which is then pushed further into the interior. The tip of the guidewire is required to have appropriate flexibility and rigidity. Currently, a core made of superelastic wire and covered with polyurethane is often used. When choosing a branch, one with greater rigidity is easier to handle. Care must be taken when handling as the vessel wall may be calcified and become brittle, or poking at the branch may perforate the blood vessel. In addition, operability may be impaired due to friction with the catheter section, and rotation transmission may become difficult due to bending into a complicated shape. In other words, guidewires are required to have torque transmission properties, kink resistance, and low friction properties. Guide wires can be classified into coil types and plastic types. The coil type has a metal core, and the outside of the core at the tip is covered with a metal coil. The core material is mostly type 316L stainless steel, while recently Co-based alloys are also available. In addition to stainless steel, the tip part is also made of Ni–Ti alloy. The plastic type uses the same material as the coil type for its core and is covered with a polymer, as shown in Fig. 4.10.

Guide wires and catheters have made it easier to diagnose minute lesions in blood vessels, making it possible to embolize cerebral aneurysms and treat intravascular stents as described later. It is expected that products that are easier to use and safer will be developed in the future. Current directions of development include making the diameter of the catheter even smaller while maintaining its strength and stiffness, reducing the friction of the catheter, and coating it with polymers to ensure lubricity between the catheter and the blood vessel wall. In the future, it is expected that the

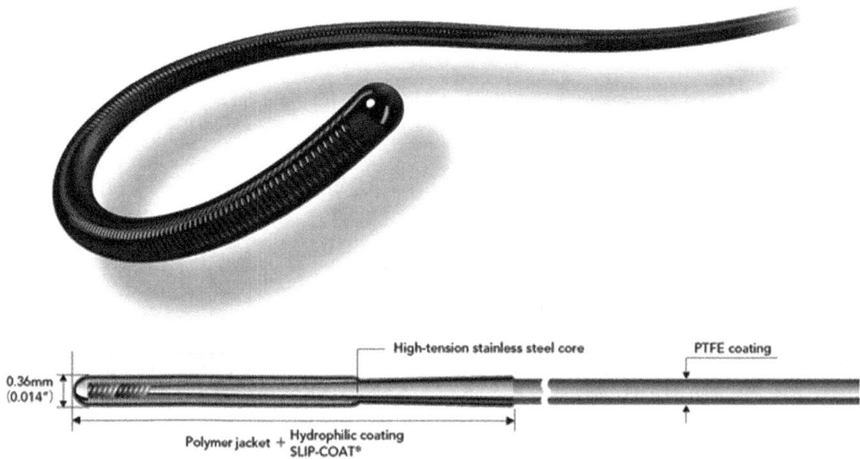

Fig. 4.10. Appearance and structure of guide wire for PTCA (Reprinted from the homepage of Asahi Intec Co. Ltd. with permission.).

shape of the tip can be controlled outside the body, and applications such as shape memory alloys and heat-responsive materials are being considered.

4.4.2 Stent and Stent Graft

Stent

Angina pectoris is a disease in which the coronary arteries that supply oxygen and nutrients to the heart become narrow due to arteriosclerosis, making it difficult for blood to pass through. Surgical treatments such as blood vessel replacement have been used to treat angina pectoris, while in recent decades, endovascular treatment techniques using guide wires and catheters have become mainstream. Endovascular treatment includes balloon treatment and stent treatment. A stent is a cylindrical metal product with a mesh structure, classified into various types depending on its material, implantation method, structure, etc. There are tubular stents made by cutting a metal tube with a laser, coil stents made from a single metal wire, and ring stents made by repeatedly joining short coils. Each type has characteristics such as expandability and flexibility, used depending on the site of use and disease. Currently, tubular stents and coil stents are the mainstream. There is a commentary on coronary artery stents (Butany et al. 2005).

Balloon therapy is a method that applies catheter testing technology called coronary angiography, including percutaneous coronary angioplasty, percutaneous transluminal coronary angioplasty (PTCA), coronary artery intervention, and percutaneous coronary intervention (PCI). In balloon therapy, first a very thin catheter (balloon catheter) with a balloon attached to the tip is inserted into the narrowed coronary artery using a guide wire, and this balloon is inflated to widen the narrowed coronary artery. Then, the balloon catheter is removed and blood flow is resumed (Fig. 4.11). Stent treatment is an application of this balloon treatment. A stent is a small mesh-patterned tube made of metals. This is delivered to the narrowed area of the blood vessel and inflated with a balloon used in balloon therapy. Balloon therapy only uses a balloon to widen the arteriosclerotic area. On the other hand, when a stent is used to widen the arteriosclerotic area, the stent plays a role in preserving the internal structure, making it possible to reliably widen the blood vessel (Fig. 4.12). Pelvic arteriography appearing vascular stenosis and securing blood flow by stent placement is shown in Fig. 4.13. An implanted stent cannot be removed. Even if balloon therapy enlarges the stenotic area, 30 to 40% of patients will experience “restenosis,” in which the blood vessel narrows again. It usually occurs within 3 mon after treatment, and if there is no restenosis 3 mon after surgery, it is considered to have been largely cured. On the other hand, stent therapy can compensate for the drawbacks of balloon therapy, reducing the restenosis rate to around 20%. Restenosis tends to occur within 6 mon, which is longer than with balloon therapy, and the time to determine cure is also delayed.

Self-expanding type stents require elasticity, so Ni–Ti superelastic alloys are mainly used; balloon expanding types require plasticity, so stainless steel and Co-based alloys are mainly used. In addition, radial support force or stiffness is required to counteract the contraction of the adventitia that occurs over time. In addition, since X-ray contrast properties are required, the use of metals is essential. For devices that

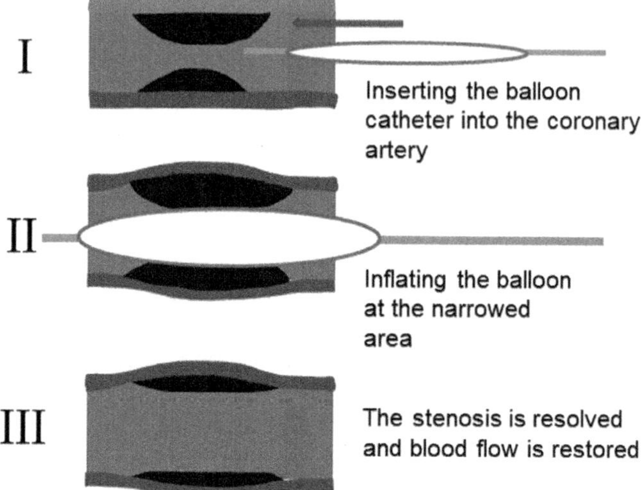

Fig. 4.11. Treatment of vascular stenosis with balloon catheter (Provided by Dr. Akio Kishida, Tokyo Medical and Dental University.).

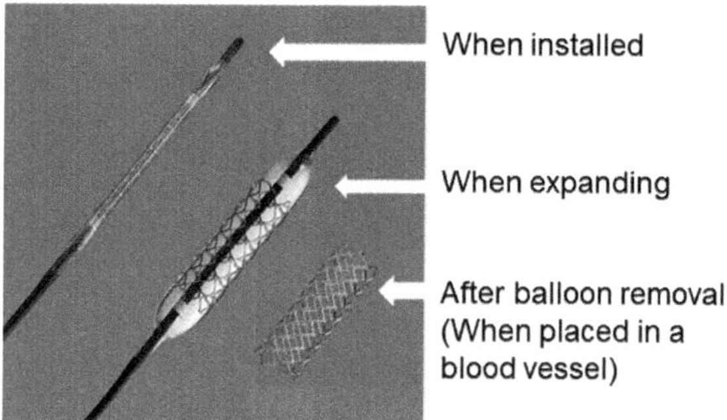

Fig. 4.12. Mechanism of widen the blood vessel using a stent (Provided by Cordis Japan G.K.).

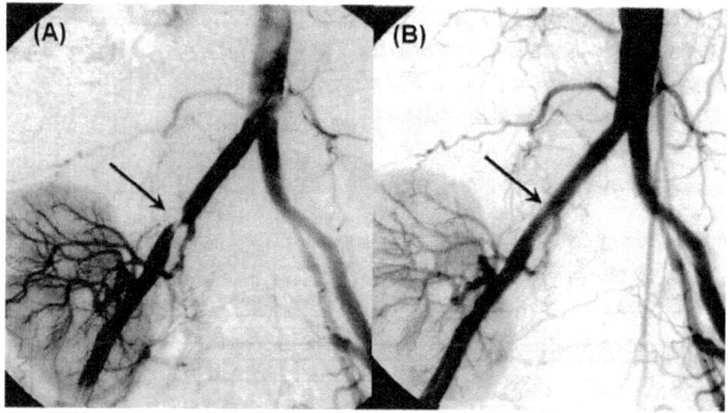

Fig. 4.13. Pelvic arteriography appearing vascular stenosis (A) and securing blood flow by stent placement (B) (Japanese Study Group of Metallic Stent & Graft 2000.).

directly affect life support, such as stents, the emphasis is on the extension of life rather than the toxicity of the material. Elasticity is also necessary for deformation along the blood vessel wall and blood vessel followability. Therefore, stents are manufactured from metals based only on mechanical properties. The mechanical properties of stents have been summarized (Tambaca et al. 2011).

Balloon-expandable stents are primarily used to dilate coronary arteries and require corrosion resistance, so type 316L stainless steel has been used from the beginning. According to the standard corresponding to type 316L stainless steel (ASTM F138-19 2020), the tensile strength is 490 MPa. Currently, the use of Co-based alloys has become mainstream, and the Co–Ni–Cr–Mo alloy (commercial name MP35N) (ASTM F562-22 2022) is used, and its tensile strength exceeds 1600 MPa, Young's modulus of 232 GPa, excellent in both elastic retention and corrosion resistance. It is used together with Co–Cr–W–Ni alloy (commercial name L-605) (ASTM F90-23 2023) for stents. In recent years, the use of Co-base alloys has been increasing. Ta is highly malleable and has good contrast properties because it is a heavy metal, which is easily oxidized and becomes passivated with a passive film of Ta_2O_5. Therefore, Ta is very stable and does not corrode in the human body. Because of its low magnetic susceptibility, it has the advantage of reducing artifacts in MRI imaging. On the other hand, self-expanding stents are used in other arteries, such as those in the lower extremities, and utilize the superelastic features of Ni–Ti alloy (ASTM F2063-18 2018). This is because arteries in the lower limbs undergo large deformations due to movements such as knee bending, and there is a risk of damaging blood vessels and the like due to plastic deformation of the stent.

Stent Graft

A stent graft is a device used to treat aortic aneurysms in which the aorta has locally enlarged. A stent graft has a self-expanding metal skeleton (stent) joined to an artificial blood vessel (graft), and its ends are placed in normal blood vessels near the aortic aneurysm, allowing blood to flow through the artificial blood vessel. It reduces the blood flow and blood pressure load on the aneurysm. In recent decades, the number of treatments using stent grafts has increased due to their minimally invasive nature. For artificial blood vessels, polyester nonwoven fabric or stretched porous polytetrafluoroethylene (ePTFE) is used (Fig. 4.14). When Ni–Ti alloys are used for the stent portion, the Ni–Ti alloys can suffer from severe pitting and crevice corrosion (Heintz et al. 2001).

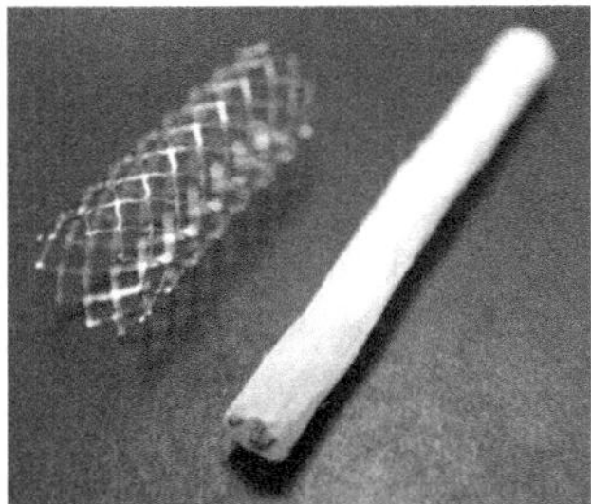

Fig. 4.14. Examples of bare and covered stents (Provide by Dr. Akio Kishida, Tokyo Medical and Dental University.).

Drug Eluting Stent

Drug eluting stents (DES), in which the surface of the stent is coated with a drug, have rapidly become popular to prevent restenosis of coronary arteries. Clinical trials began at the end of 1999 for DES, a coronary artery stent coated with a drug that inhibits cell proliferation, and it attracted a lot of attention when it was suggested that it had the potential to eradicate restenosis. Once the results of various clinical trials are obtained, the frequency of revascularization of the target lesion, including the stent margin, being required is less than 5%, and it may become a definitive treatment method for direct treatment of coronary artery lesions. Compared to radiation therapy, which requires a large-sale equipment, DES is technically the same as conventional stent placement, and is a treatment method that is gentle for both the surgeon and the patient, making it the most promising treatment at present.

First-generation DESs are coated with sirolimus to coat a drug, which have the effect of suppressing smooth muscle cell proliferation and inflammatory cell infiltration. One DES is coated with the anti-tumor drug Paclitaxel. In second generation DES is coated with a primer non-absorbable poly(xylylene chloride), and an intermediate layer of two non-absorbable polymers poly(ethylene-co-vinylacetate), PEVA, and poly(n-butyl methacrylate), PBMA. It has a three-layer structure in which PBMA and sirolimus are mixed in a ratio of 2:1, and then top coated with PBMA for sustained release. The coating is approximately 10 μm thick and is designed to release sirolimus over a period of 30-42 d. Another DES is coated with paclitaxel mixed with poly(styrene-b-isobutylene-b-styrene), which is also non-absorbable. The coating thickness is just under 20 μm. Once released, these DES gained a high market share in a short term, and are now considered the first choice for coronary artery treatment. Remaining challenges for stent treatment include improving the success rate of chronic complete occlusion, preventing peripheral embolization and side branch occlusion, and eradicating stent thrombosis.

The DES segment dominated the market for coronary stents and held the largest revenue share of over 66.0% in 2021. The continued advancement and launch of the new devices are important factors in strengthening DES's dominance as the preferred device for PCI procedures. The competitors in the market continue to develop and launch technologically advanced DES. In comparison to the previous generation devices, these newer-generation DES provide greater stent integrity, higher deliverability, and lower complication rates (Global Market Insights 2023b).

4.4.3 Cerebral Aneurysm Clip and Embolization Coil

The typical treatment method for cerebral aneurysms that causes subarachnoid hemorrhage is craniotomy (clipping), in which the root of the aneurysm is occluded with a cerebral aneurysm clip, completely blocking blood flow through the aneurysm, and endovascular treatment (coil embolization) in which a catheter is inserted into the blood vessel to the root of the aneurysm and a Pt coil is sent to fill the inside. Metallic biomaterials are used in both treatments.

Cerebral Aneurysm Clip

In the clipping procedure, in order to access the aneurysm, a part of the skull is first removed through a craniotomy, brain tissue is removed, and the blood vessels where the brain aneurysm is located are identified. The neck of the aneurysm (the border between the aneurysm and normal blood vessels) is then closed with a small metal clip to prevent blood from flowing into the aneurysm (Fig. 4.15). This prevents the cerebral aneurysm from rupturing and further eliminates the risk of rupture by coagulating the blood within the aneurysm. A Co–Cr–Ta–Ni alloy and a Co–20Cr–16Fe–15Ni–7Mo alloy called Elgiloy (ASTM F1058-16 2017) are used, while Ti–6Al–4V ELI is used to reduce MRI artifacts (ASTM F136-13(2021)e1 2021). Type 630 stainless steel and type 631 stainless steel are also used, but they have fallen out of use with the spread of MRI.

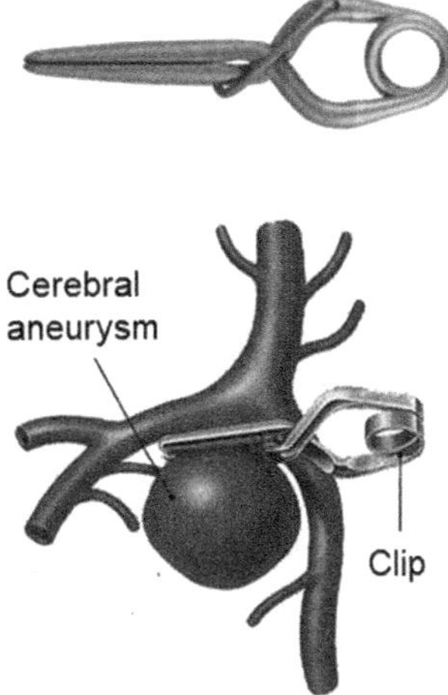

Fig. 4.15. Cerebral aneurysm clip.

Embolization Coil

In coil embolization, when an aneurysm is diagnosed in a cerebral blood vessel, a Pt (ASTM B561-94 2018) coil is transported with a catheter, expanded within the aneurysm, and the aneurysm is filled to prevent bleeding due to rupture of the aneurysm. This allows the blood within the aneurysm to coagulate and prevent bleeding (Fig. 4.16). The treatment method of placing a Pt coil inside a cerebral aneurysm was developed in the late 1980s (Guglielmi et al. 1992). The coil needs to be flexible enough to be visible under X-ray fluoroscopy and to match the shape of the aneurysm, so Pt is used. The coil is attached to a delivery wire that passes through the micro-catheter to reach the aneurysm. This delivery wire allows the physician to move the coil in and out of the brain aneurysm until it is placed in the correct position. These systems are called Guglielmi detachable coil (GDC) systems, named after their inventor. This method is widely used today, but Pt coils generally have low blood coagulation ability, so they must be tightly packed to avoid creating spaces within the aneurysm. However, if the coil is packed too tightly, there is a risk that the

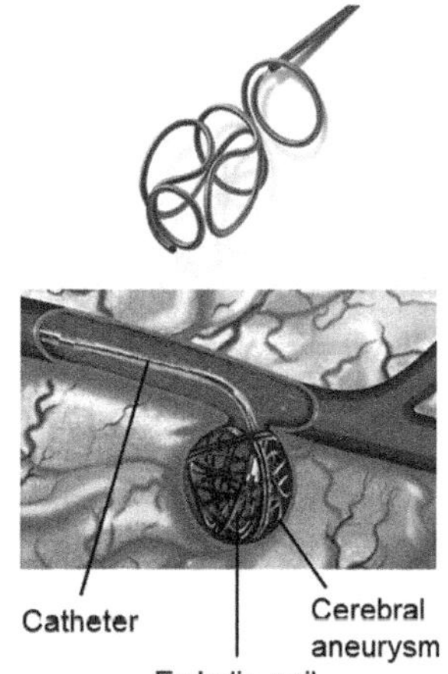

Fig. 4.16. Cerebral aneurysm embolization coil.

aneurysm will rupture, so the surgeon's skill and experience are required. To solve these problems, attempts have been made to improve the coil surface by modifying the blood-coagulating properties by wrapping cotton-like Pt fibers around the coil. In addition, since Pt coils do not have the ability to adhere to blood vessels, the aneurysms that can be targeted are limited to so-called balloon-shaped aneurysms with small diameters and large interiors.

4.4.4 Artificial Heart, Pacemaker, and Artificial Valve

Pace Maker

Electrical stimulation artificially increases the membrane potential of cardiac muscle cells, causing cardiac contraction through its propagation; by doing this periodical stimulation, the heart rate can be controlled. A pacemaker consists of a pulse generator that generates electrical stimulation and an electrode lead that transmits the electrical stimulation to the heart (Fig. 4.17). The pulse generator consists of a battery and the electrical circuitry required for pacing, sealed in a housing consisting of CP Ti or type 316L stainless steel. Lithium batteries are currently used. The electrode lead contacts the myocardium, a polymer-coated conductor, and a connector that connects to the pacemaker housing. Co–Cr–Ni–Mo–Fe alloy (Elgiloy) or Ni–Co alloy is used for the conductor part, and CP Ti or Pt–90Ir alloy is used for the electrode part. For these parts, materials have been selected based on their electrical properties rather than their mechanical properties. In other words, the resistance value is inversely proportional to the surface area of the electrode, so if the surface area is small, pacing can be performed with a weak current, which saves power, while the sufficient surface area for recording intracardiac potentials improves the S/N ratio. The material and shape must be selected in consideration of pacing and sensing efficiency, battery life, and durability. Current pacemakers have an electrode surface area of 10 to 12 mm^2, a single lead resistance of about 75 to 150 Ω, and a lifespan of about 10 to 12 yr.

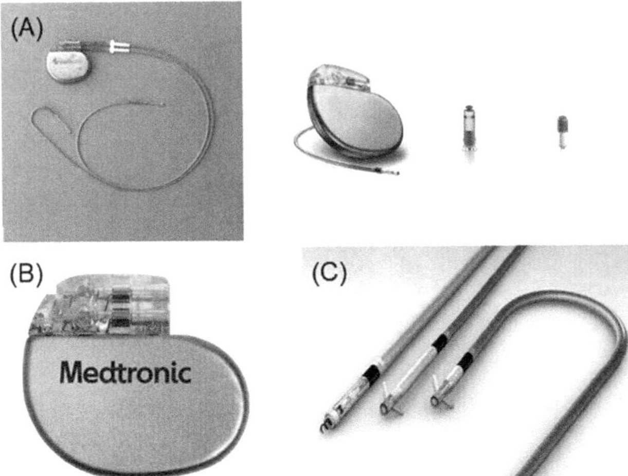

Fig. 4.17. Pacemaker. (A) Exterior, (B) main body, and (C) electrode part (Provided by Medtronic Co. Ltd.).

Metals are used for impellers in continuous flow pumps, housing members that house the pump mechanism, and connecting members between blood pumps and blood vessels. Stainless steel such as type 304 was initially used, but now almost Ti–6Al–4V ELI alloy is used.

Implantable Cardioverter Defibrillator

Similar to a pacemaker, an implantable cardioverter defibrillator (ICD) is a device that controls heart beats. An ICD is a device that uses high-energy shocks to eliminate ventricular fibrillation (arrhythmia) when it occurs. The method of implanting a defibrillator and the placement of its leads are generally similar to those of a pacemaker, but the electric shock occurs when ventricular fibrillation requires a large amount of energy, so the battery may run down faster than a pacemaker. In addition to ventricular fibrillation, defibrillators and newer devices have the ability to perform low-energy pacing for tachyarrhythmia as well as pacing for bradycardia arrhythmia.

Artificial Valve

Artificial valves are used for replacement surgery to treat heart valve disease. The patient's defective valve is removed and replaced with a new artificial valve. Artificial valves can be broadly divided into "mechanical valves" and "biological valves", and mechanical valves use artificial materials. As shown in Fig. 4.18, the current mainstream of mechanical valves is the bileaflet valve, which has a structure that opens and closes with two half-moon-shaped leaflet plates made mainly of pyrolite carbon (carbon fiber). Ti–6Al–4V alloy is used for the frame (valve seat).

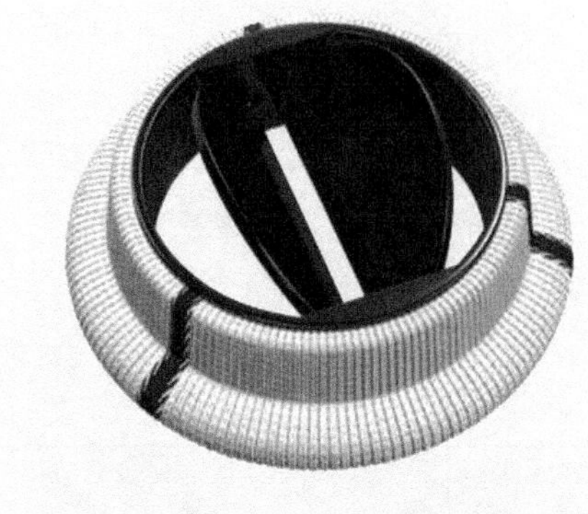

Fig. 4.18. Artificial heart valve (Provided by LivaNova Japan K.K. with Courtesy of CORCYM Srl.).

4.5 Dentistry

4.5.1 Outline

In dental treatment, when a part of a tooth or the tooth itself is lost, materials play an important role in replacing the missing part. Treatments for restoring teeth (coronal restorations) and replacing missing teeth (prosthetics) use metals, polymers, ceramics, or a combination of these materials in an appropriate manner, depending on the needs of each case. Custom-made dental technology is usually used. Furthermore, metals also play an important role in treatments of dental implants and orthodontics. This section provides an overview of major dental devices using metals. There are also classic textbooks for use as dental materials (Anusavice 2003, Powers and Sakaguchi 2006).

4.5.2 Restorations

When the form or function of the crown (the part of the tooth exposed in the oral cavity) is partially impaired due to caries or trauma, crown restoration using artificial materials is performed. Restoration methods vary depending on the extent of the defect and the need for restoration. When the area of the defect is relatively small and localized, such as on the occlusal surface of the molars (the biting surface of the back teeth) or the adjacent surface of the front teeth, a composite material consisting of a polymer and glass fillers is used to fill the cavity,[1] and is then cured after being molded. A method of filling with Au foil was also used, while dental amalgam is a typical molded filling material using metal. In dental amalgam restorations, cavities are filled with plastic amalgam[2] paste mixed with Ag–Sn or Ag–Sn–Cu alloy powders and Hg. After hardening, surface finishing is performed by polishing. Amalgam filling restorations have been widely used clinically since ancient times due to their excellent therapeutic effects and ease of operation. However, there are drawbacks

[1] The defect area where the lesion has been removed and an appropriate shape has been given.

[2] An alloy composed of Hg and other metals.

such as Hg in the environment, discoloration, and breakage, so composite resins have been developed that adhere to teeth and have excellent esthetics, which is currently used (see Subsection 9.2.8).

Crown restoration performed by bonding a cast metal made outside the oral cavity with dental cement is called cast restoration. A restoration that fits into a medial (surrounded by tooth substance) cavity formed in a tooth is called an "inlay." Class I inlays are limited only to the occlusal surface, class II inlays include one adjacent surface, and examples include the MOD inlay[3] (Fig. 4.19), which includes both distal and adjacent surfaces. In addition, a restoration that is used to cover a tooth with a relatively large defect in tooth structure is called a "crown," and is generally manufactured using a casting method. Partially covered crowns that cover part of the crown include three-quarter crowns and four-fifths crowns, and those that cover the entire crown are called "full crown" (Fig. 4.19). Additionally, in order to enable restoration with a crown, a method called abutment construction is often used to replace the missing tooth structure. If the defect is relatively small, a molded filling material is used, but if the defect extends to the root canal, a prefabricated post or a metal core made by casting is used.

In cast crown restoration, the carious part is first removed, and the tooth structure is shaved (formation) and supplemented (lining) to prepare the form suitable for restoration. In the next stage, impressions of the dentition to be restored and opposing dentition are taken, and the occlusal relationship is recorded (occlusal recording). A plaster model is made based on the obtained impression and occlusal relationship, and a wax pattern (wax model) is prepared on this model. This wax pattern is invested in a heat-resistant mold material and burned to create a mold, and molten alloy is cast into the mold. The dental casting method is a type of lost wax process that has been industrialized as a precision casting method. Finally, the cast body is adjusted on the model, polished, and bonded with dental cement in the oral cavity. The thickness of the cement layer when bonding a dental crown restoration to the tooth structure is on the order of several tens of micrometers, and extremely high precision is required in dental casting. If the cement layer is too thick, the exposed cement layer will begin to disintegrate, and bacteria will enter from food, drink, and saliva, causing secondary caries and falling off of the cast. In order to achieve high casting accuracy, silica (SiO_2) such as quartz or cristobalite is used as the base material of the mold, and the

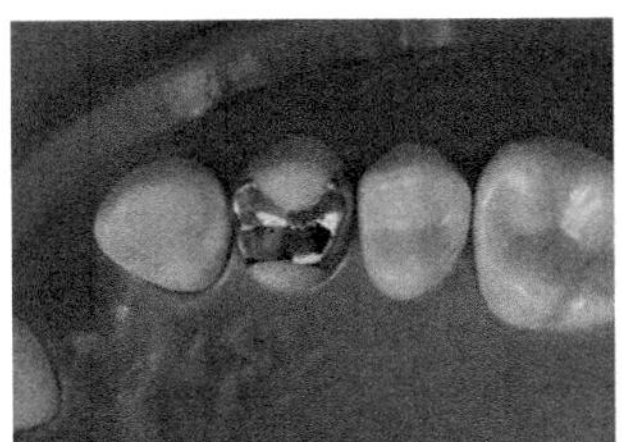
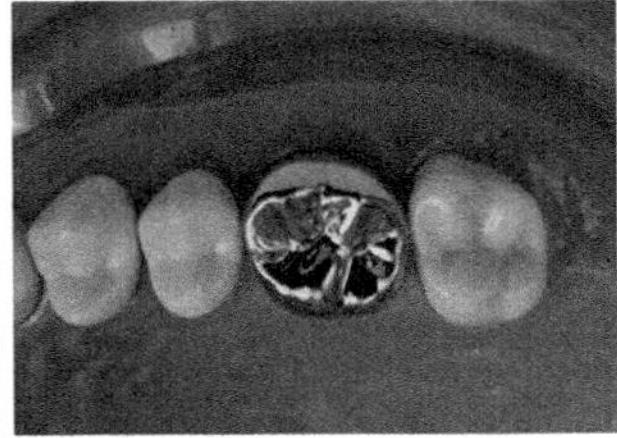

Fig. 4.19. MOD inlay (left) and full crown (right) (Provided by GC Co.).

[3] Inlay covering medial, occlusal, and distal.

casting shrinkage of the alloy is compensated for by the hardening expansion and heating expansion of the mold material.

Full crowns include not only metal-only crowns, but also veneer crowns that use tooth-colored hard resin or porcelain for parts of the cast crown (such as the labial surface) to improve esthetics. For veneers with these composite structures, the adhesive strength and durability of the two components are important factors, and for the former hard resin veneer, the adhesion is adjusted according to the type of alloy. A primer (pretreatment agent) for bonding in veneer crown has been developed. In the veneer crowns, the porcelain combines by baking onto the surface of the cast crown, and elements are added to the alloy to form an oxide film that increases the baking strength of the porcelain. At the same time, the melting point of the metal must be increased to inhibit the deformation during the firing. On the porcelain side, the firing temperature is lowered to ensure that the alloy does not deform, and the coefficient of thermal expansion is increased to a level slightly smaller than that of the alloy to prevent crack initiation at the interface due to shrinkage during cooling after firing of porcelain (see Subsection 9.2.5). Recently, porcelain inlays and all-porcelain crowns (all-ceramic crowns), which do not use metal at all, have also come into use. Restoration using cast alloys requires casting precision, and Au–Ag–Cu–Pd–Pt alloys are used (see Subsection 9.2.3).

4.5.3 Prosthodontics

When teeth are lost due to periodontal disease, caries, trauma, etc., prosthetics are used to restore form and function using artificial materials. The prosthetic method is selected depending on the degree of the defect, intraoral conditions, etc. When one to several teeth are missing, a bridge (Fig. 4.20) is a method to restore form and function by connecting two to several teeth as abutment teeth (teeth used to support and maintain the denture). In the case of relatively small bridges, a one-piece casting method is sometimes used, while especially in cases involving many teeth, the bridge is cast in several parts and brazed with a brazing alloy or laser welding. The part corresponding to the defect is replaced with an artificial tooth called a pontic, and its shape is determined depending on the location, taking into consideration cleanability, functionality, aesthetics, etc. Aesthetics is an important factor for anterior teeth, so hard resin veneers and porcelain-fused crowns are used (metal-ceramics crown).

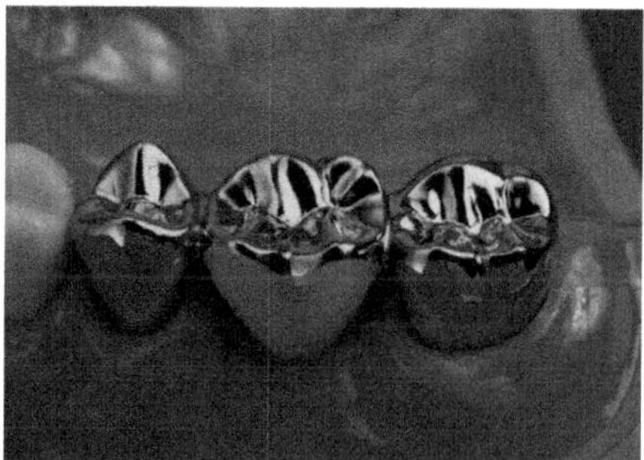

Fig. 4.20. Bridge (Provided by GC Co.).

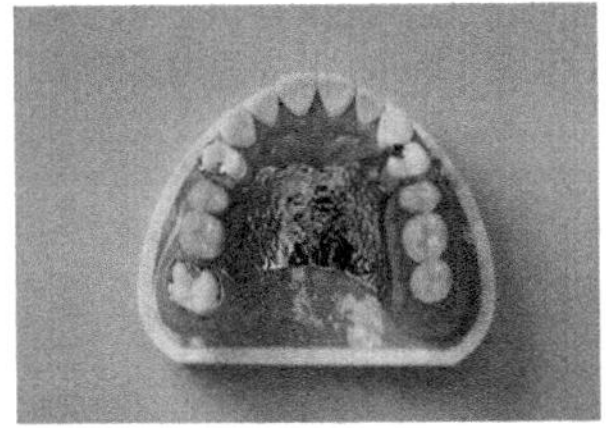 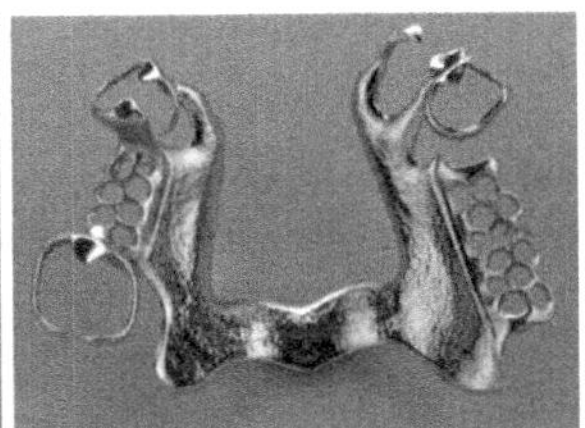

Fig. 4.21. Partial denture (left) and its metal flame consisting of Ti-6Al-7Nb alloy (Provided by GC Co.).

In addition, new bridge restoration technique removing only small amount of teeth has been developed that use adhesive resin to strengthen the adhesive force of the luting cement.

A removable denture is a prosthesis that morphologically compensates for tooth loss and the accompanying decline in surrounding tissues, and aims to restore functionality and esthetics. A partial denture is used when there are remaining teeth (Fig. 4.21). Partial denture designs vary widely depending on factors such as the number and placement of remaining teeth, and the type of retainer. Metal-based dentures consist of metal skeleton of the denture base to increase strength and wear feeling, and are generally manufactured using precision casting. Retention device to prevent dentures from falling off is "clasp", which is metal wire fixing around the abutment teeth. The removable denture exert a retaining force through a combination of parts that are attached to the abutment teeth and parts that are built into the denture. There are two types of clasps: wire clasps made by bending alloy wire and cast clasps made by casting. In addition, Co–Cr–Mo alloy is used for the denture base.

Magnetic attachments have also been developed that use the attractive force of magnets for retention. The magnets include Sm–Co alloys and Ne–Fe–B alloys. Yokes equipped in dentures are attracted to the magnetic force of the magnets and cover the magnet that is made of ferritic magnetic stainless steel (type 444, type XM27, and type 447J1) with excellent corrosion resistance. Shield ring and spacer consist of type 316L stainless steel.

4.5.4 Dental Casting Alloys

Dental casting alloys are widely used in dental treatments such as crown restoration and defective prosthetics, and they must have sufficient mechanical properties (strength, elongation, etc.) suitable for each application, excellent corrosion resistance, and no toxicity. In addition, properties such as non-irritant properties, excellent castability, and good compatibility are required. Previously, standards were established for each alloy system, while an international unified standard came into effect in 2006 (ISO 22674 2022). In this standard, dental metallic materials are classified into six types based on their mechanical properties, and their standards and uses are summarized in Table 4.2.

Au alloy for dental casting (Au–Ag–Cu alloy) refers to an alloy containing 60% or more of Au and 75% or more of Au + Pt group elements (Pt and Pd). It exhibits excellent corrosion resistance, as well as excellent castability, compatibility, and malleability, and is classified into types 1 to 4 based on its properties. Type 1 (soft)

Table 4.2. Type number, 0.2% offset yielding strength, elongation to fracture, elastic modulus, and purpose of metallic materials for dental restorations and prosthodontics.

Type	0.2% Offset yield strength (MPa)	Elongation to fracture (%)	Elastic modulus (GPa)	Purpose
0	-	-	-	Intended for low stress bearing single-tooth fixed restorations, e.g., small veneered one-surface inlays and veneered crown. Note: Metallic materials for metal-ceramic crowns produced by electroforming or sintering belong to Type 0.
1	≥ 80	≥ 18	-	Intended for low stress bearing single tooth fixed restorations, e.g., veneered or unveneered on-surface inlays and veneered crown.
2	≥ 180	≥ 10	-	Intended for single tooth fixed restorations, e.g., crowns or inlays without restriction on the number of surfaces.
3	≥ 270	≥ 5	-	Intended for multiple unit fixed restorations, e.g., bridges.
4	≥ 360	≥ 2	-	Intended for appliances with thin sections that are subject to very high forces, e.g., removable partial dentures, clasps, thin veneered crowns, wide-span bridges or bridges with small cross-sections, bars, attachments, and implant retained superstructures.
5	≥ 500	≥ 2	≥ 150	Intended for appliances in which parts require the combination of high stiffness and strength, e.g., thin removable partial dentures, parts with thin cross-sections, and clasps.

Co–Cr alloys and Ni–Cr alloys have limited elastic modulus, so they are used in thin Type 5 frames and metal floors

The CP Ti of dental implants and casting ingots is about Type 2 or Type 3.

is indicated for simple inlays, type 2 (medium-hard) for complex inlays and crowns, type 3 (hard) for crowns and bridges, and type 4 (super-hard) for denture bases and bridges. Types 3 to 4 are often used for a wide range of applications. Addition of Cu has the effect of decreasing the melting point, increasing mechanical strength, and imparting heat treatment hardenability, but corrosion resistance decreases. In addition, Au alloys (types 3 and 4), Pt additives, and Au–Ag–Pd alloys can be hardened by heat treatment.

The composition of Co–Cr alloy for dental casting is Co: 40–70%, Cr: 20–30%, Ni: 0–20%, Mo: 0–10%, etc., and its mechanical properties are equivalent to type 5. It is used in cases where a large load is applied and high rigidity is required, such as metal frames and clasps for fixed dentures.

Due to its stable passive film, CP Ti has excellent corrosion resistance and tissue compatibility, and has properties suitable as a metal for biological applications, such as low specific gravity and light weight. However, its high melting point and

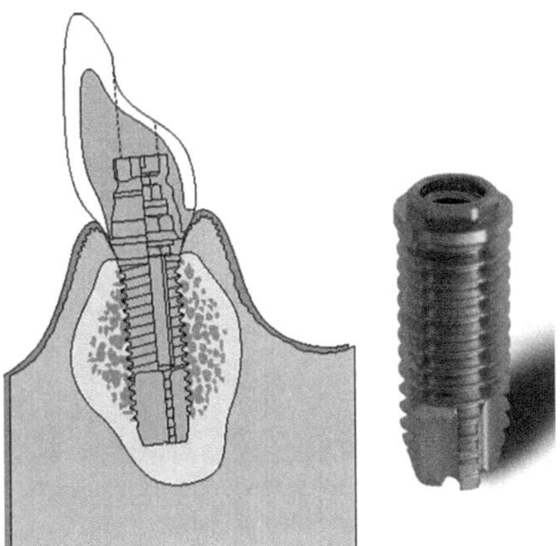

Fig. 4.22. Dental implant (Provided by GC Co.).

high reactivity with oxygen in the melting atmosphere and mold material made it difficult to apply it to dental casting. In spite of the above situation, research and development in dental casting technology has led to the development of specialized casting machines and investment materials, which are now in practical use. CP Ti has a wide range of mechanical properties, from soft to slightly hard, depending on its purity (1 to 4 types), and is used in denture bases, crowns, bridges, etc. In addition, the Ti–6Al–7Nb alloy has excellent biosafety, high strength, and good operability, and is now being used clinically.

4.5.5 Dental Implant

Dental implants are artificial materials that are implanted within the oral cavity to replace missing teeth. Dental implants are classified into intramucosal, subperiosteal, endodontic, and intraosseous implants depending on their location, while currently intraosseous implants (Fig. 4.22) are the mainstream and this method has become widely used clinically. CP Ti, which has excellent biocompatibility, is mainly used as the material for the fixture implanted in the alveolar bone and has good osseointegration with no fibrous intervening between it and the bone tissue. In addition, implant surface is sometimes roughened or pored to improve bone bonding or coated with bioceramics such as HA, which has osteoconductive property. In dental implant treatment, an abutment is established using a fixture placed in the bone as a base, and a type of prosthesis with a crown, bridge, or denture called a superstructure is fixed to this abutment. Dental implants consist of CP Ti or Ti alloys because they need to be connected to the jawbone.

4.5.6 Orthodontics

In orthodontic treatment, the elasticity or superelasticity of metal wires is primarily used as the orthodontic force to move teeth to the desired position. The metal wires consist of stainless steel, Co–Cr alloy, Ni–Ti alloy, Ti–Mo alloy, etc. In particular, Ni–Ti alloy wire, which utilizes superelasticity, is widely used clinically because it continuously exerts orthodontic force suitable for tooth movement.

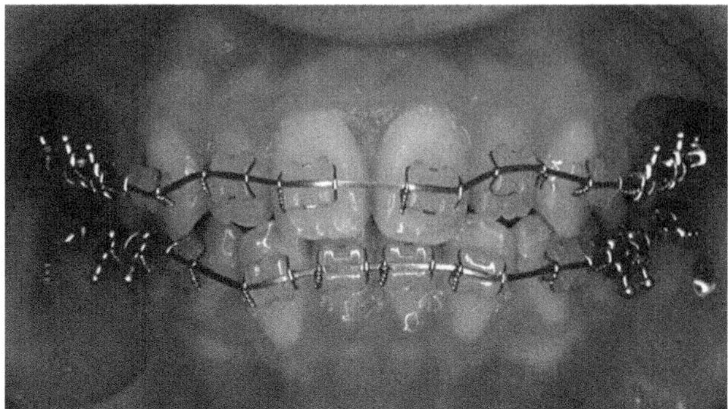

Fig. 4.23. Ni–Ti alloy superelastic archwire for orthodontics (Provided by Dr. Keiji Moriyama, Tokyo Medical and Dental University.).

Archwires shaped to follow the teeth dentition have circular, rectangular and bundle cross-sectional shapes, which are fixed to brackets bonded to the labio-buccal surfaces of the teeth (Fig. 4.23). In addition, various devices are used in orthodontic treatment to move teeth and dentition; for example, an expansion device that uses screws and thick wire to widen narrowed maxillary teeth, an arch wire device that consists of an elastic wire and hook brazed to the wire, and a resin denture base combined with a labial guide wire, clasp, and elastic wire. Various types of retainers are also used to prevent tooth recurrence after the tooth has been moved to the correct position. Various orthodontic devices generally use bent Co-based alloy or stainless steel wire.

4.5.7 Endodontics and Dental Surgery

As the degree of caries progresses and bacteria reach the pulp (soft tissue containing nerves and blood vessels) in the center of the tooth, in order to save the tooth, the infected pulp must be removed and the root where the pulp was located must be removed. Mechanical and chemical expansion and cleaning of the wall around the tube becomes necessary. In this type of endodontic treatment, the instruments used for mechanical root canal enlargement are dental reamers and files (Fig. 4.24). Dental reamers and files used in endodontic treatment have been widely made of stainless steel. In recent years, a motorized root canal formation method using a superelastic Ni–Ti alloy file (Fig. 4.24), which enables good root canal formation

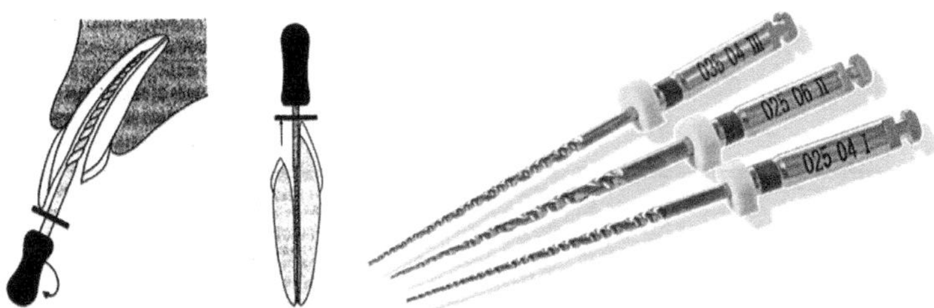

Fig. 4.24. Schematic illustrations of endodontic treatment and Ni–Ti alloy superelastic endodontic files (Provided by MANI Co.).

even in curved root canals, has been used clinically and is attracting attention. The static and dynamic cyclic fatigue resistance of contemporary Ni–Ti endodontic files with different kinematic, metallurgic, and design features are investigated (Thu et al. 2020). In addition, the phase composition, phase transformation temperatures, bending property, and cyclic fatigue resistance of different heat-treated Ni–Ti rotary files with the same tip diameter and taper at room and body temperatures are evaluated (Kasuga et al. 2023).

A bone plate similar to that used in orthopedic surgery is used to fix bone fragments in jaw fractures and jaw correction surgery, while a smaller miniplate is often used in oral surgery. In the past, stainless steel was used, but now CP Ti and Ti alloys are the mainstream. After adjusting the bend to follow the bone surface, it is fixed to the bone fragment with a screw. Other types of maxillofacial reconstructive surgery include dental implants and various reconstruction plates.

4.5.8 Adhesion of Polymers to Metals in Dentistry

Metal restorations and prostheses such as inlay, crown, and bridge must be retained in a fixed position in a mouth. For this purpose, dental cements are used: glass ionomer cements, zinc phosphate cements, polyacrylate cements, resin-based cements, etc. In particular, resin-based cements generate chemical adhesion between tooth and metal. Cements based on resin composites are now used for cementation of crown and bridges and direct bonding of orthodontic brackets to enamel. Polymer-based filling, restorative, and luting materials are specified (ISO 4049 2019). Resin cements based on methyl methacrylate (MMA) have been available since 1952 for the use of cementation of inlays, crowns, etc. Resin composite for crown and resin was invented in early 1970s. Cementation of alloy restorations is performed with self-cured composite cements. Two-paste systems are adopted for self-cured composite cements. One paste mainly consists of a diacrylate oligomer diluted with lower-molecular-weight dimethacrylate monomers. The other consists of silanated silica or glass. Peroxide-amine is used for the initiator-accelerator. Although many efforts had been made to use industrial adhesives such as epoxy resins and cyanoacrylate as dental adhesives, adequate adhesion is not achieved under the extreme conditions of the oral cavity. Much effort has been expended to achieve adhesion between artificial compounds and tooth substances. A new dental adhesive that meets the requirements stated above was synthesized (Takayama et al. 1978). The dental adhesives contained 4-methacryloxyethyl-trimellitic anhydride (4-META) as an adhesive monomer with MMA. An adhesive containing a dimethacrylate monomer bis-glycidyldimethacrylate (Bis-GMA) and phosphate monomers was synthesized (Omura et al. 1983). 4-META is an ethyl anhydride of trimellitate acid and hydroxyethyl methacrylate and has both hydrophilic and hydrophobic groups. The 4-META cement is formulated with MMA monomer and acrylic resin filler and is catalyzed by tributylborane (TBB). Another adhesive resin cement is phosphonate cement supplied with two-paste system, containing bis-glycidyldimethacrylate (Bis-GMA) resin and silanated quartz filler. Phosphonate molecule is very sensitive to oxygen, so a gel is provided to coat the margins of a restoration until setting has occurred. One of the main problems in dental adhesion techniques is that bonds between adhesives and metals are strong in

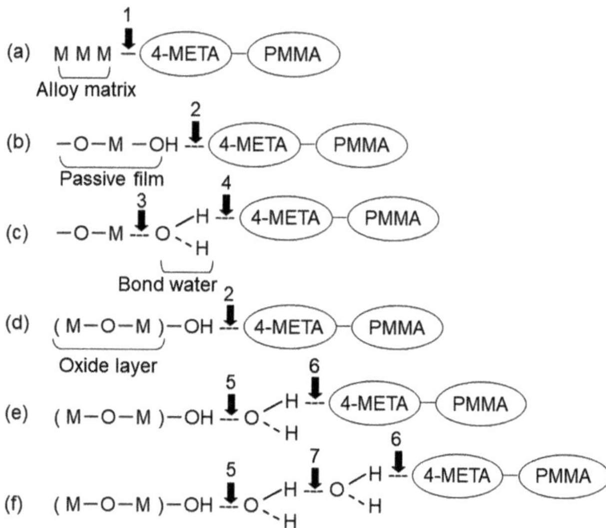

Fig. 4.25. Suggested adhesion model of PMMA resin containing 4-META on as polished (a, b, and c) and oxidized (d, e, and f) surface of metals: M is metal atom, dashed line is hydrogen bond. The chemical bonds which are similar in bonding strength are labeled by the same number at the bonding position (Ohno 2006).

a dry environment and weaken in a wet environment. For example, there are clinical reports of dental adhesion bridges fracturing off from teeth after extended use, and this has led to a loss of confidence in dental adhesion techniques. Hence, a major problem awaiting solution in dentistry is the durability of bonding joints exposed to water. Researches on dental adhesives are well reviewed somewhere (Ikemura and Endo 2010). Figure 4.25 shows the possible adhesion mechanism models of 4-META: Models (a), (b), and (c) are for the as-polished surface and models (d), (e), and (f) are for the oxidized surface.

The adhesion of 4-META resin to Co–Cr and Ni–Cr alloys is examined by tensile test with and without thermally induced stress (Ohno et al. 1986a). The resin bond to the as-polished surface of Co–Cr and Ni–Cr alloys is stronger than that of the oxidized surfaces. The thermal cycles causes clear differences in the surface states that affected the adhesion. The effect of a thick water layer adsorbed on the top of oxide surfaces on the bonding ability of 4-META resin is examined with a Co–Cr alloy and type 304 stainless steel (Ohno et al. 1986b). The bonding ability of the 4-META resin to the dehydrated oxide layer surface is excellent when adhesion procedures are performed in an atmosphere excluding water vapor.

Generally, joints of dental adhesive resin bonded to dental alloys weaken in a wet environment through adhesion is strong in a dry environment. Durability of the adhesion in a wet environment, such as the oral cavity, is predominantly important in the bonding of dental adhesive materials to teeth and dental alloys. The water content penetrated to the interface is calculated from the solution to Fick's second equation (Ko and Wightman 1988).

4-META adheres to hydroxyl groups on metal surface as explained already and noble metals and noble metal alloys have smaller number of hydroxyl groups on their surfaces. Therefore, the bonding strength of 4-META with noble metals and precious alloys is weaker than base metal alloys. The resins bond independently to dental noble metal alloys because they have low chemical affinity for the noble metals.

4.6 Endoscope, Surgical Robot, and Imaging Equipment

Endoscopes are mainly based on optical technology such as fibers. Abdominal surgery devices use high-frequency waves to make incisions and ultrasonic waves to stop bleeding. The tip body and water supply hole are made of stainless steel, but the type of steel is not disclosed. Probably type 304 or type 316L stainless steel are used. Stainless steel is also the main component material for surgical robots. The metals used in advanced contrast imaging equipment such as CT, MRI, and positron emission tomography (PET) are used in structures that support the object, except for electrical circuits and strong magnetic field generation parts, similar to normal equipment.

References

Anusavice, K.J. 2003. Phillips' Science of Dental Materials, 11th ed. Sanders, St. Louis, MO, USA.

ASM Handbook, Vol. 23. 2023. Materials for Medical Devices. ASM International, Materials Park, OH, USA.

ASM Handbook, Vol. 23A. 2023. Additive Manufacturing in Biomedical Applications. ASM International, Materials Park, OH, USA.

ASTM B561-94(2018). 2018. Standard Specification for Refined Platinum. ASTM International, West Conshohocken, PA, USA.

ASTM F90-23. 2023. Standard Specification for Wrought Cobalt-20Chromium-15Tungsten-10Nickel Alloy for Surgical Implant Applications (UNS R30605). ASTM International, West Conshohocken, PA, USA.

ASTM F136-13(2021)e1. 2021. Standard Specification for Wrought Titanium-6Aluminum-4Vanadium ELI (Extra Low Interstitial) Alloy for Surgical Implant Applications (UNS R56401). ASTM International, West Conshohocken, PA, USA.

ASTM F138-19. 2020. Standard Specification for Wrought 18Chromium-14Nickel-2.5Molybdenum Stainless Steel Bar and Wire for Surgical Implants (UNS S31673). ASTM International, West Conshohocken, PA, USA.

ASTM F562-22. 2022. Standard Specification for Wrought 35Cobalt-35Nickel-20Chromium-10Molybdenum Alloy for Surgical Implant Applications (UNS R30035). ASTM International, West Conshohocken, PA, USA.

ASTM F1058-16. 2017. Standard Specification for Wrought 40Cobalt-20Chromium-16Iron-15Nickel-7Molybdenum Alloy Wire, Strip, and Strip Bar for Surgical Implant Applications (UNS R30003 and UNS R30008). ASTM International, West Conshohocken, PA, USA.

ASTM F2063-18. 2018. Standard Specification for Wrought Nickel-Titanium Shape Memory Alloys for Medical Devices and Surgical Implants. ASTM International, West Conshohocken, PA, USA.

Butany, J., K. Carmichael, S.W. Leong and M.J. Collins. 2005. Coronary artery stents: identification and evaluation. J. Clin. Pathol. 58: 795–804.

Charnley, J. 1961. Arthroplasty of the hip. A new operation. Lancet 1: 1129–1132.

Global Market Insights. 2023a. Spinal implants and devices market size, share & trend analysis by product, by technology, by surgery type, by procedure type (discectomy, laminotomy, foraminotomy), by region, and segment forecasts, 2023–2030. https://www.gminsights.com/industry-analysis/spinal-implant-market?gclid=Cj0KCQjwx5qoBhDyARIsAPbMagAi_wMgDthCPrOxEpEJ0SFF_OaLPH6s5dR4biFvDL5-9fPD0B9F2EkaAmo_EALw_wcB

Global Market Insights. 2023b. Coronary stents market size, share & trends analysis report by product (bare metal stents, drug eluting stents, bioresorbable vascular scaffold), by region, and segment forecasts, 2022–2030. https://www.gminsights.com/industry-analysis/coronary-stents-market?gclid=Cj0KCQjwx5qoBhDyARIsAPbMagAXz8uIK-DUMMOoFDrq89ley0TmWLZpFMMhAnsDteQJljJKa6o412EaAuXNEALw_wcB

Grand View Research. 2023. Joint Reconstruction Devices Market Size, Share & Trends Analysis Report By Technique (Joint Replacement, Osteotomy, Arthroscopy, Resurfacing, Arthrodesis), By Joint Type (Knee, Hip, Shoulder), By Region, And Segment Forecasts, 2023 –2030. https://www.grandviewresearch.com/industry-analysis/joint-reconstruction-devices-market

Guglielmi, G., F. Viñuela, G. Duckwiler and J. Dion. 1992. Endovascular treatment of posterior circulation aneurysms by electrothrombosis using electrically detachable coils. J. Neurosurg. 77: 515–524.

Heintz, C., G. Riepe, L. Birken, E. Kaiser, N. Chakfe, M. Morlock et al. 2001. Corroded Nitinol wires in explanted aortic endografts: An important mechanism of failure? J. Endovasc. Ther. 8: 248–253.

Ikemura, K. and T. Endo. 2010. A review of our development of dental adhesives –Effects of radical polymerization initiators and adhesive monomers on adhesion. Dent. Mater. J. 29: 109–121.

Ishihara, K. 2015. Highly lubricated polymer interfaces for advanced artificial hip joints through biomimetic design. Polym. J. 47: 585–597.

Ishimoto, T., Y. Kobayashi, M. Takahata, M. Ito, A. Matsugaki, H. Takahashi et al. 2022. Outstanding *in vivo* mechanical integrity of additively manufactured spinal cages with a novel "honeycomb tree structure" design via guiding bone matrix orientation. Spine J. 22: 1742–1757.

ISO 22674:2022. 2022. Dentistry–Metallic materials for fixed and removable restorations and appliances, International Organization for Standardization, Geneva, Switzerland.

ISO 4049:2019. 2019. Dentistry–Polymer-based restorative materials, International Organization for Standardization, Geneva, Switzerland.

Japanese Study Group of Metallic Stent & Graft. 2000. Current status and progress of metallic stent III. pp. 150–151.

Kasuga, Y., S. Kimura, K. Maki, H. Ueno, S. Omori, K. Hirano et al. 2023. Phase transformation and mechanical properties of heat-treated nickel-titanium rotary endodontic instruments at room and body temperatures. BMC Oral Health 23: 825.

Ko, C.U. and J.P. Wightman. 1988. Experimental analysis of moisture intrusion into the Al/Li-polysulfone interface. J. Adhesion 25: 23–29.

Kyomoto, M., T. Moro, M. Miyaji, M. Hashimoto, H. Kawaguchi, Y. Takatori et al. 2009. Effects of mobility/immobility of surface modification by 2-methacryloyloxyethyl phosphorylcholine polymer on the durability of polyethylene for artificial joints. J. Biomed. Mater. Res. 90A: 362–371.

Lan, R.I., Y. Ren, X. Wei, L.Z. Tang, N.A. Shah, L. Xu et al. 2021. Synergy between vitamin E and D-sorbitol in enhancing oxidation stability of highly crosslinked ultrahigh molecular weight polyethylene. Acta Biomater. 134: 302–312.

Market Research Report. 2023. Spinal Implants and Devices Market Size, Share & Trend Analysis by Product, by Technology, by Surgery Type, By Procedure Type (Discectomy, Laminotomy, Foraminotomy), by Region, and Segment Forecasts, 2023–2030. Grand View Research. https://www.grandviewresearch.com/industry-analysis/spinal-implants-spinal-devices-market#.

Matsugaki, A., M. Ito, Y. Kobayashi, T. Matsuzaka, R. Ozasa, T. Ishimoto et al. 2023. Innovative design of bone quality-targeted intervertebral spacer: accelerated functional fusion guiding oriented collagen/apatite microstructure without autologous bone. Spine J. 23: 609–620.

McAfee, P.C., I.D. Farey, C.E. Sutterlin, K.R. Gurr, K.E. Warden and B.W. Cunningham. 1989. Device-related osteoporosis with spinal instrumentation. Spine 14: 919–926.

Ohno, H., Y. Araki and M. Sagara. 1986a. The adhesion mechanism of dental adhesive resin to the alloy—relationship between Co-Cr alloy surface structure analyzed by ESCA and bonding strength of adhesive resin–. Dent. Mater. J. 5: 46–65.

Ohno, H., Y. Araki, M. Sagara and Y. Yamane. 1986b. The adhesion mechanism of dental adhesive resin to the alloy –Experimental evidence of the deterioration of bonding ability due to adsorbed water on the oxide layer. Dent. Mater. J. 5: 211–216.

Ohno H. 2006. A study on adhesion of adhesive resin to dental alloys. Ph.D. dissertation, Graduate School of Engineering, Yokohama National University. p. 35.

Omura, I., J. Yamauchi, Y. Nagase and F. Uemura. 1983. Japanese Published Unexamined Patent Application. 58-21607. Japan Patent Office, Tokyo, Japan.

Oonishi, H., Y. Takayama and E. Tsuji. 1992. Improvement of polyethylene by irradiation in artificial joints. Radiat, Phys. Chem. 39: 495–504.
Powers, J.M. and R.L. Sakaguchi [eds.]. 2006. Craig's Restorative Dental Materials, 20th ed., Mosly, St. Louis, MO, USA.
Precedence Research. 2023. Artificial Joints Market (By Type: Cemented joints, Non-cemented joints; By Material Type: Ceramics, Alloy, Oxinium, Other Material; By Application: Artificial Knee Joints, Artificial Hip Joints, Artificial Joints of the Shoulder, Other Application; By End User: Prosthetics clinics, Hospitals, Rehabilitation center, Others) - Global Industry Analysis, Size, Share, Growth, Trends, Regional Outlook, and Forecast 2023-2032. https://www.precedenceresearch.com/artificial-joints-market
Rony, L., R. Lancigu and L. Hubert. 2018. Intraosseous metal implants in orthopedics: A review. Morphologie 102: 231–242.
Schmalzried, T.P., T.J. Grogan, P.A. Neumeier and F.J. Dorey. 1991. Metal removal in a pediatric population: benign procedure or necessary evil. J. Pediat. Orthop. 11: 72–76.
Sin, D.C., Kei and H.L.X. Miao. 2009. Surface coatings for ventricular assist devices. Expert Rev. Med. Dev. 6: 51–60.
Szczęsny, G., M. Kopec, D.J. Politis, Z.L. Kowalewski, A. Łazarski and T. Szolc. 2022. A review on biomaterials for orthopaedic surgery and traumatology: from past to present. Materials 15: 3622.
Takeyama, M., S. Kashibuti, N. Nakabayashi and E. Masuhara. 1978. Studies on dental self-curing resins (17)—Adhesion of PMMA with bovine enamel or dental alloys. J. Jpn. Soc. Dent. Appar. Mater. 19: 179–185.
Tambaca, J., S. Canic, M. Kosor, R.D. Fish and D. Paniagua. 2011. Mechanical Behavior of fully expanded commercially available endovascular coronary stents. Tex. Heart Inst. J. 38: 491–501.
Tapscott, D.C. and C. Wottowa. 2023. Orthopedic Implant Materials. StatPearls [Internet], Treasure Island, FL, USA.
Thu, M., A. Ebihara, K. Maki, N. Miki and T. Okiji. 2020. Cyclic fatigue resistance of rotary and reciprocating nickel–titanium instruments subjected to static and dynamic tests. J. Endodont. 46: 1752–1757.

CHAPTER 5

Degradation and Current Problem of Metallic Biomaterials

5.1 Introduction

Materials inevitably deteriorate sooner or later due to chemical and mechanical environmental factors in the human body. If material destruction, shape change, or component dissolution occurs due to deterioration, it becomes necessary to retrieve or replace the medical device. In the case of implant devices, surgery for retrieval or replacement imposes a large burden on the patient, so it is important to prevent deterioration during use. The biological environment that affects the durability of metals is summarized in Fig. 5.1. When metals corrode, metal ions are released and corrosion products are generated. In addition, if the mechanical properties are poor, fatigue will occur and wear debris will be generated at the sliding parts. Metal ions and wear debris cause toxicity, and severe corrosion and fatigue cause failure. In particular, screwed parts are considered to be the initial point for fretting fatigue. Metallic biomaterials themselves do not exhibit toxicity such as allergies. However, metal ions released by corrosion or corrosion products such as oxides, hydroxides, salts, and complexes may become toxic when they bind to biomolecules, cells, or organs and inhibit biological functions. In addition, when wear debris and metal ions are incorporated into living tissues, they cause metallosis. Metallosis is a condition in which loosening of an artificial joint, local necrosis of surrounding tissues, and fibrous tissue formation occur due to corrosion of metals and generation of wear debris. The tissue may be black-colored and show a metallic luster. Metal ions and wear debris not only accumulate in the living tissues around the implant, but are also carried into body fluids, and some are dissolved in the urine and excreted. Although there are many studies on the carcinogenicity of compounds containing metal elements, little is known about the carcinogenicity of metallic biomaterials themselves. International Agency for Research on Cancer (IARC), The World Health Organization (WHO) states that there is no evidence that orthopedic metallic implants are carcinogenic, and in particular, there is no evidence that pure Cr, stainless steel, CP Ti, or Ti alloys is carcinogenic (IARC 1999). Metals currently used for medical purposes are not carcinogenic in other situations, although caution must be taken in environments where a large amount of wear debris are generated.

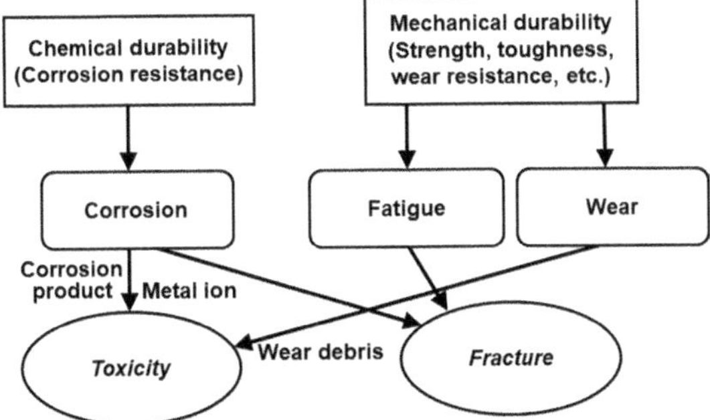

Fig. 5.1. Toxicity and fracture caused by the lack of chemical and mechanical durability of metals. Lack of corrosion resistance generates metal ions and corrosion products and lack of wear resistance generates wear debris that may induce toxicity. Severe corrosion and fatigue of a material cause fracture of the material.

This chapter explains the problems that may occur when metals are used as medical devices, such as infections, MRI artifacts, metal allergies, corrosion, frictional wear, fracture, and stress shielding.

5.2 Biological Environment

The electrolyte concentrations of body fluids are summarized in Table 5.1. The concentrations of chloride ions in serum and interstitial fluid are 113 and 117 mEq L^{-1}, respectively, which is about 1/3 of the concentration in brine and a seriously corrosive environment for metals. Body fluids contain various amino acids and proteins that influence metallic corrosion (Merritt and Brown 1998, Williams et al. 1988, Hanawa et al. 2004) because they are electrolytes. In addition, the concentration of dissolved oxygen in venous blood is 1/4 that of air and in intercellular spaces 1/80-1/4 that of air (Black 1984), which accelerates the corrosion of metals. Changes in the pH of body fluids are small because the fluids are buffered solutions and the pH usually

Table 5.1. Electrolyte concentrations per 1-L water (mEq).

Electrolyte	Extracellular fluid		Intracellular fluid
	Serum	Interstitial	
Na^+	152	143	14
K^+	5	4	157
Ca^{2+}	5	5	-
Mg^{2+}	3	3	26
Cl^-	133	117	-
HPO_4^{2-}	2	2	113 (PO_4^{3-})
SO_4^{2-}	1	1	-
HCO_3^-	27	27	10
Organic acid	6	6	-
Protein	16	2	74

remains between 7.0 and 7.35 (Black 1984). The pH of the hard tissue into which a material is implanted decreases to approximately 5.2 and then recovers to 7.4 within 2 wk (Hench and Ethridge 1975). However, the local pH may change according to the dissociation of protein in the body fluid and the isoelectric point of protein (usually 5–7). The pH in an oral cavity may decrease to about 2 if carbonated drinks and some foods are ingested. The cell and bacteria is also a kind of electrically charging body that may influence the corrosion of metals. Materials implanted in the human body are intermittently stressed with loads due to weight and action (Table 5.2) (Black 1984). In particular, materials in the lower extremities are intermittently loaded with stress several times heavier than the body weight. In addition, loading is repeated in tremendous cycles. Such loads are applied in the chemical environment described above. Chemical and mechanical factors affecting degradation of metals are summarized in Fig. 5.2.

Table 5.2. Load applied to each part of the human body and number of repetitions (Data from Black, J. 1984. Biological Performance of Materials: Plenum, New York, USA).

Load	
Cancellous bone	0–4 MPa
Compact bone	0–40 MPa
Artery wall	0.1–0.2 MPa
Cardiac muscle	0.02–0 MPa
Skeletal muscle (maximum)	40 MPa
Tendon (maximum)	400 MPa
Number of repetition	
Myocardial contraction	5×10^6–4×10^7/yr
Finger joint movement	10^5 – 10^6/yr
Walking	2×10^6/yr

5.3 Degradation of Materials in the Human Body

When biomaterials and medical devices/artificial organs (dental implants, artificial bones, artificial blood vessels, etc.) are implanted in the body, they come into contact with body fluids and adsorption of water molecules, component electrolyte ions, and proteins. Thereafter, cells adhere to them to form tissues (Fig. 5.3). "Biocompatibility" has been defined as the property of a material to exhibit its performance without interfering with this series of processes. In this process, physical and electrochemical signals due to the presence of the material and its micro-dissolution are transmitted to the living body, thereby defining the response of the living body to the material. Although basic research to elucidate the mechanism of biocompatibility was actively conducted for a time, it was difficult and stalled due to the complex biological phenomena. On the other hand, the promotion of tissue formation on materials that could show immediate results for clinical application and result, and the research subject has shifted to developing surface treatment technology. As a result, this research to elucidate the interaction is gradually diminished. Therefore, even now, the

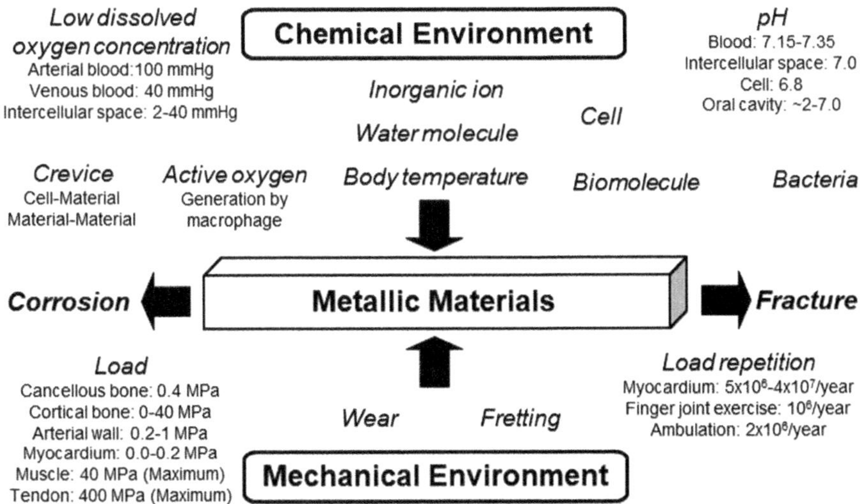

Fig. 5.2. Chemical and mechanical factors affecting the degradation of metals in the human body. Each factor degrades the metal in a complex manner.

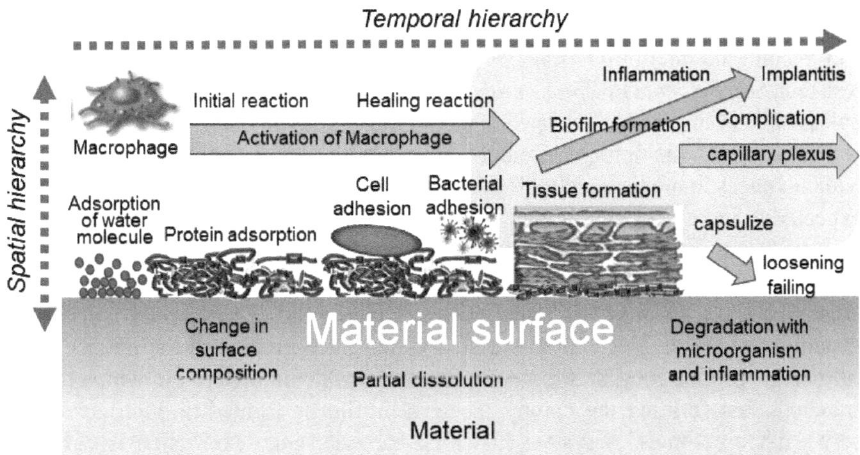

Fig. 5.3. Reactions at the surface of a material implanted into the human body (Reprinted with permission from Frontiers Media S.A. open access, Hanawa. 2019. Front. Bioeng. Biotechnol. 7: 170.).

interfacial reactions between material surfaces and living tissues are only discussed on a weak scientific basis. Furthermore, the material-cell/tissue interface is often a special environment, such as the flow of body fluids (in blood vessels and lymphatic vessels), high pressure conditions, and repetitive shear stress (in joints and tooth roots during occlusion). In addition, infection/inflammation caused by macrophages due to biofilm formation cannot be discussed from the perspective of signal transduction that originates from materials. The above phenomena, which should be understood as a series of processes, have been studied individually, and no progress has been made in constructing a unified theory.

5.4 Infectious Disease

When bacteria adhere to the surface of biomaterials, it causes osteolysis and bone destruction around the material, resulting in loosening of the implant devices. In particular, since there are many bacterial groups in the oral cavity, it is impossible to avoid the adhesion of bacteria to dental restoration/prosthetic materials and dental implants. Although the musculoskeletal system in the human body is basically a sterile field, if bacteria settle around implants used in the orthopedics, it not only causes destruction of the surrounding bones and joints, but also causes damage to elderly people with no systemic reserves. This can lead to serious symptoms such as sepsis. If the infection becomes prolonged and an abscess forms around the implant, it becomes necessary to retrieve the entire implant, which is foreign to the body. It has been reported that the risk of bacterial contamination of implant during the perioperative period of hip arthroplasty surgery reaches 30% (Maathius et al. 2005). Infection control in the use of biomaterials is becoming more and more important as the number of surgeries using biomaterials increases. Furthermore, with the increase in the elderly population in recent years, the number of infected cases increases, and the emergence of resistant bacteria that are ineffective against antibiotics is becoming more prominent. The bacteria that frequently cause infections in orthopedics are the *Staphylococcus aureus* and *Staphylococcus epidermidis*, Gram-positive *cocci*. These strains become resistant (unresponsive to existing antibiotics) and become methicillin-resistant *Staphylococcus aureus* (MRSA) and methicillin-resistant *Staphylococcus epidermidis* (MRSE), and infection cannot be controlled unless special antibiotics are used. The number of cases where this is not possible is increasing. As the number of elderly people with various complications increases with advances in medical technology, the number of cases of refractory infections is expected to increase in the future.

Bacterial growth around metallic biomaterials begins with airborne bacteria adhering to the metal surface. *Pseudomonas aeruginosa*, *Staphylococcus aureus*, *Staphylococcus epidermidis*, oral *streptococcus*, and *Escherichia coli* secrete exopolysaccharaide glucocalyx and sticky substance mucoid to the outside of the cells while proliferating on the surface of the metallic biomaterial to which they are attached, first forming the colony. Then, a biofilm is formed through coadhesion between the colonies. A system in which bacterial gene expression is controlled according to the density of bacteria attached to the surface of a metallic material is called quorum sensing (QS). The formed biofilm also has special channels that take in nutrients, and once formed, the biofilm does not disappear easily. In addition, administered antibiotics are not only inhibited by the biofilm that has formed and their ability to penetrate into the infection nest is reduced, but exopolysaccharides also mask bacterial antigens. In this way, bacteria adhere to foreign substances and continue to survive in the body for a long term without being eliminated by phagocytes, which are responsible for immunity.

The thickness of biofilm formed on metal surfaces varies depending on the bacterial species. On stainless steel and Ti alloy surfaces, pyogenic bacteria such as *Staphylococcus epidermidis* form very thick biofilms that are difficult to peel

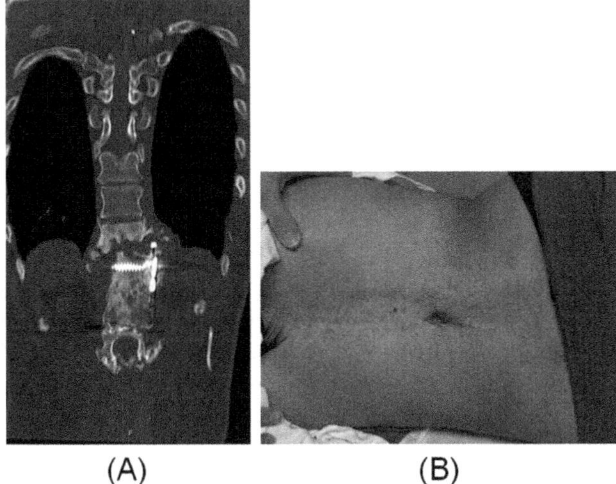

Fig. 5.4. (A) Case of infection after spinal instrumentation surgery. CT images show progressing bone destruction and osteolysis not only around the spinal implant but also in the vertebral body (arrow). (B) A fistula with continuous pus discharge is seen on the skin on the surgical site. (Provided by Dr. Manabu Ito, National Hospital Organization).

off, whereas *Mycobacterium tuberculosis* forms thin biofilms that are easy to peel off (Ha et al. 2005). This is why many spinal instrumentation surgeries have been performed for tuberculous spondylitis, and relatively good clinical results have been reported. On the other hand, in many cases of infections caused by MRSA, the infection cannot subside unless the artificial joint or spinal implant (Fig. 5.4) inserted into the body is retrieved. This is the reason why there are negative opinions about spinal reconstruction surgery using metallic biomaterials for purulent spinal infections. Infections after implantation of metallic biomaterials, which are caused by inactive bacteria, often do not show significant clinical symptoms in the early stages, and diagnosis and appropriate treatment tend to be delayed, while osteolysis around the implant may occur at the beginning of treatment. In many cases, implant failure progresses, eventually causing loosening or movement of the implant, which becomes a major clinical problem.

The thickness and ease with which biofilms form on the surface of metallic biomaterials vary depending on the type of the material. Biofilms formed on Ti alloys are thinner than on stainless steel and tend to peel off easily with antibiotics, so it has been reported that Ti alloys are more advantageous in fighting infections (Adachi et al. 2007). However, the ease of bacterial adhesion is closely related to the surface charge, pH, metal ions, surface treatment, etc. of the metallic biomaterial (MacKintosh et al. 2006). At present, CP Ti has no antibacterial properties against *Staphylococcus aureus* but has antibacterial properties against *Escherichia coli*. Pure metals that have antibacterial properties against *staphylococci* include Co, Ni, Cu, Zn, Zr, Mo, and Pb. On the other hand, CP Ti, Co, Ni, Cu, Zn, Zr, Mo, and Pb have antibacterial properties against *E. coli* (Miyano et al. 2007). The creation of new metallic biomaterials with antibacterial properties is a major future challenge.

5.5 MRI Artifact

The number of patients with various implants is increasing, and in the widely used magnetic resonance imaging (MRI) examination, the influence of medical tools on patients and their images is a medically important issue (Noda et al. 2022). In fact, when applying for approval of clips for cerebral arteriovenous malformation surgery, an evaluation of the effect on MRI examinations is required. MRI compatibility evaluation items for medical devices such as implants include displacement force and torque caused by magnetic fields, heating by radio frequency (RF), and image artifacts, while MRI artifacts caused by metallic devices in particular are proportional to the magnetic field strength of the MRI equipment. There are concerns about the effects of the recent increase in the magnetic fields of MRI.

MRI is a method of irradiating electromagnetic waves (high-frequency magnetic fields) in a strong static magnetic field inside a scanner to generate magnetic resonance signals from hydrogen nuclei to create images. Therefore, images that reflect water and fat, which are the main molecules in living body that contain hydrogen, can be obtained. Hydrogen nuclei have spin angular momentum of rotational motion and an associated magnetic moment. The precession of this so-called spin generates a magnetic resonance signal, whose resonant frequency is proportional to the magnetic field strength. The static magnetic field of MRI is required to be uniform. When the static magnetic field is disturbed by a medical device such as an implant, the alignment (phase) of the generated magnetic resonance signals is disrupted, causing artifacts such as defects and distortions in MR images (Fig. 5.5). Most tissues in living body are diamagnetic with negative susceptibility and are dominated by the

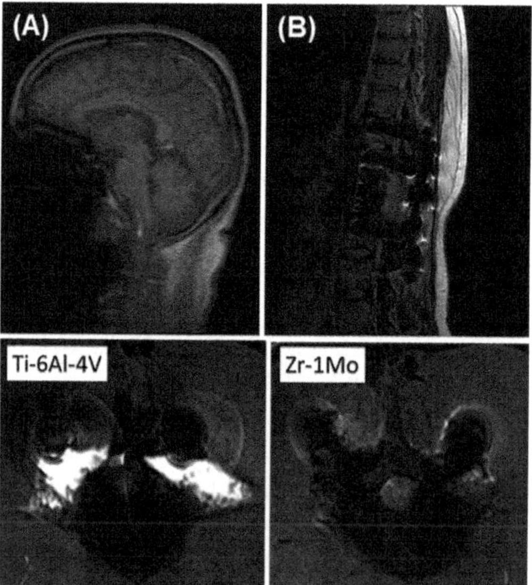

Fig. 5.5. MRI artifact caused by (A) dental restorations consisting of metals and (B) spinal fixation devices. Bottom pictures are the comparison of MR images through a 3T-MRI equipment between Ti-6Al-4V and Zr-1Mo alloys. Less artifact in the Zr-1Mo alloy clearly appearing vertebral canal. (Provided by Dr. Toru Yamamoto, Hokkaido University).

magnetism of water, which is the main constituent molecule. Therefore, if an object with a magnetic susceptibility different from that of tissue exists in a living body, it will disturb the static magnetic field. Since the magnetic susceptibility of air (almost zero) is also different from that of tissue, the magnetic field is disturbed even in areas where air exists in the body, such as the sinuses, and artifacts occur. Such artifacts are called magnetic susceptibility artifacts because they occur when there is a substance with a magnetic susceptibility different from that of the tissue.

As the static magnetic field strength of an MRI device increases, the magnetic resonance signal increases and the signal-to-noise ratio (SNR) improves, so MRI devices are increasingly using higher magnetic fields. On the other hand, when the magnetic field is distorted, the frequency of the magnetic resonance signal is dispersed, and the degree of this dispersion increases in proportion to the static magnetic field strength, so the effect of magnetic field distortion on MR images is more pronounced in high-field MRI systems. Metals currently used for medical purposes are easily magnetized in the strong magnetic field environment of MRI equipment, causing artifacts and hindering contrast imaging. In order to prevent artifacts caused by metal magnetization that interfere with MRI imaging, it is necessary to create metals with low magnetic susceptibility or diamagnetic properties. In addition, as surgery under open MRI contrast is becoming more common, similar properties are required for surgical procedures, therapeutic instruments, and equipment. When using scaffold materials for regenerative medicine, it is necessary to consider in advance the impact on MRI artifacts. Due to the spread of MRI, medical devices used in minimally invasive medicine, especially those used in the circulatory system and cerebrovascular system, are exposed to strong magnetic fields while implanted in the body, causing heat generation within the body. It is necessary to consider the safety of the motor and motion torque. Furthermore, since 3T-MRI has become popular for diagnostic purposes, artifacts occur even in Ti alloys with relatively low magnetic susceptibility. In the United States, when applying for medical device approval, it is already mandatory to evaluate MRI safety, that is, displacement force (suction force), torque, heat generation, and artifacts.

The main countermeasure against MRI artifact is to reduce phase changes due to magnetic field distortion. By shortening the echo time (TE), this phase change is reduced and the defect area is reduced. However, this also changes the contrast of the lesion, so there is a trade-off between artifacts and image contrast. Image distortion can also be improved by shortening the signal acquisition time (increasing received bandwidth (BW)) (Fig. 5.6), but this will reduce the SNR. On the other hand, when low-field MRI such as 0.2–0.4 T open MRI is used, the SNR decreases, while the rotation speed of spin precession, which is proportional to the magnetic field strength, slows down, so phase changes and artifacts are reduced. Both methods reduce artifacts, but at the expense of contrast, SNR, etc.

5.6 Corrosion

5.6.1 Corrosion of Medical Devices

Corrosion of metallic biomaterials implanted in the human body directly influences toxicity and fracture, so many studies have been conducted on corrosion, and the

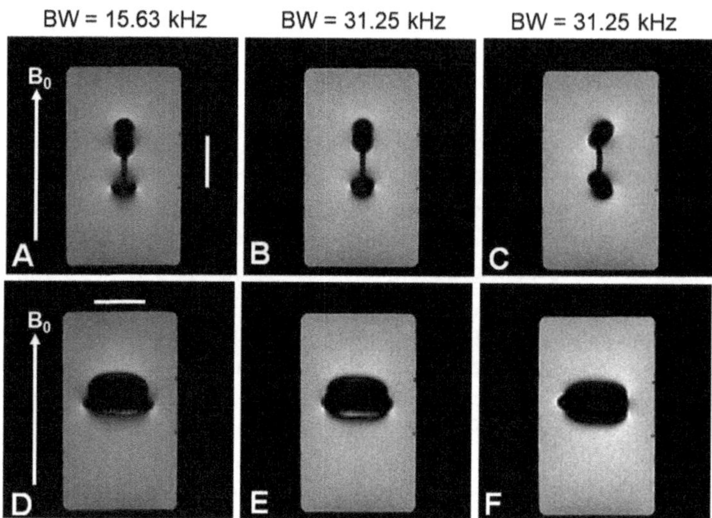

Fig. 5.6. MRI artifact caused by a metal rod. A metal specimen (Co-Cr-Mo alloy with a diameter of 5 mm and a length of 50 mm) was placed in an agar phantom parallel (A, B, and C) or perpendicular (D, E, and F) to the static magnetic field (B_0), the frequency encoding direction is set to the vertical direction (A, B, D, and E) or the horizontal direction (C and F). Images were acquired using a gradient echo pulse sequence (TE = 6.8 ms) with three types of bandwidth (BW). White bars represent the size of metal specimen. (Provided by Dr. Toru Yamamoto, Hokkaido University).

effects of biological factors on corrosion have been clarified. However, most of these studies are conducted outside the body in biologically simulated environments, *in vitro* (see Sections 3.7–3.14). Research in the *in vivo* environment mainly involves evaluation of metal ion release through animal implantation experiments or analysis of tissue around implants in humans, while there are not many examples of analysis of corrosion damage of metallic implants in the human body. This is because implants are retrieved only when there is a sufficient reason to do so, and clinicians are less interested in corroded retrievals. There is an excellent review on corrosion of metallic implants (Eliaz 2019).

5.6.2 Example of Corrosion in Dentistry

Saliva in the oral cavity has a pH of 6.2 to 7.6 and is 99.5% water, and is an electrolytic solution containing organic components such as proteins and amino acids in addition to inorganic species. However, in addition to the regular drop in pH and temperature fluctuations (0 to 60°C) caused by food intake, some of the food remaining in the oral cavity is transferred to plaque bacteria and other microorganisms as substrates for sugar metabolism. Organic acids, such as lactic acid, are produced mainly through anaerobic glycolysis. Sulfur-containing proteins may be degraded by bacteria with proteolytic enzymes, producing hydrogen sulfide that promotes tarnishing of Ag alloys (Fig. 5.7). Some of these acids are released outside the plaque and are neutralized, but much of it penetrates toward the enamel, causing a drop in pH. The interior of dental plaque, where anaerobic bacteria exist, produces organic acids and at the same time becomes an area deficient in dissolved oxygen. Therefore, if plaque

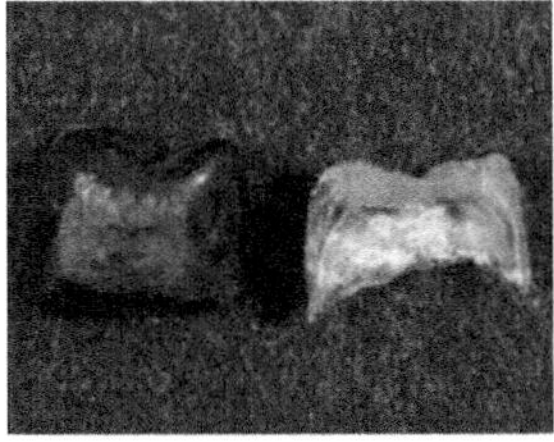
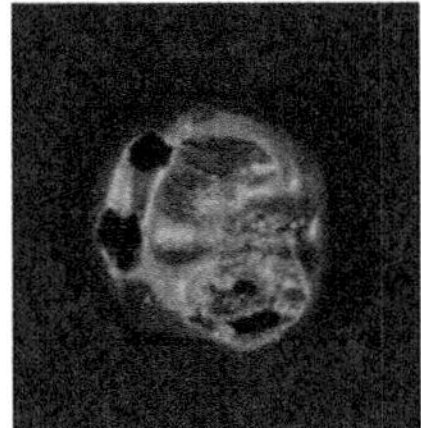
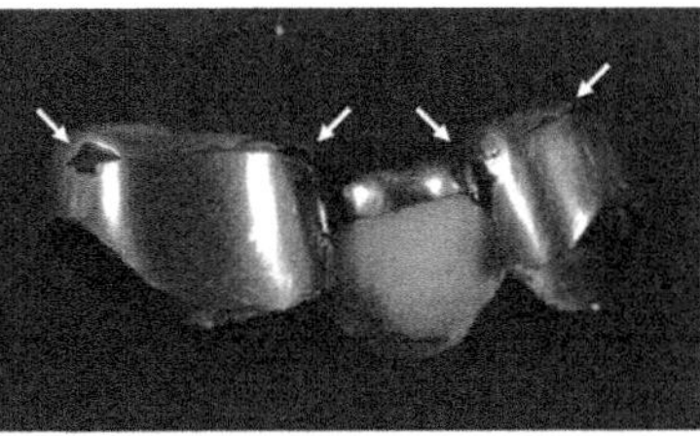

Tarnish of Ag alloy   Fretting corrosion   Galvanic corrosion of brazed part

Fig. 5.7. Tarnish and corrosion of dental restorations.

adheres to the surface of a metallic restoratives or prosthesis, dissolved oxygen may form an oxygen concentration cell and cause localized corrosion. In particular, teeth have an anatomically complex shape and are covered with sticky saliva, so gaps between adjacent teeth are likely to become breeding grounds for microorganisms, and crevice corrosion is likely to occur. Occlusal movements cause periodic stress on the restoratives or prosthesis and abrasion between the restoratives or prostheses. The maximum occlusal force at the molar region is generally equivalent to the static load of the patient's body weight, and the restoratives or prosthesis may be damaged by stress corrosion or fretting corrosion (Fig. 5.7).

In addition to the corrosive environment in the oral cavity, deterioration of metals caused due to dental techniques is also a factor that promotes corrosion. Dental alloys are formed into prosthetics by casting, brazing, cast welding, polishing, etc. In casting, alloys are generally melted together with flux in the atmosphere, and if casting is not performed properly, oxidation of the alloy, casting defects, segregation, etc., will occur even in Au and Ag alloys, decreasing corrosion resistance. Brazing is mainly used to join prostheses, and the brazed parts of prostheses that are worn in the oral cavity for a long term may be preferentially corroded due to galvanic corrosion (Fig. 5.7). To avoid this situation, it is common to use a brazing metal that has a similar potential to the base material. Cast welding is also a joining method in which dental alloys are cast around metals heated to a mold temperature of around 700°C and then joined together. In this case, in addition to contact between dissimilar metals, deterioration factors such as heating and melting are taken into consideration. In dental magnetic attachments, ferritic stainless steel keepers are cast-welded with noble metal alloys, so a noble metal alloy with a small potential difference is selected, because chromium carbide ($Cr_{23}C_6$) and σ phase in stainless steel induce intergranular corrosion. In order to minimize the precipitation of them, it is necessary to perform welding by heating for a short time.

After casting, the restoratives and prosthesis are often immersed in a corrosive solution as a metal cleaning agent and a chemically polished reagent to remove surface oxides. If such treatment is carelessly applied to a cast-welded prosthesis, crevice corrosion at the boundary of the cast joint or extreme corrosion of one metallic material due to contact corrosion of dissimilar metals will occur, so immersion should be kept in the minimum time. Mirror finishing of the prosthesis surface improves corrosion resistance, but caution should be taken when using orthodontic wires that have been subjected to passivating to increase corrosion resistance, as this will decrease corrosion resistance. When cleaning dentures and rinsing the mouth on

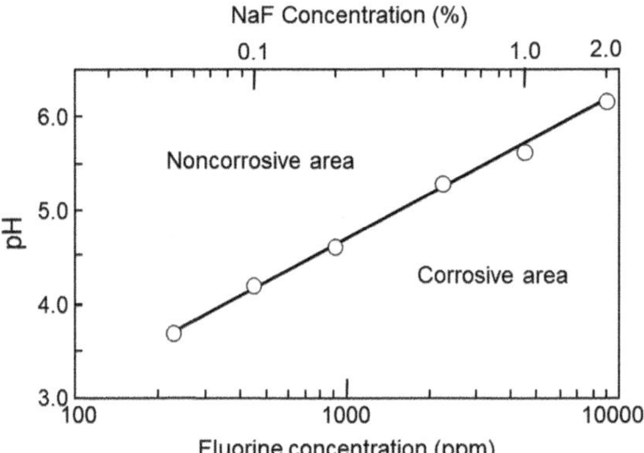

Fig. 5.8. Boundary between corroded and non-corroded areas of CP Ti in the presence of fluorine (Reprinted with permission from SAGE Publication, Nakagawa et al. 1999. J. Dent. Res. 78: 1568–1572.).

a daily basis, denture cleaners and mouth rinses containing fluoride are sometimes used, and even CP Ti and Ti alloys are at risk of corrosion (Nakagawa et al. 1999) (Fig. 5.8). In this way, when a dental alloy is worn as a prosthesis in the oral cavity for a long term, in addition to the corrosive environment in the oral cavity, multiple corrosion resistance deterioration factors overlap, so the corrosion resistance of the dental alloy in the oral cavity is affected. Therefore, it is necessary to consider the corrosion resistance of the restoratives and prosthesis rather than the corrosion resistance of the alloy itself.

5.6.3 Example of Corrosion in Orthopedics and Cardiology

Stainless steel is used in many medical devices, but suffers from pitting and crevice corrosion, which causes corrosion damage. Figure 5.9 shows the corrosion of type 316L stainless steel sternal wires that were retrieved after 22 and 30 yr of implantation. In both cases, the corrosion crevices grow along to the long axis of the wire, that is, the drawing direction (Tomizawa et al. 2006). When observing the wire before implantation, there are scratches in the drawing direction, so by removing these scratches, it is possible to delay the occurrence of corrosion. The diameter of this wire is 0.8 mm, and although the depth of the corrosion crevice does not immediately lead to fracture, metal ions equivalent to the amount of corrosion are leached into the body. Figure 5.10 shows an example of corrosion of a spinal rod (Akazawa et al. 2005). The corroded area is the contacting area with the hook, and crevice corrosion occurs between the rod and the hook. In addition, stress is constantly and repeatedly applied from the hook. Such corrosion is a constant possibility for stainless steel instruments due to the high and repeated loads in spinal fixation (Tezer et al. 2005).

There is very little data on the corrosion damage of Co-based alloys in the human body, while recently corrosion has often been investigated in relation to toxicity and metallosis (Steens et al. 2006, Afolaranmi et al. 2008).

It has been reported that 37.2% (45 of 121 cases) of self-expanding Ni–Ti stents fail within 10.7 mon (Scheinert et al. 2005). There is no doubt that fatigue is the main cause, but corrosion is also thought to be involved. An example of severe pitting and crevice corrosion in a Ni–Ti alloy used as a stent graft is shown in Fig. 5.11

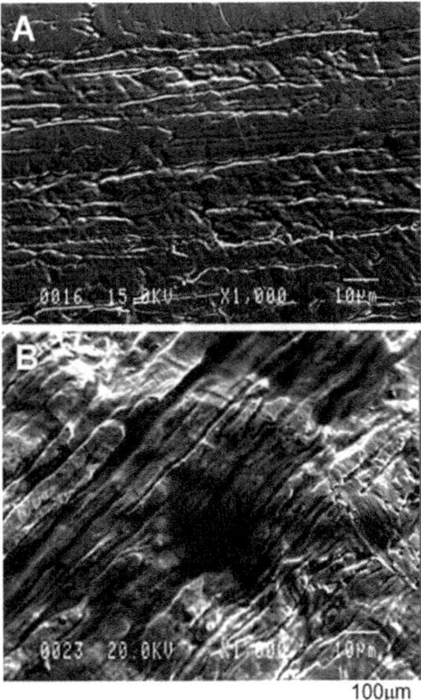

Fig. 5.9. Corrosion of sternal wire consisting of type 316L stainless steel in the human body during 22 yr (A) and 30 yr (B) after implantation. Corrosion crevices grow along drawing direction.

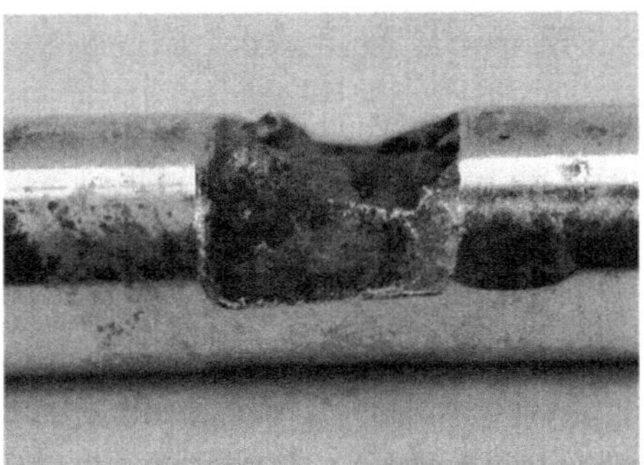

Fig. 5.10. Crevice corrosion of spinal fixation rod consisting of type 316L stainless steel (Reprinted with permission from Elsevier, Akazawa et al. 2005. J. Orthop. Res. 10: 200–205.). Hook is contacted at the corroded site.

(Heintz et al. 2001). This seems to be the result of accelerated corrosion due to the crevice between the metal and the artificial blood vessel. Stents are sometime made of stainless steel or Ni–Ti alloys, and as long as these are used, this type of corrosion is unavoidable.

5.7 Metal Allergy

Metal allergy is one of the toxicities exhibited by metallic biomaterials (Chen and Thyssen 2018). Regarding metals practically used for medical devices, there are almost no reports of toxicity other than metal allergy. This is a natural result since the material has been thoroughly tested and approved for safety. Therefore, in this book, only metal allergy as an issue of toxicity in metallic biomaterials is focused on.

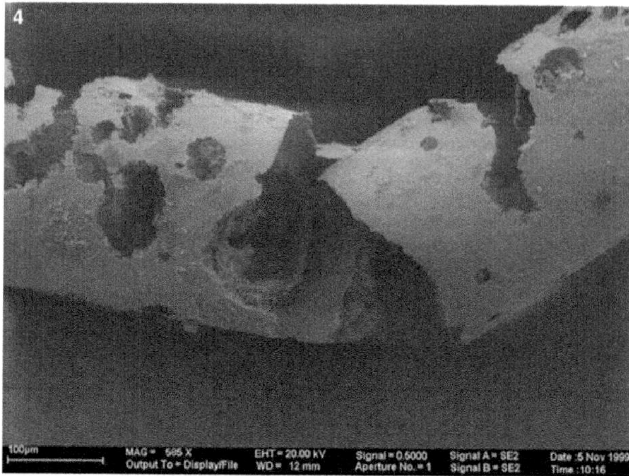

Fig. 5.11. Serious corrosion observed in Ni-Ti alloy used as stent graft for 6 mon (Reprinted with permission from SAGE publication, Heintz et al. 2001. J. Endovasc. Ther. 8: 248–253.).

Metal allergy is classified as type IV allergy (cellular immune type/delayed type). A few hours to a few days after contacting the metal, redness, swelling, and eczema appear on the affected area and the whole body. Symptoms of allergies are usually caused by metallic restorations in dentistry. Figure 5.12 shows an example of metal allergy. Dermatitis, rash, oral lichen planus, and pustular inflammation caused by metal allergy can significantly interfere with daily life even in mild cases, and once they develop, they can last for 20 to 30 yr or even a lifetime in severe cases. Metals, which are causative substances, are widely present in the living environment, including not only dental restoration alloys and ornaments, but also household goods, sporting goods, musical instruments, soap, pigments, and leather. Cases in which allergies are suspected to be caused by cardiac pacemakers or bone plates are often reported. Prevention and treatment methods for metal allergy have not yet been established, and current treatment is symptomatic. In particular, there are many reports of allergies due to dental restorations, because the oral environment is often acidic unlike orthopedic devices that are fully implantable, there is a lot of corrosion due to the drop in pH.

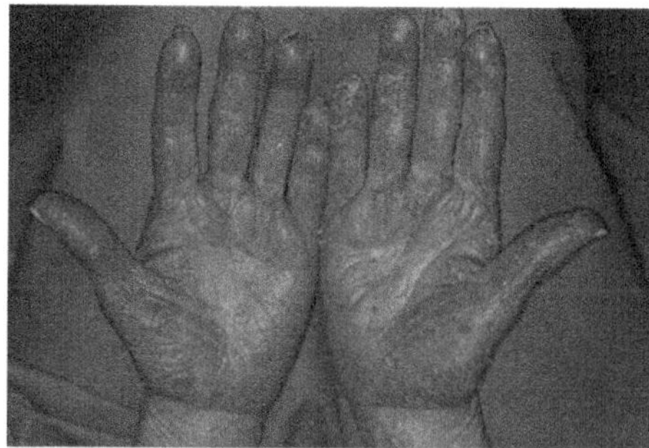

Fig. 5.12. Example of inflammation due to metal allergy (Provided by Dr. Hideya Hamano, Tokyo Medical and Dental University).

Allergy tests include internal medicine, general biochemical tests, allergy blood tests, and patch tests. Patch test is effective for identifying allergen metals. The high positive rate of each metal in recent dentistry is in this order: Ni, Hg, Co, Pd, Cr, Sn, Mo, Pt, Au, Cu, In, Zn, Ir, V, Mn, Ti, Fe, Al, Ab, Ba, Ag, Nb, and Rh (Hamano et al. 1998). Recently, among 925 patients (i.e., excluding those scheduled to undergo dental implant surgery (n = 300)), nearly one-half (44.0%) show a positive response to any metal element in the patch test. The positive rates were as follows: Ni (22.5%), Pd (14.8%), and Zr (11.5%). Almost one-half (42.3%) of the patients have diseases associated with metal allergy (Kitagawa et al. 2019). Allergy due to Ni has always been the most reported, and cases of Pd have been increasing in recent years in northern Europe. Ni allergy is particularly serious in Europe, where 10–15% of women and 1–2% of men are sensitized (Nielsen and Menne 1992, Liden and Carter 2001). As a countermeasure against Ni allergy caused by ornaments and coins, the EU Directive (1999/C 205/05) is issued in 1999, and in accordance with European Standard (EN 1811 2023), a dissolution test using artificial sweat (0.5%NaCl, 0.1% lactic acid, 0.1% urine acid in pure water adjusting 6.5 of pH with ammonia) prohibits the use of earring eluting more than 0.2 $\mu g\ cm^{-2}\ week^{-1}$ of Ni and other products eluting more than 0.5 $\mu g^{-2}\ week^{-1}$ of Ni.

5.8 Friction Wear

5.8.1 Wear of Medical Devices

Two objects sometimes come into contact, such as between the femoral head and socket or between the stem and bone cement in artificial hip joints and between bone fixation plates and screws. At these contacting areas, load fluctuations due to walking cause wear. Metals are used in these constituent materials, and as a result, loosening, wear debris, and release of metal ions occur. These phenomena cause various problems such as pain, inflammation and necrosis of surrounding tissues, and metal allergies. Therefore, by improving the wear resistance of metallic biomaterials, the amount of generated wear debris can be suppressed, and by capturing them, biological disadvantages can be kept to a minimum.

5.8.2 Wear Mechanism

Types of wear are generally classified into adhesive wear, abrasive wear, corrosion wear, and fatigue wear. Adhesive wear can be divided into severe wear, which occurs at the beginning of the wear test, and mild wear, which occurs later. In severe wear, metallic luster is observed on the worn surface. In mild wear, the wear marks appear black color, and the wear occurs through oxides, resulting in relatively mild wear. Abrasive wear includes two-body abrasive wear and three-body abrasive wear. The former is wear between two objects, while in the latter, a third object formed by the wear between the two objects enters the interface between the two objects, further accelerating the wear. In corrosive wear, metals are corroded by gases or liquids containing corrosive components, and corrosion products are easily peeled off by friction. Fatigue friction is wear in which the metal surface undergoes fatigue failure and peeling due to repeated friction. Other examples include delamination wear, in which cracks initiate and propagate on the metal due to plastic deformation, causing fretting wear between two objects (LaBerge 1998).

5.8.3 Wear Property of Metals

Among the typical metallic biomaterials, such as stainless steels, Co–Cr–Mo alloys, and Ti alloys, Ti alloys have the worst wear resistance and Co–Cr–Mo alloys have the best wear resistance. Therefore, Co–Cr–Mo alloys are used for the sliding parts of artificial hip joints and knee joints. Ultra high molecular weight polyethylene (UHMWPE) is often used in sockets for artificial hip joints, and the amount of wear on UHMWPE is the least when Co–Cr–Mo alloys are used for the mating material (Dobbs and Scales 1983). In artificial hip joints, both the femoral head and socket are usually made of Co–Cr–Mo alloys. Figure 5.13 shows the amount of wear of sockets and balls made of similar materials such as type 316L stainless steel, Co–Cr–Mo alloy, Ti alloy, and CP Ti. The combination of Co–Cr–Mo alloys is advantageous, as the amount of wear is the least for both. This result is obtained by the method explained in Section 3.5.

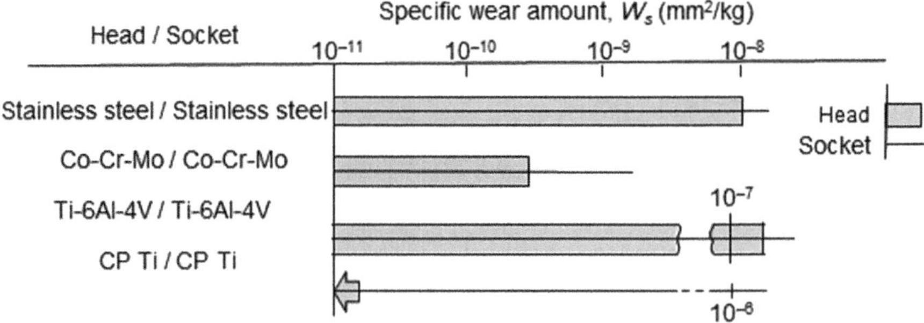

Fig. 5.13. Total wear amount of both socket and ball made of the same materials such as type 316L stainless steel, Co-Cr-Mo alloy, Ti alloy, and CP Ti when wear test was performed (Provided by Dr. Mitsuo Niinomi, Tohoku University).

5.9 Fracture

5.9.1 Outline

Metallic implant devices are often used in situations where high loads are applied repeatedly. Therefore, fatigue properties are important for fracture of metallic biomaterials. However, in addition to simple fatigue failure, for example, when a bone plate and screw are combined, fretting fatigue can significantly reduce the durability of the implant device. Fracture toughness is also considered a problem when the implant device fractures under a single load. Since the above-mentioned fracture occurs in the living body, it is necessary to elucidate the destructive phenomenon in the *in vivo* environment. However, since this is difficult, it is necessary to elucidate the destructive phenomenon in an environment that simulates the *in vivo* environment. Most of the destruction of artificial joints appears in hip and knee joints. Among born fixation devices, intramedullary nails, bone screws, plates, and screws are most frequently fractured, and intramedullary nails tend to be the most frequently fractured. See Section 3.3 and 3.4 to understand more about this item.

5.9.2 Fatigue Fracture

Fatigue occurs when loads are repeatedly applied. Fatigue is a phenomenon in which a material fractures due to repeated stress or strain. In metals, it occurs at a stress of 1/2 to 1/3 of the ultimate tensile stress, and generally does not involve macroscopic plastic deformation. 80% of metal fracture accidents are related to fatigue. Cracks initiate due to repeated stress. The crack propagates gradually as the stress amplitude is repeated, and fractures when the non-cracked part can no longer withstand the stress. As shown in Fig. 5.14, the fractured surface due to fatigue shows striation, where grooves line up parallel to each other as the crack propagates. The striation interval indicates the distance that a crack propagates with one stress amplitude. It is possible to analyze the applied stress from the direction and spacing of the striations. Through the fatigue test, the stress (strain)—number of fractures curve (S-N curve) shown in Fig. 5.15 was obtained, and the stress that does not cause fracture even after 10^7 repeated loads is usually considered the fatigue strength. Fatigue strength is an extremely important value that forms the basis of medical device design. Factors that promote fatigue include corrosion and fretting (a phenomenon in which small amplitude movements occur repeatedly at metal contact parts such as screw fasteners). Figure 5.16 shows a bone fixation plate and the stem of an artificial hip joint that were fractured in a human body.

Fatigue fracture occurs by repeated stress, plastic deformation, intrinsic slip band to form on the metal surface, and crack initiation and propagation in this area. In normal ductile fatigue fracture, the vicinity of the fatigue crack initiation site exhibits a relatively smooth fracture surface, then a stable crack propagation region with striation is formed. If the crack propagates further, a fracture occurs under a single load. An unstable crack propagation region (rapid rupture region) with a fracture surface similar to the surface is formed, leading to fracture. Furthermore, fatigue fracture occurs at a maximum cyclic stress that is considerably lower than the tensile strength. The fatigue ratio, which is the ratio of fatigue stress (fatigue limit) to tensile stress, is excellent for Ti alloys and is approximately 0.5 to 0.6. However, if there are locations where stress concentration is likely to occur, such as corners,

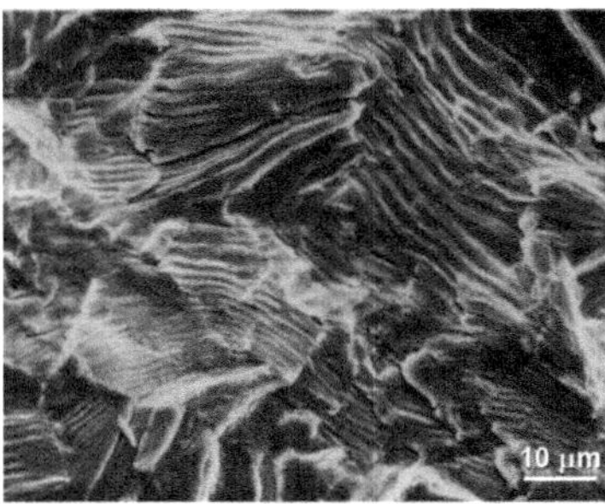

Fig. 5.14. Fatigue fractured surface of CP Ti (Reprinted with permission from ASM International, *ASM Handbook*. 1987. 20.). Striation pattern is observed on the surface that is an important indicator to analyze the fracture mechanism.

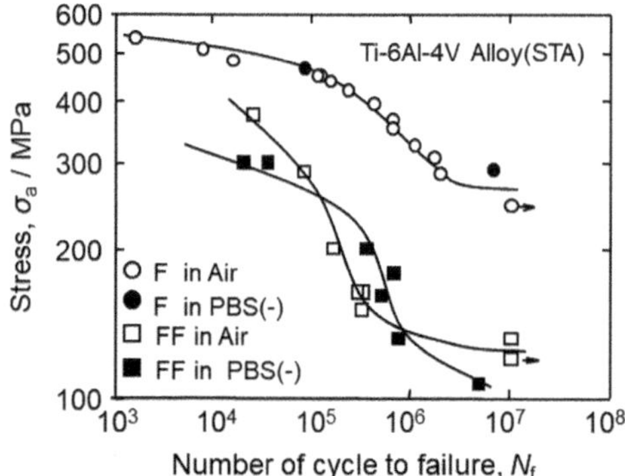

Fig. 5.15. Stress-number of cycles to failure curve (S-N curve) of Ti-6Al-4V alloy in air and phosphate buffered saline (PBS). F: fatigue. FF: fretting fatigue. (Provided by Dr. Norio Maruyama, National Institute for Materials Science). Fretting fatigue strength is much lower than fatigue strength.

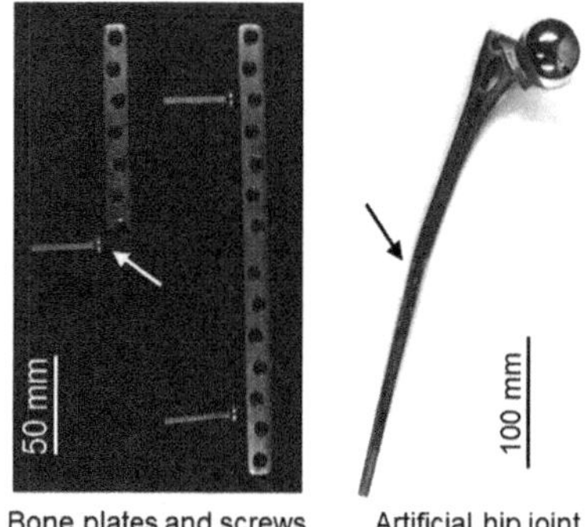

Fig. 5.16. Examples of fractured bone fixator and artificial hip joint in the human body (Provided by Dr. Norio Maruyama, National Institute for Materials Science.).

notches, or defects, such locations are likely to become fatigue crack initiation sites. Therefore, notch fatigue strength is also an important factor for metallic biomaterials. Regarding fatigue crack propagation after fatigue crack initiation, care must be taken because the influence of the microstructure on crack propagation resistance differs depending on whether the crack is short or long. This tendency is remarkable in $\alpha+\beta$ type Ti alloys; the resistance to the propagation of small cracks is higher when the microstructure is fine. On the contrary, the resistance to the propagation of long cracks is higher when the microstructure is coarse, becomes lower. The ratio of micro-fatigue crack propagation life to the total fatigue life is quite large, and increasing the micro-fatigue crack propagation resistance is extremely effective in improving the total fatigue life (Akahori et al. 2000).

Fatigue fracture is, of course, not only caused by inappropriate design, but is also often caused by problems with the material. In other words, in order to prevent fatigue failure, it is important to appropriately control the manufacturing process, microstructure, surface morphology, etc., of the material. Surface morphology is important because fatigue cracks usually initiate from the surface. If the surface finish is rough or the surface is uneven due to poor finishing accuracy, such areas become sources of stress concentration and reduce fatigue strength. Such deterioration of surface quality occurs not only due to defects in the manufacturing process of the material, but also when the implant surface is scratched by a surgical instrument or the like during surgery. In this regard, the static and dynamic cyclic fatigue resistance of contemporary Ni–Ti endodontic files with different kinematic, metallurgic, and design features is investigated (Thu et al. 2020).

5.9.3 Fatigue Fracture in Living Tissue and Simulated Body Fluids

Type 316L stainless steel suffers from corrosion fatigue in simulated body fluids (Niinomi et al. 1996). It has also been reported that the fatigue strength of Co–Cr–Mo alloys decreases in simulated body fluids and Ringer's solution (Kumar et al. 1985). In the case of Ti-6Al-4V ELI alloy, corrosion fatigue does not occur in normal simulated body fluids. In addition, the fatigue strength of Ti alloys does not decrease even in the rabbit body under uniaxial loading fatigue conditions, but the fatigue strength decreases in a simulated body fluid with reduced dissolved oxygen under rotating bending fatigue conditions. Since there is little dissolved oxygen in living bodies, it is thought that corrosion fatigue occurs in Ti alloys under bending stress conditions in living bodies or simulated body fluids. Under bending fatigue conditions, the passive film formed on the Ti alloy surface is likely to be ruptured, and the low oxygen concentration takes time to regenerate the passive film, leading to corrosion fatigue. Furthermore, it has been reported that when macrophage adheres to the surface of CP Ti, it generates active oxygen and causes corrosion, as shown in Fig. 2.25 (Mu et al. 2000). Therefore, under conditions where active oxygen is generated, corrosion fatigue may occur on Ti alloys.

5.9.4 Fretting Fatigue

Fretting fatigue occurs when minute fluctuations occur between two objects, such as between a plate and a screw or between the head and stem of an artificial hip joint where repeated stresses are superimposed. It is known that the fretting fatigue strength of metals decreases to 1/2 to 1/3 of the normal fatigue strength. In fretting fatigue, sliding occurs between two objects, which causes wear and debris. As the sliding distance increases, the fretting fatigue strength tends to decrease, so reducing the sliding distance leads to suppressing the decrease in the fretting fatigue strength. Regarding the initiation of fretting fatigue cracks, the prediction accuracy of damage models can be improved by incorporating micro models describing plasticity effects, wear effects, and inclusion of slip amplitude by determining empirical constants under fretting conditions (Bhatti and Wahab 2018). Fatigue/fretting fatigue behavior in a simulated body fluid is given in Fig. 5.15 for Ti–6Al–4V alloy. The relationship between the tensile stress and the fatigue strength/fretting fatigue stress of metallic biomaterials at 10^7 cycles in air and in a simulated body fluid is discussed (Maruyama 2010). For all of the materials tested, the fatigue stress at 10^7 cycles is similar in air and in a simulated body fluid. The fatigue stress is closely correlated to the tensile strength: the fatigue strength increases with increasing tensile strength. However, a correlation is not observed between the fretting fatigue stress at 10^7 cycles and the fatigue stress or the tensile strength (Fig. 5.17). The decrease in the fretting fatigue

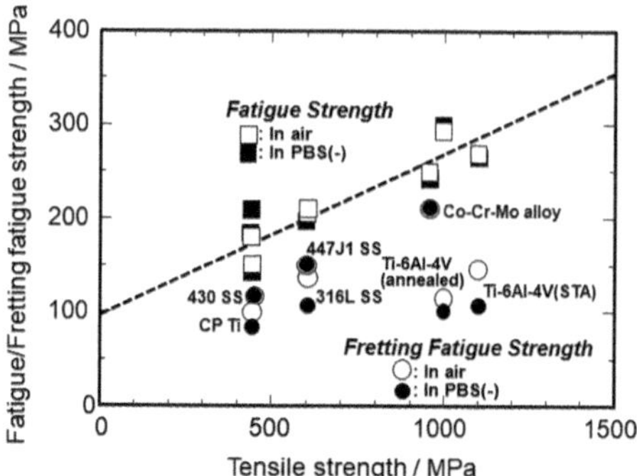

Fig. 5.17. The relationship between the tensile strength of each material and the fatigue/fretting fatigue strength in air and PBS (Provided by Dr. Norio Maruyama, National Institute for Materials Science.). Fretting fatigue strength does not relate to the tensile strength, while fatigue strength is proportional to the tensile strength.

limit relative to the normal fatigue limit is the largest for the Ti–6Al–4V alloy and the smallest for the Co–Cr–Mo alloy. This result is related to the excellent friction and wear resistance of the Co–Cr–Mo alloy. Furthermore, it is clear that the fretting fatigue limit of all materials except the Co–Cr–Mo alloy is lower in phosphate buffered saline (PBS) than in air. This is because fretting causes corrosion crevice to be formed, and fretting promotes corrosion.

5.9.5 Fracture under Single Load

Metal implants will fracture if subjected to a single overload due to violent movement. To avoid this, a material with a good balance between strength and ductility and excellent fracture toughness is required. Since metals are ductile materials, they usually exhibit ductile fracture when subjected to a single load. However, it is necessary to watch brittle fracture due to changes in the microstructure, applied load rate, corrosion, etc. Control of microstructure is extremely important because the presence of inclusions, grain boundary precipitates, etc., can cause brittle fractures such as grain boundary fractures and cleavage fractures. Furthermore, since the living body is a corrosive environment, if corrosion occurs due to long-term use or cracks initiate due to fatigue or wear, fracture toughness will decrease. It is also important to evaluate dynamic fracture toughness because the fracture toughness of metals generally decreases under impact loads. Even if there is a modified layer on the implant surface due to surface hardening to improve wear resistance, one needs to be careful as the surface modified layer becomes a stress concentration source and reduces the fracture resistance of the metal.

5.9.6 Fracture by Human Error

Metals that exhibit sufficient fatigue strength and corrosion resistance are considered safe against fracture. However, because the elongation to fracture of $\alpha+\beta$ type Ti alloy is relatively small, there have been reports of fractures in components that are deformed by the surgeon in the operating room, such as spinal rods and maxillofacial

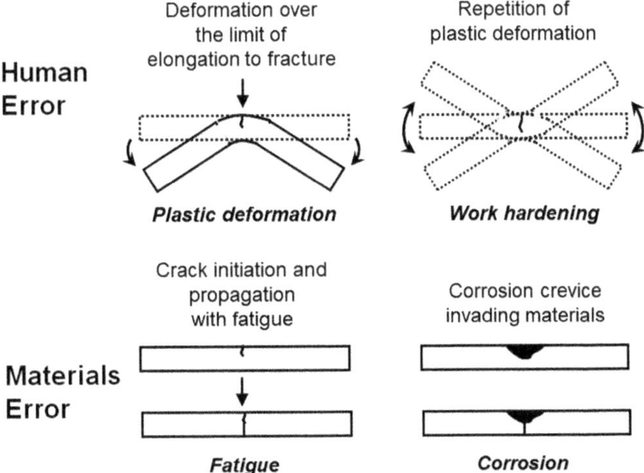

Fig. 5.18. Causes of fracture in implant materials. Human error may occur by deformation exceeding elongation to fracture and work hardening by repeated deformation.

prosthesis plates made of $\alpha+\beta$ type Ti alloy. This occurs when deformation exceeds the elongation to fracture, and cracks initiate. In another case, the plastic deformation operation is failed and plastic deformation is repeated again that induces work hardening to decrease ductility (Fig. 5.18). Similar operations may be performed when metals are used as scaffolding materials, so it is necessary to know about the phenomena that occur when metals are deformed, such as plastic deformation and work hardening.

5.10 Stress Shielding

As shown in Fig. 5.19, in the bone fixation plate and the stem of an artificial hip joint, the Young's modulus of the metal is much larger than that of the cortical bone, so the

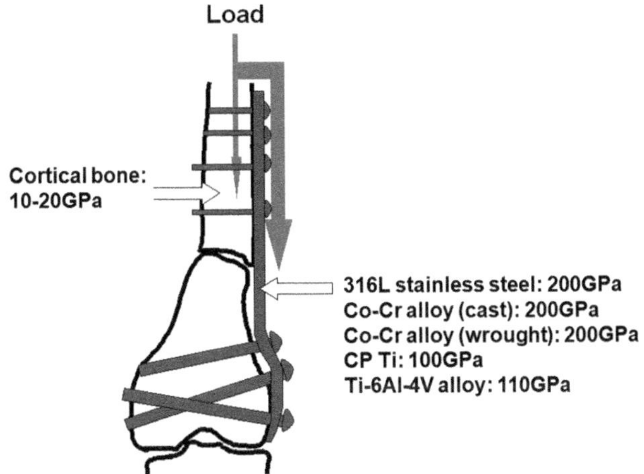

Fig. 5.19. Stress shielding to cortical bone with lower Young's modulus by receiving a load by bone fixation plate with larger Yong's modulus. The same phenomenon usually occur in artificial hip joints.

metal receives the applied load. Therefore, bone resorption due to lack of mechanical stimulation (stress shielding) has been reported because the load is not conducted to the bone. In order to prevent the stress shielding, β-type Ti alloys with a low elastic modulus have been developed. Ti–29Nb–13Ta–4.6Zr alloy, Ti–12Cr, and Ti–Nb–Sn alloy are effective to prevent stress shielding (Niinomi et al. 2016, Kunii et al. 2019). In addition, when used as a fixture of a dental implant, an alloy with a low elastic modulus can be expected to absorb occlusal pressure and prevent the direct load conduction to the maxilla and mandible. When a metal is used as a scaffolding material, it is necessary to pay attention to the difference in the elastic modulus of the surrounding tissue and the metal.

References

Adachi, K., T. Tsurumoto, A. Yonekura, S. Nishimura, S. Kajiyama, Y. Hirakata et al. 2007. New quantitative image analysis of staphylococcal biofilms on the surfaces of nontranslucent metallic biomaterials. J. Orthop. Sci. 12: 178–184.

Afolaranmi, G.A., J. Hirakata, R.M.D. Meek and M.H. Gra. 2008. Release of chromium from orthopaedic arthroplasties. Open Orthop. J. 2: 10–18.

Akahori, T., M. Niinomi, K. Fukunaga and I. Inagaki. 2000. Effects of microstructure on the short fatigue crack initiation and propagation characteristics of biomedical α/β titanium alloys. Metall. Mater. Trans. 31A: 1949–1958.

Akazawa, T., S. Minami, K. Takahashi, T. Kotani and T. Hanawa. 2005. Corrosion of spinal implants retrieved from patients with scoliosis. J. Orthop. Res. 10: 200–205.

ASM Handbook, Vol.12. 1987. Fractography, p.20. ASM Handbook 9th Ed., ASM International, Materials Park, OH, USA.

Bhattti, N.A. and M.A. Wahab. 2018. Fretting fatigue crack nucleation: A review. Tribol. Int. 121: 121–138.

Black, J. 1984. Biological Performance of Materials: Plenum, New York, USA.

Chen, J.K. and J.P. Thyssen [eds.]. 2018. Metal Allergy. Springer, Berlin, Germany.

DIN EN 1811:2023-04. 2023. Reference test method for release of nickel from all post assemblies which are inserted into pierced parts of the human body and articles intended to come into direct and prolonged contact with the skin. Deutsches Institüt für Normung, Berlin, Germany.

Eliaz, N. 2019. Corrosion of metallic biomaterials: a review. Materials 12: 407.

Ha, K.Y., Y.G. Chung and S.J. Ryoo. 2005. Adherence and biofilm formation of Staphylococcus epidermidis and Mycobacterium tuberculosis on various spinal implants. Spine 30: 38–43.

Hamano, H., K. Uoshima, W.P. Miao, T. Masuda, M. Matsumura, H. Kitazaki et al. 1998. Investigation of metal allergy to constituent elements of intraoral restoration materials. Kokubyo Gakkai Zasshi 65: 93–99.

Hanawa, T., Y. Kohyama, S. Hiromoto and A. Yamamoto. 2004. Effects of biological factors on the repassivation current of titanium. Mater. Trans. 45: 1635–1639.

Hanawa, T. 2019. Titanium-tissue interface reaction and its control with surface treatment. Front. Bioeng. Biotechnol. 7: 170.

Heintz, C., G. Riepe, L. Birken, E. Kaiser, N. Chakfe, M. Morlock et al. 2001. Corroded nitinol wires in explanted aortic endografts : an important mechanism of failure? J. Endovasc. Ther. 8: 248–253.

Hench, L.L. and E.C. Ethridge. 1975. Biomaterials-the interfacial problem. Adv. Biomed. Eng. 5: 35–150.

IARC, WHO. 1999. IARC Monograph on the Evaluation of Carcinogenic Risks to Humans, Vol. 74, Surgical Implants and Other Foreign Bodies, International Agency for Research on Cancer, World Health Organization, Lyon, France.

Kitagawa, M., S. Murakami, Y. Akashi, H. Oka, T. Shintani, I. Ogawa et al. 2019. Current status of dental metal allergy in Japan. J. Prosthodont. Res. 63: 309–312.

Kumar, P., A.J. Hickl, A.I. Asphahani and A. Lawley. 1985. Properties and characteristics of cast, wrought, and powder metallurgy (P/M) processed cobalt-chromium-molybdenum implant materials.

pp. 30–56. *In*: Fraker, A.C. and C.D. Griffin [ed.]. ASTM STP 859. American Society for Materials and Testing, Philadelphia, PA, USA.
Kunii, T., Y. Mori, H. Tanaka, A. Kogure, M. Kamimura, N. Mori et al. 2019. Improved osseointegration of a TiNbSn alloy with a low Young's modulus treated with anodic oxidation. Sci. Rep. 9: 13985.
LaBerge., M. 1998. Wear. pp. 364–405. *In:* Black, J. and G. Hastings [eds.]. Handbook of Biomaterial Properties, Chapman & Hall, London, UK.
Liden, C. and S. Carter. 2001. Nickel release from coins. Contact Dermutitis 44: 160–165.
Maathius, P.M., D. Neut, H.J. Busscher, H.C. van der Mei and J.R. vanHorn. 2005. Perioperative contamination in primary total hip arthroplasty. Clin. Orthop. 433: 136–139.
MacKintosh, E.E., J.D. Patel, R.E. Marchant and J.M. Anderson. 2006. Effects of biomaterial surface chemistry on the adhesion and biofilm formation of Staphylococcus epidermidis *in vitro*. J. Biomed. Mater. Res. 78A: 836–842.
Materials Handbook. 1987. Materials Handbook, 9th Ed., p. 20. ASM International, Materials Park, OH, USA.
Maruyama, N. 2010. Fatigue and fretting fatigue behavior of metallic biomaterials. Mater. Sci. Forum 638–642: 618–623.
Merritt, K. and S.A. Brown. 1998. Effect of proteins and pH on fretting corrosion and metal ion release. J. Biomed. Mater. Res. 22: 111–120.
Miyano, Y., K. Koyama, K.R. Sreekumari, Y. Sato and Y. Kikuchi. 2007. Evaluation of antibacterial ability of some pure metals. Tetsu-to-Hagane 93: 57–65.
Mu, Y., T. Kobayashi, M. Sumita, A. Yamamoto and T. Hanawa. 2000. Metal ion release from titanium with active oxygen species generated by rat macrophages *in vitro*. J. Biomed. Mater. Res. 49: 238–243.
Nakagawa, M., S. Matsuya, T. Shiraishi and M. Ohta. 1999. Effect of fluoride concentration and pH on corrosion behavior of titanium for dental use. J. Dent. Res. 78: 1568–1572.
Nielsen, N.H. and T. Menne. 1992. Allergic contact sensitization in unselected danish population. Acta Derm. Venereol 72: 456–460.
Niinomi, M., T. Kobayashi, O. Toriyama, N. Kawakami, Y. Ishida and Y. Matsuyama. 1996. Fracture characteristics, microstructure, and tissue reaction of Ti-5Al-2.5 Fe for orthopedic surgery. Metall. Mater. Trans. 27A: 3925–3935.
Niinomi, M., Y. Liu, M. Nakai, H.H. Liu and H. Li,. 2016. Biomedical titanium alloys with Young's moduli close to that of cortical bone. Regen. Biomater. 3: 173–185.
Noda, C., B.A. Venkatesh, J.D. Wagner, Y. Yoko Kato, M. Jason, J.M. Ortman et al. 2022. Radio Graph. 42: E102–E103.
Scheinert, D., S. Scheinert, J. Sax, C. Piorkowski, S. Braunlich, M. Ulrich et al. 2005. Prevalence and clinical impact of stent fractures after femoropopliteal stenting. J. Am. Coll. Cardiol. 45: 312–315.
Steens, W., G. Foerster and A. Katzer. 2006. Severe cobalt poisoning with loss of sight after ceramic-metal pairing in a hip—a case report. Acta Orthop. 77: 830–832.
Tezer, M., U. Kuzgun, A. Hamzaoglu, C. Ozturk, F. Kabukcuoglu and M. Sirvanci. 2005. Intraspinal metalloma resulting in late para-paresis. Arch. Orthop. Trauma Surg. 125: 417–421.
Thu, M., A. Ebihara, K. Maki, N. Miki and T. Okiji. 2020. Cyclic fatigue resistance of rotary and reciprocating Ni–Ti instruments subjected to static and dynamic tests. J. Endodont. 46: 1752–1757.
Tomizawa, Y., T. Hanawa, D. Kuroda, H. Nishida and M. Endo. 2006. Corrosion of stainless steel sternal wire after long-term implantation. J. Artif. Organ 9: 61–66.
Williams, R.L., S.A. Brown and K. Merritt. 1988. Electrochemical studies on the influence of proteins on the corrosion of implant alloys. Biomaterials 9: 181–186.

CHAPTER 6

Titanium and Titanium Alloys

6.1 Introduction

Ti materials, such as commercially pure Ti (CP Ti) and Ti alloys, are widely used in medicine and dentistry because of their large corrosion resistance, large specific strength, and high performance in medicine and dentistry (Brunette et al. 2001). Their good interfacial and chemical compatibility against tissues are well known based on substantial evidence from basic research and high clinical performances. The main reason why Ti materials have achieved excellent result as medical implant materials is their high corrosion resistance within the body. Furthermore, the low specific gravity and high specific strength are effective for large orthopedic implants. In addition, the Young's modulus of α+β-type Ti alloy (100-111 GPa) is half those of type 316L stainless steel (200 GPa) and Co–Cr–Mo alloy (approximately 220 GPa), which is a large advantage to prevent stress shielding in bone plates and stems of artificial hip joints in orthopedics. On the other hand, the mass magnetic susceptibilities of Ti (31.9×10^{-9} m^3 kg^{-1}) and Ti–6Al–4V ELI alloy (39.8×10^{-9} m^3 kg^{-1}) are much smaller than that of Co–Cr–Mo alloy (94.5×10^{-9} m^3 kg^{-1}), as well as stainless steels, decreasing the influences of magnetic resonance imaging (MRI), such as motion, attraction force, torque, heat generation, and artifacts. This property is significant, because MRI is commonly used for medical examination. Although much circumstantial evidence of biological reactions has been accumulated regarding the reason why Ti materials have the best tissue compatibility among metals, it is clear that the essential principle lies with Ti materials themselves. Although the principle behind this is not completely clear, at the end of this chapter, the possible principle of biocompatibility based on the surface properties of Ti materials is explained. A conprehensive handbook on Ti (ASM Handbook Vol. 2 2023) should be used as reference. In this chapter, contents of open-access review papers by the present author (Hanawa 2019, 2022) are used as sections.

6.2 History of Application to Medicine

The history of the application of CP Ti and Ti alloys to medicine and dentistry is summarized in Table 6.1. The first report on CP Ti for medicine appeared in 1940, and excellent bone compatibility was found to be based on an animal test

Table 6.1. History of Ti materials' application to medicine and development of Ti alloys.

Year	Material	Circumstance	References
1940	CP Ti	Confirmation of equivalent biocompatibility as stainless steel and Co–Cr alloy with animal test	Bothe et al. 1940
1940	CP Ti	Success of smelting by Kroll process	Kroll 1940
1948	CP Ti	Launching industrial production	
1951	CP Ti	Confirmation of both soft and hard tissues compatibility with animal test	Leventhal 1951
1957	CP Ti	Confirmation of non-toxicity with long-term implantation	Beder 1957
1959	Ni–Ti	Development of shape memory alloy in USA	Buehler at al. 1963, Wang et al. 1965
1960	CP Ti	Excellent results in artificial joints	Williams 1982a
1960's	CP Ti	Marketing as surgical implants in UK and USA	
1970's	Ti–6Al–4V	Diverting aircraft material to orthopedic implants	
1978	Ti–Cu–Ni	Trial of dental casting	Waterstrat et al. 1978
1980	Ti–5Al–2.5Fe	Development in Europe	
1982	CP Ti	Development of investment material and casting machine for dental casting	Miura and Ida 1988
1985	Ti–6Al–7Nb	Development in Switzerland	Semlitsch and Staub 1985
1993	Ti–13Nb–13Zr	Development in USA	
1993	Ti–12Mo–6Zr–2Fe	Development in USA	Wang et al. 1993
1996	Ti–15Mo	Development in USA	Zardiackas et al. 1996
1988	Ti–29Nb–13Ta–4.6Zr	Development in Japan	Kuroda et al. 1988
Around 2000	Ti–15Mo–5Zr–3Al	Development in Japan	Kobe Steel Rao and Houska 1979
Around 2000	Ti–6Al–2Nb–1Ta–0.8Mo	Development in Japan	Okazaki 2001
2004	Ti–15Zr–4Nb–4Ta	Development in Japan	Ozaki et al. 2004
After 2000	β-metastable alloys based on TRIP and TWIP	Development in mainly China	Marteleur et al. 2012, Ahmd et al. 2016, Brozek et al. 2016, Zhan et al. 2016, Zhang et al. 2017, Lai et al. 2018

(Bothe et al. 1940). Thereafter, the compatibility with bone and soft tissue of rabbits (Leventhal 1951), noncytotoxicity due to excellent corrosion resistance in biological environments, and excellent biocompatibility in dogs (Beder et al. 1957) were reported. The large-scale industrial manufacturing process for Ti achieved in the last half 1940s made it possible to conduct many studies for medical applications, revealing excellent biocompatibility in long-term animal testing (Williams 1982a). Thereafter, the usefulness of CP Ti was widely recognized by the last half of the 1960s through clinical evaluation (Williams 1982a, b, Pillar and Weatherly 1982).

However, to avoid the fracture of CP Ti in the human body, an aerospace Ti–6Al–4V alloy was diverted to artificial joints and bone fixators (Williams 1982a, b, Pillar and Weatherly 1982). Thereafter, V- and/or Al-free $\alpha+\beta$-type Ti alloys and β-type Ti alloys with low Young's modulus have been developed. Since V shows cytotoxicity, the V in Ti–6Al–4V alloy was replaced by Nb, which is a safe element, to develop a new $\alpha+\beta$-type Ti–6Al–7Nb alloy (Semlitsch and Staub 1985). Other $\alpha+\beta$-type alloys, Ti–6Al–2.5Fe alloy and Ti–6Al–2Nb–1Ta–0.8Mo alloy, were developed in 1970s (Rao and Houska 1979, Anon 1994).

On the other hand, β-type Ti alloys for medical use have been developed. Ti-13Nb-13Zr alloy (nearly β) has been developed in the United States. Various β-type alloys, Ti–12Mo–6Zr–2Fe alloys (Wang et al. 1993), T–15Mo (Zardiackas et al. 1996), and Ti–15Mo–2.8Nb–0.2Si–0.28O (Fanning 1996), have been developed in the United States. Ti–15Mo–5Zr and Ti–15Mo–5Zr–3Al alloys (Rao and Houska 1979) and Ti–15Zr–4Nb–4Ta alloy (Okazaki 2001) have been developed. The history of the development of β-type Ti alloys is well summarized elsewhere (Niinomi 2019). Young's modulus could decrease to 40–60 GPa in a β-type alloy.

Since 2000, a new wave of the development of Ti alloys has been generated. The design of Ti alloys through twinning-induced plasticity (TWIP) and transformation-induced plasticity (TRIP) has been attempted, making it possible to develop novel β-metastable Ti alloys (Marteleur et al. 2012, Ahmd et al. 2016, Brozek et al. 2016, Zhan et al. 2016, Zhang et al. 2017, Lai et al. 2018, Baltatu et al. 2021). The TRIP and TWIP concepts were first invented in the field of steels and applied to Ti alloys through Ni–Ti shape memory alloy. It is possible that this design will be applied to biomedical alloys in the near future.

In dentistry, CP Ti has been successfully used for dental implants since 1965 (Waterstrat et al. 1978), and the excellent hard-tissue compatibility is well-known. A magnesia-system investment material and argon-arc casting machine were developed in 1982, followed by the development of various dental casting systems for dental restoratives (Miura and Ida 1988).

Researchers are continually developing new titanium alloys for medical devices. New designs have been attempted based on d-electron alloy design theory (Kuroda et al. 1988) and the TRIP and TWIP concept. Recently, Ti-based high entropy alloy has been investigated to gain new mechanical and chemical properties (Nakano 2022).

6.3 Mechanical Property of Commercially Pure Titanium (CP Ti)

Ti has a characteristic of having a high affinity with other elements and a high solubility of other elements, such as O and C. Ti is an active metal, as evidenced by its high affinity with other elements, and is associated with the following advantages from the perspective of application to biomaterials.

(1) A stable passive film is rapidly reformed in the biological environment.
(2) Even if Ti ions are released into living tissues, they are immediately oxidized. On the other hand, the activity of Ti element is also closely related to the following issues in the material production process.
(3) It is difficult to reduce the cost of the smelting process.
(4) It is difficult to reduce the content of impurities such as oxygen.

Pure Ti is composed of hcp crystals (α phase) at ambient temperatures, but is composed of bcc crystals (β phase) over 882°C. Genuine pure Ti does not exist, because Ti easily dissolves O, C, and N and contains them as impurities. Ti containing these impurities is described as CP Ti. CP Ti is classified into 4 grades, according to its impurity content and the resulting mechanical properties (Table 6.2) (ISO 5832-2 2018). The higher the grade number, the higher the impurity, tensile strength, and offset yield stress and the lower the elongation (Fig. 6.1). In other words, CP Ti is a type of alloy, from the viewpoint of the definition of an alloy and the general effects of alloying. CP Ti is used for maxillofacial prosthetic plates, mniplates, dental Implants, dental restoratives, and dental denture bases. Sometimes, CP Ti containing more impurities than grade 4 displays almost the same strength as Ti alloys. Since the tensile strength greatly increases with cold working, bone screws that are exposed to a large load are sometimes made of CP Ti.

Table 6.2. Compositions and mechanical properties of commercially pure titanium (CP Ti) (Data from ISO 5832-2:2018. 2018. Implants for surgery, Metallic materials, Part 2: Unalloyed titanium. International Organization for Standardization, Geneva, Switzerland).

Element	**Grade 1**	**Grade 2**	**Grade 3**	**Grade 4**
	Composition (mass%)			
Fe	< 0.15	< 0.2	< 0.25	< 0.3
O	< 0.18	< 0.25	< 0.35	< 0.45
N	< 0.03	< 0.03	< 0.05	< 0.05
H	< 0.0125	< 0.0125	< 0.0125	< 0.0125
C	< 0.1	< 0.1	< 0.1	< 0.1
Ti	Balance	Balance	Balance	Balance
Mechanical property				
Ultimate tensile strength(MPa)	275–412	343–510	481–618	> 550
0.2% offset yield strength (MPa)	170	275	380	> 440
Elongation to fracture (%)	> 27	> 23	> 18	> 15
Young's modulus (GPa)	114			

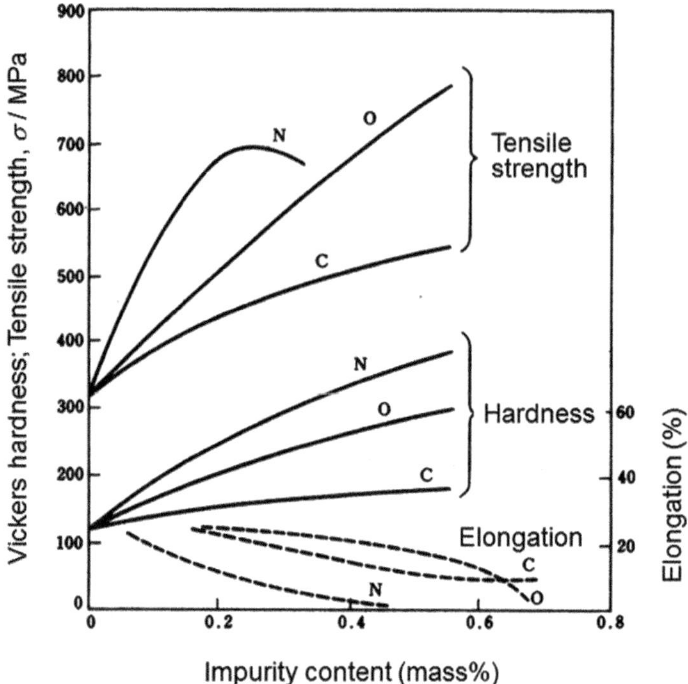

Fig. 6.1. Changes in Vickers hardness, tensile strength, and elongation to fracture of Ti with impurity contents.

6.4 Crystal Structure of Titanium Alloys

Ti is a high melting point metal and has an allotropic transformation of α phase (hexagonal close-packed structure, hcp) to β phase (body-centered cubic structure, bcc) at 882°C. Sinceβ transformation temperature (β trunsus) varies greatly depending on the alloy system, combined with the high solubility of other elements in Ti, it is possible to control the microstructure of the alloy through a variety of alloy designs, working, and heat treatments, and it can show a wide range of mechanical properties as a biomaterial.

As shown in Fig. 6.2, when alloying elements are added to Ti, a two-phase region of α+β appears. When alloying elements are α stabilizing elements, the β transus increases and α phase region expands on the equilibrium phase diagram. Beta stabilizing elements decreases the β transus and expands the β phase region. Neutral elements change the β transus slightly that is classified as a neutral element. Alloying elements have also been classified using a more detailed Ti–X binary alloy phase diagram that includes the formation of intermetallic compounds (ASM Handbook Vol. 2 2023). Equation (6-1) has been proposed as the contribution of various elements to the β transus (Ouchi 1994).

$$\beta \text{ transus } (^\circ\text{C}) = 886 + 147.7[\text{O}] + 20.4[\text{Al}] + 161.8[\text{C}] + 294.3[\text{N}] - 19.8[\text{Fe}] \\ -10.3[\text{Mo}] - 4.1[\text{Zr}] - 8.4[\text{Nb}] - 13.1[\text{V}] - 30.8[\text{Ni}] - 23.0[\text{Co}] \\ -15.7[\text{Mn}] - 17.0[\text{Cr}] - 0.2[\text{Sn}] - 8.5[\text{Cu}] \text{ (mass\%)} \quad (6.1)$$

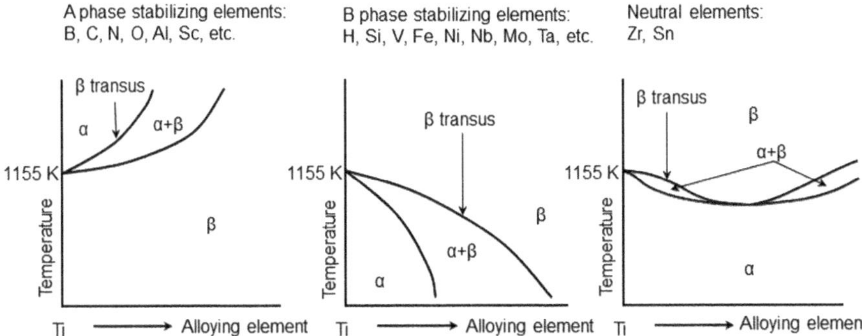

Fig. 6.2. Classification of alloy types based on Ti-X binary phase diagram.

Table 6.3. Metastable phase in Ti alloys.

<table>
<tr><th>Phase</th><th>Crystal structure</th><th>Generation condition</th></tr>
<tr><td>ω</td><td>Hexagonal system</td><td>Metastable phase formed from β phase.
Athermal ω phase: formed by quenching.
Thermal ω phase: formed by aging. Cause of brittleness.
Stress induced ω phase: formed by working.</td></tr>
<tr><td>α'</td><td>Hexagonal system
(Hexagonal closed packing)</td><td rowspan="2">Martensite phase: formed from β phase by quenching or stress induced transformation due to working.
α' phase: formed in alloys containing relatively small amount of β stabilized elements.
α'' phase: formed in alloys containing relatively large amount of β stabilized elements and decreasing M_s temperature.</td></tr>
<tr><td>α''</td><td>Orthorhombic system</td></tr>
</table>

In addition to the equilibrium phases, α and β, Ti alloys also have metastable phases shown in Table 6.3. All of these appear during the transformation process from β phase to α phase. The α" phase is known to have a significant impact on the functionality and mechanical properties of Ti alloys, such as being related to shape memory and superelasticity.

Table 6.4 lists standardized medical Ti alloys. Ti materials can be classified into α-type, α+β-type, and β-type depending on their constituent phases. The area near the boundary between α type and α+β type is sometimes called the near-α type, and the area near the boundary between the β type and α+β-type is sometimes called the near-β type. Figure 6.3 shows the classification of Ti alloys according to the concentration of β-stabilizing elements. Alfa type Ti alloys are a single α phase at room temperature, such as CP Ti and Ti–5Al–2.5Sn alloys. The α+β-type is an alloy with a composition that is in the α+β two-phase region at room temperature and has a martensite initiation temperature (M_s) above room temperature. There are two types of β-type: metastable β-type and stable β-type. On the equilibrium diagram, the metastable β type is in the α+β two-phase region at room temperature, while quenching at a temperature above the β transus suppresses the formation of martensite and α phase, resulting in a metastable β single phase region.

Table 6.4. Titanium materials for medical implants specified by ISO and ASTM.

Structure	Material	ISO		ASTM	
α type	CP Ti	5832-2:2018	Grade 1 Grade 2 Grade 3 Grade 4	F67-13	Grade 1 Grade 2 Grade 3 Grade 4
α+β type	Ti-6Al-4V	5832-3:2021 (Wrought)		F1108-21 (Cast) F1472-20a (Wrought)	
	Ti-6Al-4V ELI			F136-13 (Wrought)	
	Ti-6Al-7Nb	5832-11:2014 (Wrought)		F1295-16	
	Ti-3Al-2.5V			F2146-01	
Near β type	Ti-13Nb-13Zr			F1713-08	
Β type	Ti-15Mo-5Zr-3Al	5832-14:2019 (Wrought)			
	Ti-12Mo-6Zr-2Fe			F1813-21	
	Ti-15Mo			F2066-18	
	Ti-35Nb-7Zr-5Ta			STP37547S	
Intermetallic compound	NiTi (Ni:54.5-57.0)			F2063-05	

Alfa+β-type Ti alloys, represented by Ti–6A–4V alloy, have excellent heat treatability and are relatively easily strengthened from medium to high strength by controlling the size of α and β grains and the transformed structure. Although Ti–6A–4V alloy has poor cold workability, it has an excellent balance of mechanical properties and heat treatability, so it is widely used as the main α+β-type Ti alloy for medical applications. Although there is no problem from the viewpoint of medical device application, the toxicity of Al and V contained in Ti-6Al-4V alloy is often regarded as a concern. Therefore, Al- and V-free α+β type Ti alloys such as Ti–6Al–7Nb alloy and Ti–15Zr–4Nb–4Ta alloy containing neither Al nor V have been developed.

Beta-type Ti alloy has the following characteristics.

I. Strength greater than α+β-type Ti alloy can be obtained through heat treatment.
II. Better cold workability than α+β-type Ti alloy due to its bcc structure.
III. Lower elastic modulus than CP Ti and α+β-type Ti alloy.

The low elastic modulus of β-type Ti alloys has attracted attention since the 1990s, when simulations and animal experiments showed that low Young's modulus materials were effective for bone tissue compatibility and remodeling (Wang 1996, Niinomi 2002). The elastic modulus of stainless steel and Co–Cr–Mo alloys is over 200 GPa and those of CP Ti and α+β-type Ti alloys are about 100 GPa, which are considerably higher than that of cortical bone (10 to 30 GPa). Although the optimal elastic modulus from the perspective of bone compatibility is not clear, β-type Ti alloys with low elastic modulus are being actively developed. A β-type Ti–29Nb–13Ta–4.6Zr alloy (Kuroda et al. 1988) and a Ti-Nb-Sn alloy (Fujisawa et al. 2018) show low Young's modulus of 45 and 78 GPa close to that of human cortical bone,

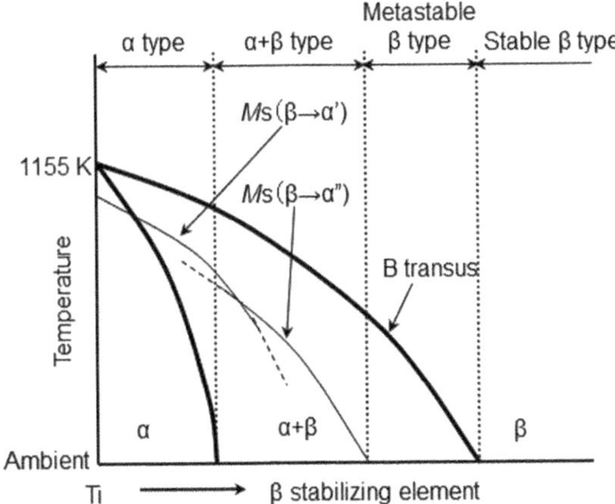

Fig. 6.3. Classification of Ti alloys according to the concentration of β-stabilizing element.

respectively. Intramedullary fixation with nails with a lower Young's modulus offers a greater capacity for fracture healing.

6.5 Mechanical Property of Titanium Alloys

Figure 6.4 shows the tensile strength and elongation to fracture of Ti alloys for medical use. As the strength increases, the elongation decreases.

In α-type Ti alloys including CP Ti, they become acicular α phase due to β processing in the temperature range above the β transus and become equiaxed α pshase due to α processing in the temperature range below the β transus or the α phase region. The process is almost the same for α+β-type Ti alloys such as the Ti–6Al–4V ELI alloy, which is typical for medical applications. However, in this case, the temperature range below the β transus is the α+β phase region, so it is α+β processing. Once an equiaxed α structure is subjected to heat treatment at a temperature above the β transus, it becomes an acicular α structure, and unless α processing or α+β processing is performed, it will not become an equiaxed α structure. Figure 6.5 shows typical optical microstructures of the equiaxed α structure and the acicular α structure of Ti–6Al–4V alloy, which is a typical α+β type alloy (Heimann and Niinomi 2020). These structures also vary depending on the process, cooling rate, etc.

Since the α+β type Ti alloy consists of two phases, the α phase and β phase, the microstructure changes significantly through heat treatment, and the mechanical properties change accordingly. Generally, solution treatment and aging treatments are applied to control the microstructure of α+β type Ti alloys. In this case, it is possible to roughly classify the mechanical properties into equiaxed α-structure and acicular α-structure. The equiaxed α structure has excellent tensile ductility, high-temperature low-cycle fatigue strength, and fatigue crack initiation resistance; the acicular α structure has excellent fracture toughness, fatigue crack propagation resistance, and creep strength, as shown in Fig. 6.6 (Lütjering and Gysler 1984). Mechanical properties such as fatigue strength and tensile strength are better when the microstructure is finer, so fracture toughness and crack growth resistance are better.

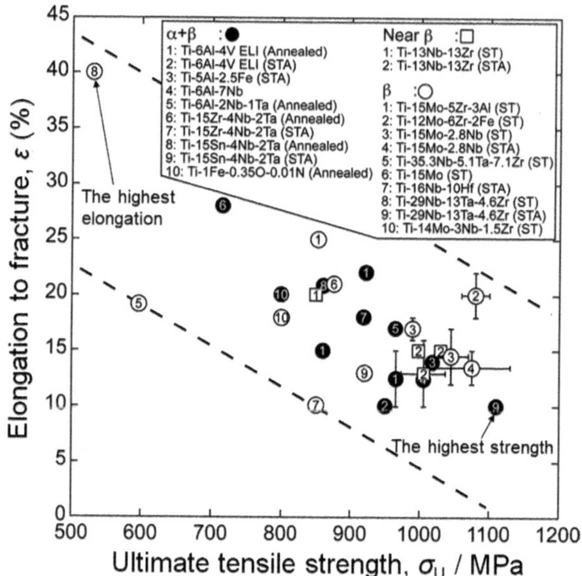

Fig. 6.4. Relationship between ultimate tensile strength and elongation to fracture of Ti alloys for medical use (Provided by Dr. Takayuki Narushima, Tohoku University.).

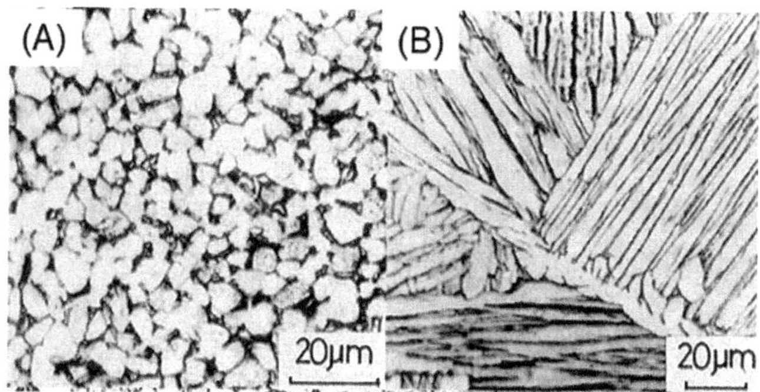

Fig. 6.5. Optical microstructure of Ti-6Al-4V alloy: (A) equiaxed α structure and (B) acicular α structure (Reprinted with permission from De Gruyter, *Materials for Medical Application* (Heimann and Niinomi: De Gruyter 2020), 75–165.).

However, in fatigue crack growth, as a typical example shown in Fig. 6.7 (Lutjering et al. 1988), the growth resistance of short cracks is better than that of long cracks, while the growth resistance of long cracks is better when the microstructure is coarse.

By high pressure tortsion (HPT) working as a kind of severe workings with 6 GPa and 5 rotations, the ultimate tensile strength of Ti-6Al-7Nb alloy increases upto 1,200 MPa, while the elongation to fracture is almost maintained (Ashida et al. 2014, 2015, 2022), as shown in Fig. 6.8. This change is due to the crystal grains becoming ultra-fine due to HPT.

In β-type Ti alloys, solution treatment turns them into a metastable β single phase at room temperature, so mechanical properties associated with microstructural control are generally governed by solution treatment and aging treatment. In other

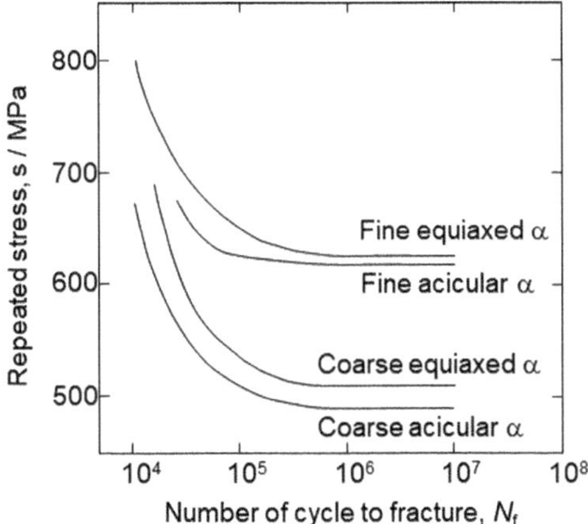

Fig. 6.6. Effect of microstructure on fatigue strength of Ti-6Al-4V alloy (stress ratio R = –1) (Reprinted with permission from Deutsche Gesellschaft für Metallkunde, *Proc. 5th International Conference on Titanium* (Lütjering and Gysler 1984), 2065–2083.).

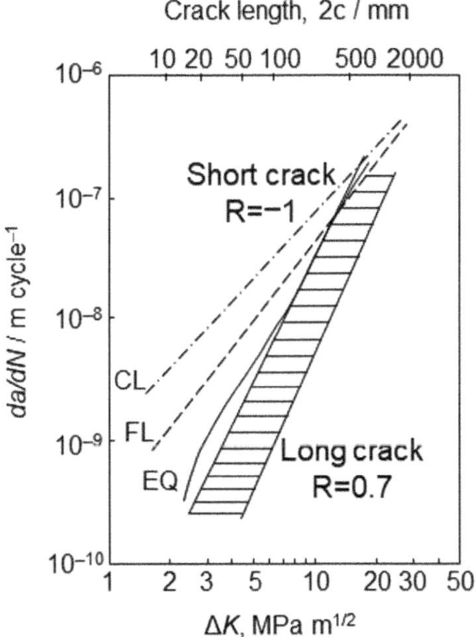

Fig. 6.7. Effect of microstructure on the relationship between short crack growth rate (*da*/*dN*) and stress intensity factor range (*Δk*) in Ti–6Al–4V alloy. Long crack growth rate is also clearly shown. CL: coarse acicular α structure, FL: fine acicular α structure, EQ: equaled α structure (Reprinted with permission from Societe Francaise de Metallurgie, *Proc. 6th World Conference on Titanium* (Lütjering et al. 1988), 71–80.).

words, in β-type Ti alloys, aging treatment after solution treatment improves strength by precipitating α and ω phases in the β phase. The ω phase includes an athermal ω phase and an isothermal ω phase. Generally, the former is formed by rapid cooling after solution treatment and the latter is formed by aging treatment, and the latter in

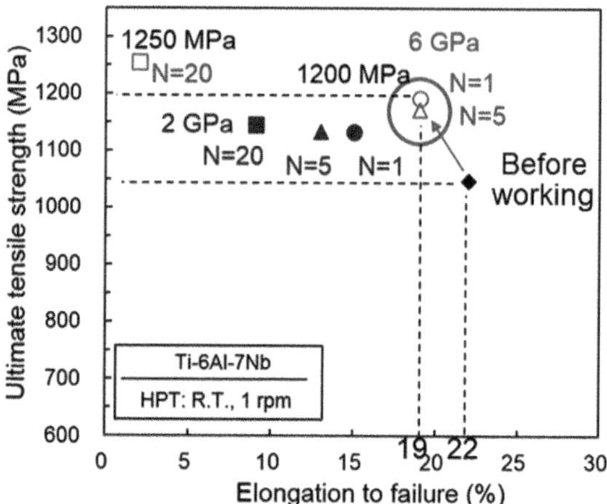

Fig. 6.8. Change in mechanical property of Ti–6Al–7Nb alloy before and after high pressure torsion processing (provided by Dr. Maki Ashida, Seikei University.).

particular causes embrittlement. Therefore, there is a tendency to avoid precipitation of the thermal ω phase, while recently there has been a movement to make effective use of this. The mechanical properties of β-type alloys are greatly influenced by the precipitated phase and also by the β grain size. The smaller the β particle size, the better the strength and elongation. Fracture toughness is better when the precipitated α phase is coarser.

The metastable β phase undergoes so-called deformation-induced transformation, which transforms into martensite due to stress or strain by being subjected to deformation. This results in superelasticity and shape memory properties. Furthermore, it is also possible to improve fracture toughness (Niinomi et al. 1990), fatigue strength (Iman and Gilmore 1983), fatigue crack growth resistance (Niinomi et al. 1993), etc. Figure 6.9 shows the S-N curves when the metastable β phase remains in the Ti-6Al-4V alloy at room temperature by quenching and when

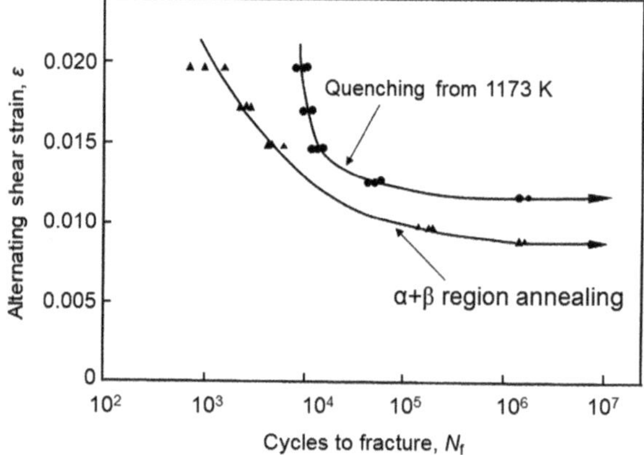

Fig. 6.9. S-N curves of Ti-6Al-4V alloy solution treated (quenched from 1173 K) and α+β region annealed (Reprinted with permission from Springer Nature, Iman and Gilmore. 1983. Metall. Trans. A 14: 233–240.).

it does not remain it by annealing (Iman and Gilmore 1983). In this case, it has been confirmed that the residual β phase undergoes martensitic transformation.

6.6 Titanium-Zirconium Alloys

The development of new Ti alloys including Ti–Zr alloys for medical devices continuously challenges researchers. Ti–13Zr–13Ta alloy (nearly β) developed in the United States (Mishra et al. 1996) is the first commercial example of Ti–Zr alloys. Recently, a Ti-Zr alloy has been comercialized as a popular dental implant, Roxolid®.

Equilibrium phase diagram of Ti–Zr binary alloy shows all proportional solid solution. However, practically the Ti–Zr alloys up to 30%Zr formed α structure, and the 40 and 50%Zr alloys formed α' structure. The Ti–40Zr alloy and the Ti–50Zr alloy exhibits significantly higher grindability than CP Ti, attributed to the α' structure in addition to the decrease in elongation (Takahashi et al. 2009). In the range of 0.02 to 0.04%O in Ti–Zr alloy, oxygen has no influence on the structure, microstructure or biocompatibility of the alloys, while causes hardening of the alloys, increasing the values of the micro hardness, and causing variation in the elasticity modulus values (Vicente et al. 2014). Ti–Zr alloy with gradient porosities is fabricated by the powder metallurgy. The production method and atomic radii of the elements used in the synthesis influences the material structure (Matula et al. 2019). The Ti–2Zr alloy exhibits higher corrosion potential and lower corrosion current density compared with Ti–1Zr and Ti–16Zr alloys. Under wet friction, wear volume loss of Ti–Zr alloy decreases with increasing Zr content (Zhang et al. 2018). Ti–Zr alloys with 50–50 mol% composition have a decreased biologic response, although the mechanical properties improved. The overall highest strength is Ti–30mol%Zr without significant decrease of biologic response (Lee et al. 2016). Ti–xZr (x = 0, 25, 50, 60, 75, and 100) alloys in mass% are abraded and kept for 300 s in water and Hanks' solution. The regenerated surface oxide film in Hanks' solution does not form calcium phosphate on themselves but forms phosphate without calcium except Ti (Hanawa et al. 1992, 2002).

Beta stabilizing effect of Zr for Ti–16Nb alloys is proved. Transformation temperature of α to β decreases about 30°C by using Zr as β stabilizer, the grain size decreases and the amount of lattice parameters and β phase increases, hardness of the base alloy increases to 412 HV from 336 HV, but no significant effect on the elastic modulus and elastic modulus stays steady at the band of 103–100 GPa (Yilmaz et al. 2018). In the case of Ti–35Nb–7Zr alloy, the relaxation peak identified is complex, since the sequence of phase transformations β→ω→α occurred, affecting the distribution of elements among the phases present. The matrix–interstitial interactions and substitutional–interstitial interactions contribute to the elasticity observed in the β phase of the alloy (Chaves et al. 2014). Ti–15Zr–7.5Mo and Ti–15Zr–15Mo alloys present tribocorrosion behavior superior to CP Ti, abrasion being the main wear mechanism. Wear volume analysis shows that the Ti–15Zr–7.5Mo presents better tribocorrosion properties, besides the higher Young's modulus (Correa et al. 2016). Ti–15Zr–10Mo alloy presents high mechanical strength and large elongation (854 ± 63 MPa and 18.7 ± 2.8 %), while Ti–15Zr–15Mo alloy exhibits better mechanical compatibility, due to its combination of low Young's modulus (75 ± 1 GPa) (Correa et al. 2020).

6.7 Corrosion Resistance of CP Ti and Titanium Alloys

Titanium is an extremely active element, causing a low standard electrode potential of −1.63 V vs. NHE in the reaction, $Ti \rightarrow Ti^{2+} + 2e^-$. This activity is the basis of the chemical properties of Ti element, such as the difficulty in smelting it, its high corrosion resistance, and safety in the human body (Fig. 6.10). The corrosion resistance of Ti is very high, in spite of the high activity of the Ti element, because Ti element immediately reacts with water molecules in aqueous solutions and moisture in the air, and forms a very thin titanium oxide film on its surface. This oxide film is immediately repaired even when it is ruptured by scratching, and thus the reaction of Ti element with the external environment is inhibited, causing the apparent inactivity of Ti materials. This property directly contributes to its corrosion resistance and its safety.

Numerous studies confirm the Ti materials' superior corrosion resistance in biological environments. CP Ti, Ti–6Al–4V alloy, Ni–Ti alloy, Co–Ni–Cr–Mo alloy, Co–Cr–Mo alloy, type 316L stainless steel, and pure Ni exhibit the strongest passivation in this order in Hanks' physiological solution at 37°C and pH 7.4 (Speck and Fraker 1980). Afterwards, anodic polarization measurements of several orthopedic implant metals and alloys, including type 316L stainless steel, Co–Cr–Mo alloy (ASTM F75-23 2023), Ni–Ti alloy, pure Ni, CP Ti, and Ti–6Al–4V alloy, are performed in Ringer's solution with and without 1% bovine serum albumin (Nakayama et al. 1990) and in Ringer's solution and rabbit (Nakayama et al. 1989), which demonstrates the excellent corrosion resistance of CP Ti and Ti–6Al–4V alloy, as shown in Fig. 6.11. Recent studies (Asri et al. 2017, Manam et al. 2017) have produced comparable results. The corrosion behaviors of the aforementioned materials have been thoroughly reviewed (Eliaz 2019). Both CP Ti and Ti–6Al–4V alloy demonstrate much lower passive currents and higher breakdown potentials without pitting *in vitro* and *in vivo*.

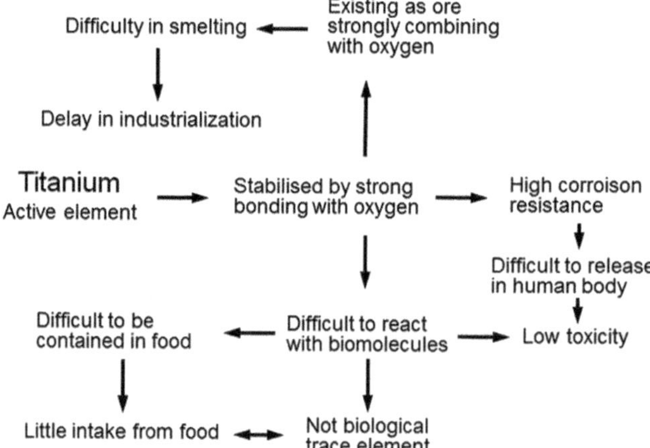

Fig. 6.10. Characteristics of Ti material generated by chemical activity of titanium element.

Despite the high corrosion resistance of Ti materials, since more than three decades, numerous researches have demonstrated that despite the absence of abrasion, a significantly greater quantity of Ti elements is detected in the surrounding tissues when Ti materials are implanted (Meachin and Wiiliams 1973, Woodman et al. 1984, Bessho et al. 1995, Ektessabi et al. 1994, 1996, Bianco et al. 1996).

The effect of amino acids and proteins on the solubility of metals is examined (Williams et al. 1988, Clark and Williams 1982). Possible Ti ion release mechanisms are examined from the perspective of the isoelectric point and the electric charge of proteins contained in body fluids (Merritt and Brown 1988). Mo, Cu, Co, and Ni ions are released when pure metal powders are immersed in saline, with or without serum albumin or fibrinogen, but Ti ions are not released and are unaffected by the presence of proteins (Bruneel and Helsen 1988). In the case of Ti–6Al–4V alloy, Ti and Al ions are released in Hanks' solution containing 2% EDTA; Ti, Al, and V ions are released in Hanks' solution containing 0.05-M sodium citrate (Ryhanen et al. 1997). Ni–Ti alloy initially releases more Ni than stainless steel immersed in a medium containing osteoblasts or fibrinogen, but the amount released decreases after 2 d (Bianco et al. 1996). As a result, metal ions are released in rabbits in the absence of wear and are detected in the rabbit's tissues, serum, and urine. Fretting corrosion depends on (the charge of) proteins; in the presence of proteins, Ni preferential dissolution increases (Merritt and Brown 1988). Biomolecules may account for the release of metal ions. Although the mechanism for the accelerated release of metal ions in the presence of amino acids and proteins has not been elucidated, an imbalance between partial dissolution and re-precipitation in the passive film may accelerate the release of ions. In other words, repassivation of a metal influences the release of ions from the metal. During the repassivation of CP Ti in aqueous solutions, inorganic ions and proteins accelerated the repassivation of CP Ti, whereas certain amino acids slowed it (Hanawa et al. 2004).

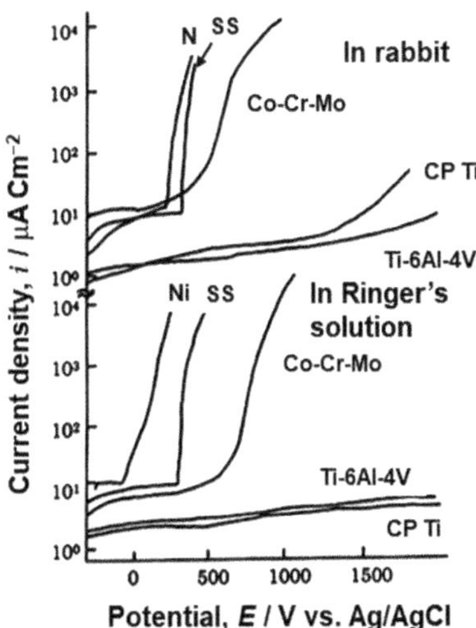

Fig. 6.11. Anodic polarization curves of CP Ti, Ti–6Al–4V alloy, Co–Cr–Mo alloy, type 316L stainless steel (SS), and pure Ni in rabbit and Ringer's solution, reproduced from the data in a reference (Reprinted with permission from Elsevier, Nakayama et al. 1989. Biomaterials 10: 420–424.).

Immunological reactions and the adhesion of macrophages (Mφ) to the surface of an implanted material identify it as a foreign body (Tang and Eaton 1993). Mφ generates active oxygen species, H_2O_2, which has a much longer lifetime and higher permeability against cell membrane than O^{2-}: H_2O_2 reaches the surface to which Mφ has adhered, and the CP Ti surface is hyperoxidized by H_2O_2 (Tangvall et al. 1989, Pan et al. 1998), which may result in the release of Ti ions. H_2O_2 reacts with the passive film on CP Ti according to the following equation (Pan et al. 1998): $Ti^{4+} + H_2O_2 \rightarrow Ti^{5+} + OH^- + OH^*$, where * represents radical. Dissolution of Ti with active oxygen generated by Mφ has been elucidated adequately (Mu et al. 2000), as shown in Fig. 2.25. On the other hand, surgical handling during implantation and wear and/or fretting are the leading causes of Ti release (Mu et al. 2002).

Regardless, despite the detection of Ti element in the surrounding tissues, the toxicity of Ti materials has hardly manifested. In the majority of instances involving the detection of released Ti elements, the chemical states of these elements are obscure. As shown in Fig. 2.29, dissolved Ti ions combine immediately with hydroxide ions and anions to stabilize the Ti element in the human body and are utilized for the reconstruction of the passive film. Therefore, the possibility of Ti surviving as ionic states and combining with biomolecules is extremely low. Consequently, Ti exhibits low toxicity.

Ti alloy fabricated by electron beam melting (EBM) has better corrosion resistance in 20% HCl solution at room temperature compared to Ti alloy fabricated by laser metal deposition (LMD) (Lavrys et al. 2022). Localized corrosion can be initiated by survival pits under sufficient conditions of the breakdown passive films. Survival probability means a quantitative probability value of the transition from metastable pit to stable pit to occur localized corrosion. The higher the survival probability constant of additive manufacturing (AM) Ti alloys, the more difficult the repassivation and the easier occurrence of localized corrosion is (Seo and Lee 2023).

6.8 Passive Film on Titanium

Except in environments of reduction, the corrosion process always results in the formation of a reaction film on metals. Potential-pH diagram (Poubaix diagram) of Ti-H_2O system at 298 K shows that the oxide state is stable in a wide region (see Fig. 2.19B). Passive film is one such reaction film, and its importance for corrosion protection is especially noteworthy. When solubility is extremely low and pores are absent, film adhesion will be strong to the substrate; the film then becomes a passive or corrosion-resistant film. A passive film has a few nanometers of thickness and is transparent. Passive film readily becomes amorphous as a result of the incredibly rapid rate at which it is formed (Revie and Uhlig 2008, Kelly 1982). For instance, a film is generated on a Ti metal substrate in approximately 1/100 s. Figure 6.12 shows the transient current density following the rupture of the passive film. In 30 ms, the current density approaches zero, indicating that the passive film is reconstructed immediately. Since amorphous films contain few grain boundaries and structural defects, they are resistant to corrosion. However, crystallization decreases corrosion resistance. Fortunately, passive films contain water molecules that promote and preserve amorphousness.

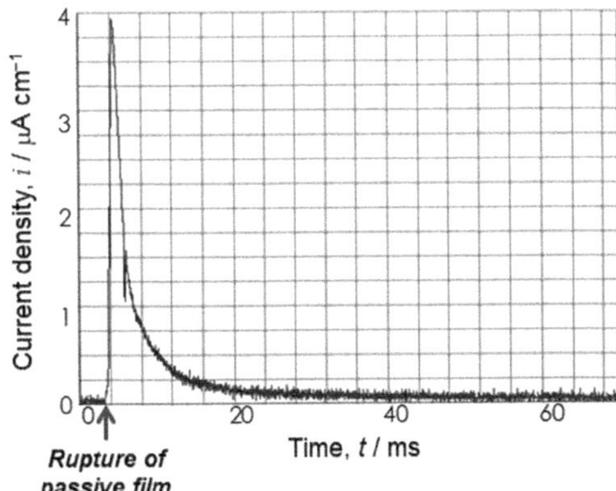

Fig. 6.12. Time transient of current density of Ti after rupturing the passive film by abrasion in Hanks' solution at 1 V vs. SCE. Positive current is generated both by ion dissolution and the formation of the passive film.

Metallic Ti naturally forms the surface oxide film on itself according to following equations. In acidic solution, the anodic reactions are:

$Ti + 2H_2O \rightarrow Ti(OH)_2 + 2H^+ + 2e^-$ (oxidation to divalence);

$Ti(OH)_2 \rightarrow TiO + H_2O$ (dehydration);

$TiO + H_2O \rightarrow TiOOH + H^+ + e^-$ (oxidation to trivalence);

$2TiOOH \rightarrow Ti_2O_3 + H_2O$ (dehydration);

$Ti_2O_3 + 3H_2O \rightarrow 2TiO(OH)_2 + 2H^+ + 2e^-$ (oxidation to tetravalence);

$2TiO(OH)_2 \rightarrow TiO_2 + 2H_2O$ (dehydration).

On the other hand, in neutral and basic solutions, the anodic reactions are:

$Ti + 2OH^- \rightarrow Ti(OH)_2 + 2e^-$ (oxidation to divalence);

$Ti(OH)_2 + OH^- \rightarrow TiOOH^- + H_2O$ (dehydration);

$TiOOH^- + H_2O \rightarrow TiOOH + e^-$ (oxidation to trivalence);

$2TiOOH \rightarrow Ti_2O_3 + H_2O$ (dehydration);

$Ti_2O_3 + 4OH^- \rightarrow 2TiO(OH)_2 + H_2O + 2e^-$ (oxidation to tetravalence);

$2TiO(OH)_2 \rightarrow TiO_2 + 2H_2O$ (dehydration).

Since a considerable portion of oxidized Ti stays in Ti^{2+} and Ti^{3+} in the surface film, the oxidation process may proceed to the end just at the uppermost part of the surface film.

Consequently, when Ti is characterized using X-ray photoelectron spectroscopy (XPS), the Ti 2p spectrum exhibits four doublets according to valence: the metallic state of Ti^0 and the oxide states of Ti^{2+}, Ti^{3+}, and Ti^{4+}, as shown in Fig. 6.13A based on previously published data (Asami et al. 1993, Eda et al. 2022). The decomposition spectrum reveals the presence of Ti^{2+} oxide within the surface oxide layer; however, Ti^{2+} formation is thermodynamically inferior to Ti^{3+} formation at the surface (Olver and Ross 1963, Beck 1973, Silverman 1982). As shown in Fig. 6.13B, the spectrum of the O 1s region contains three peaks originating from O^{2-}, hydroxide or hydroxyl groups, OH^-, and hydrate or adsorbed water, H_2O (Asami and Hashimoto 1977). Concerning the average effective escape depth of photoelectrons as determined by angle-resolved XPS measurements (see Fig. 3.16), λ was the average mean free path of Ti 2p and O 1s photoelectrons, and the effective escape depth is estimated as λ times the sine of the detection angle (Eda et al. 2022, Hanawa et al. 1998). Figure 6.14 shows the ratio of the relative oxygen concentration to that of Ti, [O]/[Ti], versus the average photoelectron escape depth. Oxygen is more abundant in the outer layer of the passive film, while Ti was more abundant in the inner layer. $[Ti^{4+}]/([Ti^{4+}]+[Ti^{3+}]+[Ti^{2+}])$ obtained using the angle-resolved technique is shown in Fig. 6.14B as the proportion of the integrated intensity of the peak attributed to Ti^{4+} relative to all of its oxide states. At small detection angles, the percentage of Ti^{4+} is high, indicating that Ti^{4+} is distributed more in the passive film's outer layer than in its inner layer. In addition, the depth profiles of the $[OH^-]/[O^{2-}]$ ratios are shown in Fig. 6.14C, which reveals that OH^- is more abundant in the passive film's outer layer. Consistent with previous research, it is evident that the passive film on CP Ti consists primarily of an extremely thin TiO_2 film with trace amounts of Ti_2O_3 and TiO, as well as water and hydroxyl groups (Kelly 1982, Hanawa et al. 1988,

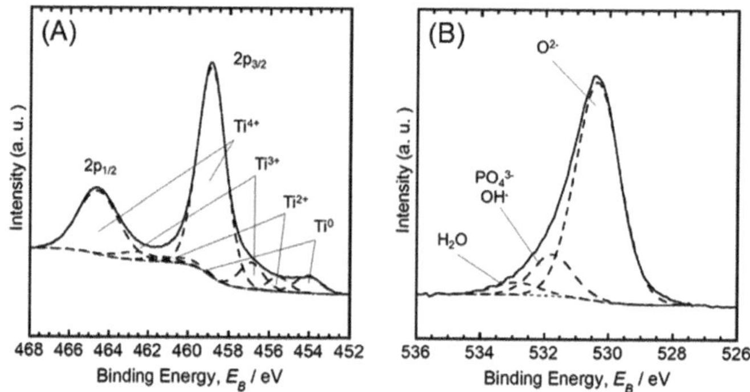

Fig. 6.13. Ti 2p (A) and O 1s (B) electron energy region spectra obtained from Ti immersed in pure water for 1 d and their de-convolutions into component peaks (Reprinted with permission from Wiley open access, Hiji et al. 2021a. Surf. Interface Anal. 53: 185–193.).

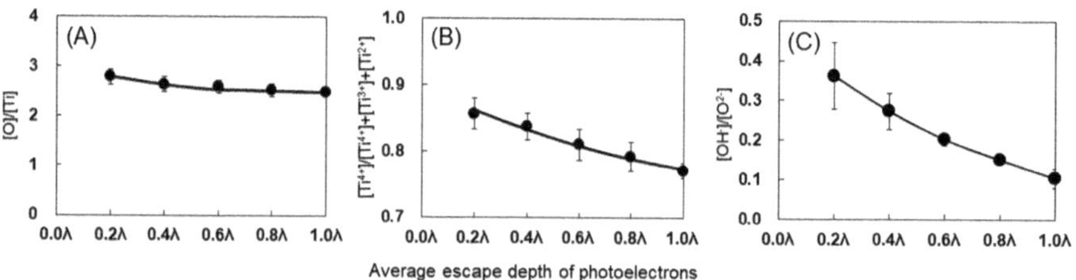

Fig. 6.14. The ratios of [O]/[Ti] (A), $[Ti^{4+}]/([Ti^{4+}]+[Ti^{3+}]+[Ti^{2+}])$ (B), and $[OH^-]/[O^{2-}]$ (C), plotted against the average escape depth of photoelectrons (n = 3). The angle-resolved technique for XPS was applied to Ti at the photoelectron detection angles of 12°, 24°, 37°, 53°, and 90°, corresponding to the detection depths of 0.2λ, 0.4λ, 0.6λ, 0.8λ, and 1.0λ, where λ was the photoelectrons' effective mean free path. The effective escape depth was estimated as λ times the sine of the detection angle. The detection angle was defined as the angle between the direction of the photoelectron path to the electron spectrometer and the specimen surface. (Reprinted with permission from Wiley open access, Eda et al. 2022. Surf. Interface Anal. 54: 892–898).

HIji et al. 2021a). This process of passive film formation has been covered elsewhere (Olver and Ross 1963). The topmost surface (~ 5.0 nm) reveals that the ratio of $[TiO_2]/[Ti_2O_3]$ is consistent with that of passivation/dissolution of electrochemical activity, and that both the structures of passivation, and dissolution are distorted due to the appearance of two different sites of Ti–O and Ti–Ti, with bound water in the topmost surface playing a crucial role in structural disorder (Wang et al. 2016). It has been determined that the composition, structure, and chemical state of the passive film are distinct from those of crystalline TiO_2 ceramics. Therefore, the adsorption kinetics of calcium and phosphate ions differ between passive films on Ti and TiO_2 ceramics (Hiji et al. 2021b).

6.9 Response of the Host Body

CP Ti shows a unique property, "osseointegration," among metals. Osseointegration is defined as follows. "The formation of a direct interface between an implant and bone, without intervening soft tissue." No scar tissue, cartilage or ligament fibers are present between the bone and implant surface. The direct contact of bone and implant surface can be verified microscopically (Brånemark et al. 1977). Osseointegration shows the excellent hard tissue (bone and tooth) property of Ti materials. This concept, osseointegration, in dental implants, generated and explosively accelerated studies on the reaction between hard tissue and Ti materials, followed by studies on surface treatment. Figure 6.15 shows example exhibiting osseointegration by CP Ti dental implant (Thomsen et al. 1997). Studies on evaluation of osteoblast calcification, histological evaluation such as bone formation, bone-contacting rate, bone bonding strength, and clinical results have demonstrated Ti materials' excellent compatibility with hard tissues. Important determinants of hard tissue compatibility are the adhesion and proliferation of osteogenic cells as a result of the surface morphology (roughness), wettability, and other characteristics. Ti materials-bone interface reaction has been characterized to demonstrate the significance of surface morphology and wettability for osseointegration (Rupp et al. 2018, Shah et al. 2018, Shah 2019). Numerous studies on the compatibility of Ti materials with hard tissues have been conducted, and detailed information is available in the literature (Brunette et al. 2001, Hanawa 2019). In orthopedics, bone screws and bone nails made of Ti alloys typically form calluses and assimilate into bone tissue after long-term implantation, causing the bone to refracture during retrieval (Sanderson et al. 1992). This is due to the fact that Ti alloys are compatible with hard tissues.

The surface of Ti implants stored for a long time after manufacturing becomes contaminated, and the bone conduction ability is depressed during storage (Art et al. 2009). The interface between Ti and bone tissue has been observed from early on at a micrometer and nanometer scale (Albrektsson and Hansson 1986, Davies et al. 1990, Listgarten et al. 1992, Sennerby et al. 1993, Murai et al. 1996, Brånemark et al. 1998, Sundell et al. 2017). Metal Ti substrate is covered by titanium oxide (a few nanometers in thickness), an amorphous layer containing proteoglycans (20–50 nm in thickness), a slender cell layer, a weakly calcified region, and bone tissue, in that order. Endeavors to observe a structure near the Ti surface have

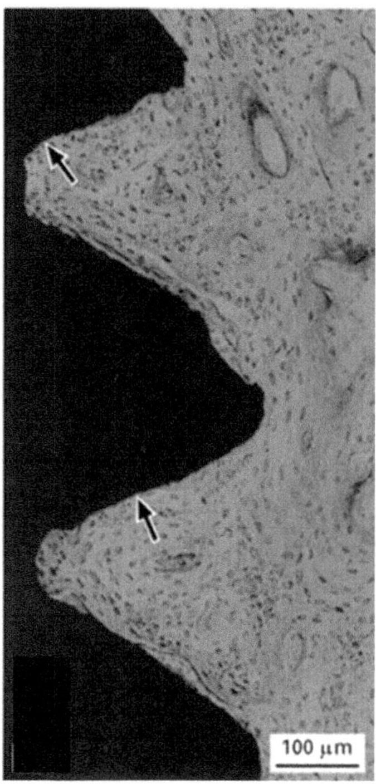

Fig. 6.15. Example of osseointegration. Optical micrograph of ground sections of CP Ti implants and tissue in proximal threads 1 mon after insertion. The proximal threads contain newly formed bone in contact with the implant surface in several locations (arrows) (Reprinted with permission from Springer Nature, Thomsen et al. 1997. J. Mater. Sci. Mater. Med. 8: 653–665.).

continued to elucidate the mechanism of osseointegration (Palmquist et al. 2010, Goriainov et al. 2014).

Bonding between metals and soft tissue is also important in abutments of dental implants, orthodontic implant anchors, transdermal devices, and screws of external fixators (see Subsection 2.14.3 and Fig. 2.33). In these devices, metals penetrate from the inside to the outside of tissues. Therefore, insufficient bonding of soft tissue makes possible the invasion of bacteria that generates inflammation, followed by loosening, movement, and falling out. In the case of dental implants, these events are known as peri-implantitis. Other medical devices completely implanted in tissues may be covered by fibrous tissue unless enough soft-tissue compatibility is shown. It is well-known that Ti materials show good soft-tissue compatibility only in the case of complete implantation, while chemical bonding of soft tissue to Ti materials is not observed. In particular, despite the significance of the adhesion of junctional epithelium to Ti in dental implants, this subject is still unresolved. Bonding of junctional epithelium to CP Ti is attempted by a mechanical anchoring with rough or grooved CP Ti surfaces at present, because chemical adhesion of soft tissue to metals is difficult (Williams 2011). On the other hand, the acid-treated CP Ti and Ti–6Al–4V alloy can easily and stably immobilize a device implanted in the mouse subcutaneous tissue (Okada et al. 2020, Wang et al. 2021). Sand blast treatment is also effective to soft tissue adhesion (Yabe et al. 2021).

A platelet adhesion test with human blood reveals that platelets easily adhered and a fibrin network formed on Ti materials (Tanaka et al. 2009). Ti materials may form thrombus easily and show low blood compatibility. Probably for this reason, CP Ti and Ti alloys except Ti-Ni alloy are not used for devices contacting blood. Recently, red-blood-cell and platelet interactions (Park and Davies 2000), wettability and hydrophilicity (Gittens et al. 2014, Albrektsson and Wennerberg 2019), increase in osteogenesis-, angiogenesis-, and neurogenesis-associated gene expression (Salvi et al. 2015), healing- and immune-modulating effect (Trindade et al. 2016), immune osteocyte-related molecular signaling mechanisms (Shah et al. 2018), and inflammation-immunological balance (Trindade et al. 2018, Albrektsson et al. 2019) have been considered as factors of osseointegration.

However, the trend of the research moved to surface treatments to accelerate bone formation and bone bonding. The reaction mechanism is usually investigated to explain the effect of the treatments and the above phenomena are explained by the surface properties of Ti materials and situational evidence. Aside from this, the surface properties causing the above phenomena must be understood. Properties of the Ti material surface that may cause osseointegration are explained in the following section.

6.10 Principle of Excellent Biocompatibility of Titanium

6.10.1 Relationship between Corrosion Resistance and Biocompatibility

Ti shows excellent corrosion resistance compared with other metals (Nakayama et al. 1989, Brunette et al. 2001, Asri et al. 2017, Manam 2017, Eliaz 2019) as shown in Fig. 6.11, inducing low toxicity. One of the reasons for the excellent biocompatibility of Ti is caused by the excellent corrosion resistance, while the corrosion resistance is not sufficient condition for the biocompatibility. Even the best corrosion-resistant metal, Au, is inferior in tissue compatibility (Thomsen et al. 1997, Chen et al. 2016). In addition, electric plating of Pt to Ti increases the corrosion resistance but depletes bone formation (Itakura et al. 1989), because a property of Ti is shielded, and the bone formation ability is prevented. These results reveal that hard tissue compatibility is not induced only by the corrosion resistance. In other words, the corrosion resistance is a necessary condition but not a sufficient condition for biocompatibility; there are other factors that contribute to biocompatibility.

6.10.2 Property as n-Type Semiconductor

As is common knowledge, TiO_2 ceramics function as *n*-type semiconductors. How does the passive film on Ti behave as a semiconductor? As shown in Fig. 6.16A, the maximum energy of the balance band, E_v, versus Fermi level energy, E_F, is determined by linearly extrapolating the peak to the baseline (Singh et al. 2016). The E_v value of anatase is approximately 0.2 eV, greater than that of rutile (Breeson et al. 2017). In the case of the passive film on Ti, the E_v are 2.8–2.9 eV in Hanks' solution and 2.8–3.0 eV in saline (Kim et al. 2022), while that in the polished Ti

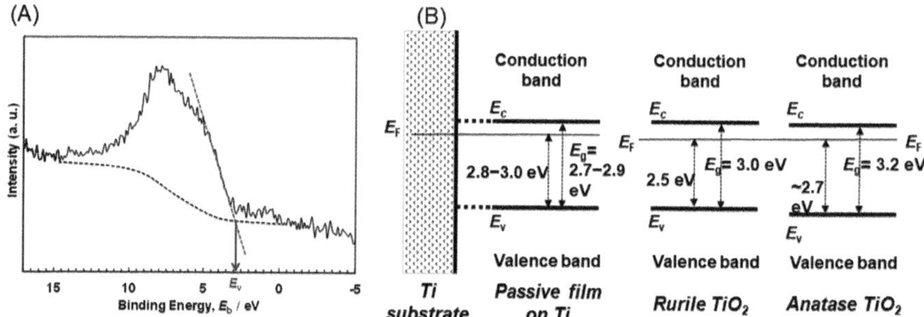

Fig. 6.16. (A) Valence band region spectra of Ti after polarization at 0 V in Hanks' soluiton for 1 h and the determination of the maximum energy of valance band, E_v. (B) Relationship among E_g, E_v, and E_F in the band structures of the passive film on Ti, rutile TiO_2, and anatase TiO_2 (Reprinted with permission from Taylor & Francis open access, Kim et al. 2022. Sci. Technol. Adv. Mater. 23: 322–331.).

without polarization is 2.8–2.9 eV; this is a higher value than that for rutile, which is 2.5 eV (Singh et al. 2016). The observed E_v value of the as-deposited TiO_2 film was 1.86 eV (Singh et al. 2016). Therefore, the E_v value for the passive film on Ti is greater than the E_v value for ceramics composed of TiO_2. Figure 6.16B shows the difference in E_v versus E_F between the passive film on Ti and TiO_2. In other words, the energy between the conduction band's minimum energy, E_c, and the passive film's E_F is less than that of TiO_2. In addition, as will be explained later, the E_g of the passive film on Ti is between 2.7 and 2.9 eV, which is significantly less than 3 eV, indicating that the property as an *n*-type semiconductor is much stronger in the passive film on Ti than in the TiO_2 ceramics.

6.10.3 Dissociation of Surface Hydroxyl Groups–Surface Electric Charge

The interface reaction between CP Ti and living tissue is governed by the passive film property of CP Ti. This passive film forms hydroxyl groups on their surfaces due to a reaction with atmospheric moisture (Boehm 1966). In aqueous solutions, such as body fluid, these hydroxyl groups dissociate to form electric charges (Boehm 1966, 1971, Parfitt 1976). At a particular pH, the electric charge becomes zero. It is dependent on the pH of the surrounding solution. This pH is defined as the zero-charge point (p.z.c.) (Fig. 6.17). The p.z.c. is specific to each oxide and serves as an indicator of acidic or basic properties (table in Fig. 6.17). In the case of TiO_2, rutile has a p.z.c. of 5.3 and anatase has a p.z.c. of 6.2 (Parfitt 1976); therefore, TiO_2 demonstrates neither an acidic nor a basic property, but rather an almost neutral property. The surface concentration of hydroxyl groups on TiO_2 is relatively high 4.9–12.5 nm^{-2} (Boehm 1971, Westall and Hohl 1980). This concentration or wettability increases when immersed in an aqueous solution. This high concentration and neutral charge promotes the adsorption of proteins, such as integrin and cytokine.

6.10.4 Dielectric Constant–Electrostatic Force

Because proteins are electrically charged objects, adsorption to a metal surface aggravates the conformation of proteins. The electrostatic force exerted by proteins

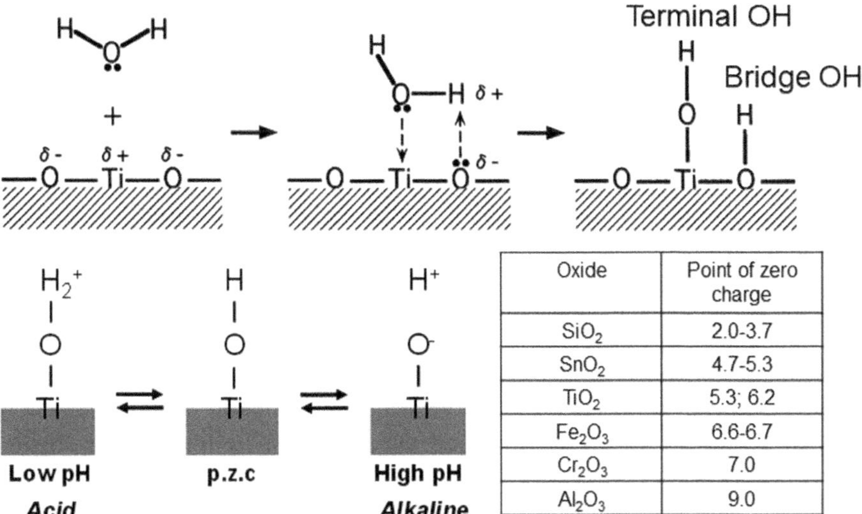

Oxide	Point of zero charge
SiO_2	2.0-3.7
SnO_2	4.7-5.3
TiO_2	5.3; 6.2
Fe_2O_3	6.6-6.7
Cr_2O_3	7.0
Al_2O_3	9.0

Fig. 6.17. Formation mechanism of surface hydroxyl groups and point of zero charge (p.z.c.) of surface hydroxyl groups on TiO_2 and their dissociation in aqueous solutions according to the pH. The p.z.c. values of metal oxides are listed in the table.

on a metal surface is determined by the relative permittivity of the passive film; the greater the relative permittivity, the lower the electrostatic force. The relative permittivity of TiO_2 is 82.1, which is significantly greater than that of other oxides and comparable to that of water (80.0) (Lide 2006). Consequently, the conformational change of protein adsorbed on TiO_2 may be minimal. On Ti, the fibrinogen adsorption layer is thicker, but the adsorption amount is less than on Au in aqueous solution (Sundgren et al. 1986a). Because CP Ti is covered by TiO_2 and Au is exposed without surface oxide, the electrostatic force on CP Ti is small compared to Au. On CP Ti, the conformational change of proteins is smaller than on Au. Proteins adsorbed on CP Ti are more natural, as shown in Fig. 6.18.

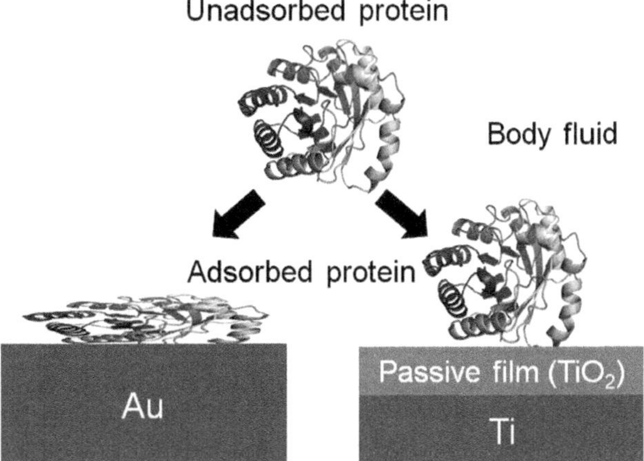

Fig. 6.18. Schematic model of change in the conformation of protein adsorbed on Au and Ti.

6.10.5 Calcium Phosphate Formation

Maintaining corrosion resistance, the passive film is macroscopically stable. From a microscopic standpoint, a passive film generally maintains a continuous process of partial dissolution and re-precipitation in the electrolyte (Kelly 1982). Consequently, the composition and chemical state are affected by the environment. In this way, the surface composition of the passive film is constantly changing in response to its surroundings. CP Ti and Ti alloys readily form calcium phosphates and sulfite and sulfide in biological environments, particularly under cell culture (Hanawa and Ota 1992, Healy and Ducheyne 1992, Serro et al. 1997, Frauchiger et al. 1999, Hiromoto et al. 2004). Recent research (Hiji et al. 2021a) has elucidated the initial formation kinetics of calcium phosphate on Ti. First, phosphate ions were incorporated, then calcium ions were incorporated to form calcium phosphate on Ti. Figure 6.19 demonstrates that calcium and phosphate were incorporated by direct reaction between the Ti substrate and calcium and phosphate ions as calcium and phosphate concentrations increased as immersion time increased from 10^3 s to 10^5 s. In addition, calcium and phosphorus are found at the interface between Ti and bone tissue (Sundgren et al. 1986b, Esposite et al. 1999, Sundell et al. 2017). Zr does not form calcium phosphate against Ti, but rather zirconium phosphate. The passive film on Ti is not fully oxidized and is relatively reactive, whereas the passive film on Zr is more stable and protective than that on Ti (Tsutsumi et al. 2009). The following subsection clearly explains these phenomena from the perspective of the band gap energy, E_g. Nb and Ta exhibit properties intermediate to those of Ti and Zr (Tsutsumi et al. 2015). Electrochemical impedance and photoelectrochemical measurements have characterized the direct interaction of calcium and phosphate ions with the passive film of Ti-6Al-4V alloy in physiological solutions (Hodgson et al. 2002), and calcium phosphate formation on Ti-6Al-4V alloy is dependent on defects in the

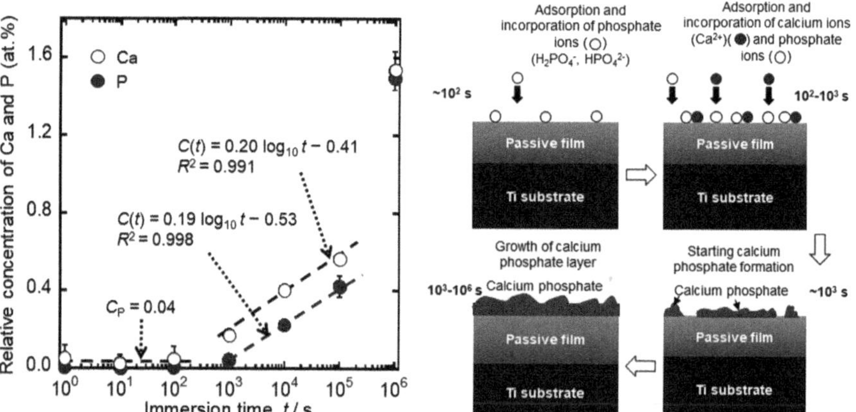

Fig. 6.19. Change in the relative concentrations of calcium and phosphorus in the surface layers on Ti immersed in Hanks' solution ($n = 3$) and illustration of the formation process of calcium phosphate on Ti in Hanks' solution and estimated reaction scheme (Reprinted with permission from Wiley open access, Hiji et al. 2021. Surf. Interface Anal. 53: 185–193.).

passive film (Chávez-Díaz et al. 2019). The ability of Ti materials to form calcium phosphate is therefore one of the reasons for its superior compatibility with hard tissues.

6.10.6 Band Gap Energy

Using the photoelectrochemical response at potentials as close as possible to the open circuit potential, the E_g values of passive films formed on CP Ti in Hanks' solution and 0.9% NaCl aqueous solution have been evaluated (Km et al. 2022). The passive film on Ti behaves like an *n*-type semiconductor with two layers: an inner oxide layer with a high E_g and an outer hydroxide layer with a low E_g. In Hanks' solution, the value of E_g in the innermost layer is between 3.3 and 3.4 eV, whereas it is significantly lower in the surface layer (2.9 eV). E_g is 3.3 eV in the innermost layer and 2.7 eV in the outermost layer of saline. As shown in Fig. 6.20, the E_g values of the outermost surfaces of passive films formed on Ti are much lower than those of TiO_2 ceramics (Kim et al. 2022). Therefore, the passive film on Ti is more reactive than the ceramic TiO_2 surface. In addition to the excellent corrosion resistance, this reactivity likely contributes to the excellent biocompatibility of Ti. Calcium phosphate forms regularly on Ti, but not regularly on TiO_2. The kinetics of calcium phosphate formation on Ti differ from those on TiO_2 crystalline ceramics (Hiji et al. 2021b).

The optical absorption edge is typically used to evaluate the E_g between the valence and conduction bands in crystalline TiO_2 ceramics. It is well known that E_g determines the reactivity of TiO_2 ceramics, and numerous efforts have been made to reduce E_g to improve their photocatalyst performance (Diebold 2003). Therefore, the E_gs of TiO_2 anatase and rutile are intensively researched for photocatalyst applications. Figure 6.21 presents a summary of the published data on TiO_2 ceramics, other metal oxide ceramics, and passive films on metals (Hanawa 2022). From the data, the optimal balance between high corrosion resistance and appropriate reactivity of Ti as a result of the passive oxide film is one of the most important reasons for the excellent biocompatibility of Ti among metals.

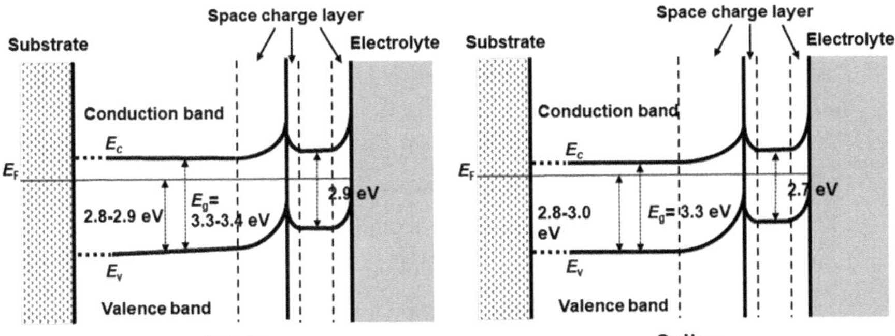

Fig. 6.20. Electronic band structures of passive films formed on Ti in Hanks' solution and saline (Reprinted with permission from Taylor & Francis open access, Kim et al. 2022. Sci. Technol. Adv. Mater. 23: 322–331.).

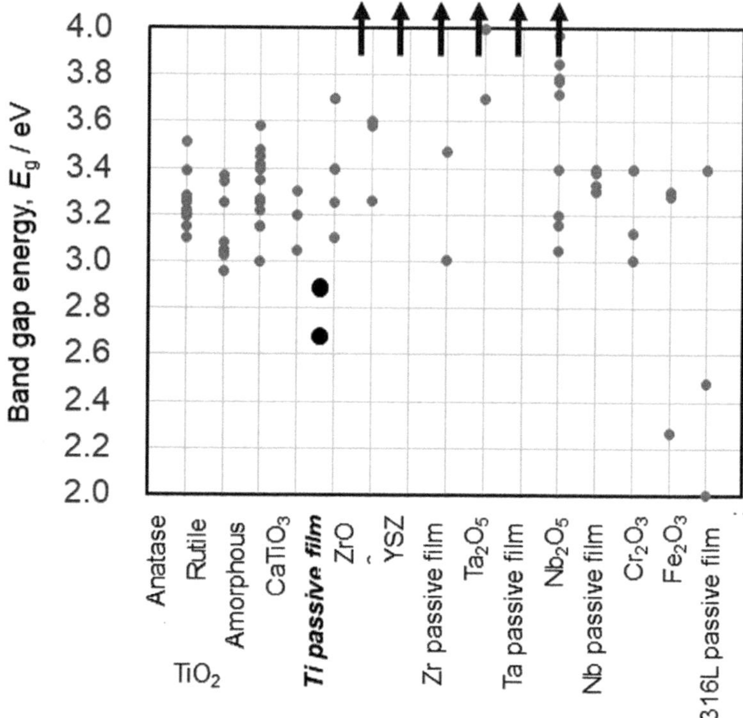

Fig. 6.21. Band gap energies of various oxides and passive films on metals. This figure is originally drawn based on band gap energy data in published papers. The band gap energy of the passive film on Ti in simulated bioliquids is relatively low that may contribute to the reactivity of Ti. (Reprinted with permission from Taylor and Francis open access, Hanawa. 2022. Sci. Technol. Adv. Mater. 23: 457–472).

According to the above review and discussion, it is possible to explain the excellent biocompatibility of Ti through the following considerations.

- The excellent corrosion resistance of Ti compared to other metals due to a macroscopically strong passive film.
- Ti ions are stabilized immediately to prevent toxicity if released into body fluids.
- Positive and negative charges are well-balanced due to the dissociation of surface hydroxyl groups on the passive film.
- Low electrostatic force of the passive film inducing a natural adsorption of proteins retaining their natural conformation.
- Excellent performance as an *n*-type semiconductor.
- Lower bandgap energy of the passive film on Ti produces optimal reactivity.
- As a result of this reaction, calcium phosphate is naturally formed.

It should be mentioned again that the optimal balance between high corrosion resistance and appropriate reactivity of Ti materials due to the passive oxide film is the most prevalent mechanism for excellent biocompatibility of Ti materials. The combination of these properties and the resulting biological response is essential to the elucidation of the biocompatibility of materials as a future spectacular subject. In future, this subject will be essential to better understand the interface phenomena between materials and host bodies using materials informatics (MI) and materials digital transformation (Material DX), because all biological and tissue reactions start from an electronic transfer of the surface.

6.11 Tasks of Titanium for Medical Application

Present problems of CP Ti and Ti alloys in medicine are summarized in Table 6.5. Ti alloys are used in orthopedics for artificial joints, bone fixators, spinal fixators, etc., receiving large mechanical stress. Bone absorption caused by stress shielding sometimes appears in bone fixators and artificial hip joints. Because load is mainly applied to the metal plate and stem, less load is applied to cortical bone by the difference in Young's modulus between metal and cortical bone (Gefen 2002). If the Young's modulus of the metal plate is similar to that of cortical bone, load is equally applied to both metal and bone to prevent bone absorption. In this sense, β-type Ti alloys showing a lower Young's modulus are more suitable than α+β-type alloys. Therefore, β-type Ti alloys consisting of Group 4 and 5 elements in the periodic table have continued to be designed and developed.

Bone screws and bone nails made of Ti alloys form calluses and assimilate to bone tissue, forming calluses, during implantation, so bone is sometimes refractured when the devices are retrieved (Sanderson et al. 1992). Therefore, when the devices must be retrieved after healing, devices made of type 316L stainless steel are selected. This assimilation occurs because of the excellent hard tissue compatibility of Ti alloys. A proper surface treatment may inhibit bone formation and bonding of Ti alloys contacting bone tissue.

In spinal surgery and maxillofacial surgery, the rod and plate of Ti alloys are sometimes bent by medical doctors in the operation room (see Section 5.10 and Fig. 5.18). These operations sometimes generate crack or fracture of Ti alloys, because the elongation to fracture of α+β-type Ti alloy (10% of Ti–6Al–4V ELI) (Brunette et al. 2001) is much smaller than that of type 316L stainless steel (40%) (ASTM A240 2023). Therefore, the strengthening of α+β-type Ti alloy while maintaining elongation is required.

The fixture part of dental implants consists of CP Ti and Ti alloys to bond alveolar bone. A Ti–Ni superelastic alloy and a Ti–Mo alloy are used as orthodontic arch wire. In particular, Ti–Ni alloy is widely used, because proper and continuous orthodontic force remains for a long time. Ti–Ni alloy is suitable for reamers and files for endodontics for bending tooth roots, while the alloy sometimes fractures by an overload with dental engines.

Corrosion of metallic implant devices implanted into the human body has been studied (Nakayama et al. 1989, Brunette et al. 2001, Alves et al. 2009, Asri et al. 2017, Manam et al. 2017, Eliaz 2019), because the corrosion is related to toxicity and fracture, whereas examples of corrosion-fracture of metal implants are few. The reason is because the retrieval case of implants is limited, and surgeons are rarely interested in corroded retrieved implants. In particular, severe corrosion cases of CP Ti and Ti alloys are rare. However, Ti used as dental restoratives is corroded by

Table 6.5. Problem to be solved in CP Ti and Ti alloys for medical use.

Problem	Material	Medical device
Stress shielding	α+β type Ti alloy	Bone plate; Stem of artificial hip joint
Adhesion to bone	Whole Ti alloy	Bone screw; Bone nail
Cracking and fracture by excessive deformation	CP Ti; α+β type Ti alloy	Spinal rod; Maxillofacial plate
Corrosion with fluoride	CP Ti; Whole Ti alloy	Dental restorative
Cytotoxicity	CP Ti; Whole Ti alloy	All devices
Peri-implantitis	CP Ti; Whole Ti alloy	Abutment of dental implant; Orthodontic implant anchor; Percutaneous device; Screw of external bone fixator

fluorine compounds contained in mouthwashes and dental pastes (Nakagawa et al. 1999). Microbial corrosion of Ti in the oral cavity has also been studied (Fukushima et al. 2017). The corrosion phenomena of metallic biomaterials are reviewed (Manam et al. 2017, Eliaz 2019), while the corrosion of Ti alloys is rare.

References

Albrektsson, T. and H.A. Hansson. 1986. An ultrastructural characterization of the interface between bone and sputtered titanium or stainless steel surfaces. Biomaterials 7: 201–205.

Albrektsson T., T. Jemt, J. Molne P. Tengvall and A. Wennerberg. 2019. On inflammation-immunological balance theory-A critical apprehension of disease concepts around implants: mucositis and marginal bone loss may represent normal conditions and not necessarily a state of disease. Clin. Implant. Dent. Relat. Res. 21: 183–189.

Albrektsson, T. and A. Wennerberg. 2019. On osseointegration in relation to implant surfaces. Clinic. Implant. Dent. Related Res. 21: 4–7.

Anon. 1994. Ti-6Al-2Nb-lTa-0.8Mo (Ti-6211). pp. 321–336. *In*: R. Boyer, G. Welsch and E.W. Collings [eds.]. Materials Properties Handbook, ASM International, Materials Park, OH, USA.

Art, W., N. Hori, M. Takeuchi, J. Ouyang, Y. Yang, M. Anpo et al. 2009. Time- dependent degradation of titanium osteoconductivity: an implication of biological aging of implant materials. Biomaterials 30: 5352–5363.

Asami, K. and K. Hashimoto. 1977. The X-ray photo-electron spectra of several oxides of ion and chromium. Corros. Sci. 17: 559–570.

Asami, K., S.C. Chen, H. Habazaki and K. Hashimoto. 1993. The surface characterization of titanium and titanium–nickel alloys in sulfuric acid. Corros. Sci. 35: 43–49.

Ashida, M., P. Chen, H. Doi, Y. Tsutsumi, T. Hanawa and Z. Horita. 2014. Microstructures and mechanical properties of Ti-6Al-7Nb processed by high-pressure torsion. Proced. Eng. 81: 1523–1528.

Ashida, M., P. Chen, H. Doi, Y. Tsutsumi, T. Hanawa and Z. Horita. 2015. Superplasticity in the Ti–6Al–7Nb alloy processed by high-pressure torsion. Mater. Sci. Eng. A 640: 449–453.

Ashida, M., M. Hanai, P. Chen and T. Hanawa. 2022. Developing manufacture and enhancing strength of Ti–6Al–7Nb alloy with heat treatment processed by high-pressure tortion. Mater. Trans. 6: 948-956.

ASM Handbook, Vol. 2. 2023. Properties and selection: Nonferrous allos and special-purpose alloys: ASM International, Materials Park, OH, USA.

Asri, R.I.M., W.S.W. Harun, M. Samykano, N.A.C. Lah, S.A.C. Ghani, F. Tarlochan et al. 2017. Corrosion and surface modification on biocompatible metals: A review. Mater. Sci. Eng. C 77: 1261–1274.

ASTM A240/240M-23. 2023. Standard Specification for Chromium and Chromium-Nickel Stainless Steel Plate, Sheet, and Strip for Pressure Vessels and for General Applications. ASTM International, West Conshohocken, PA, USA.

ASTM F75-23. 2023. Standard Specification for Cobalt–28 Chromium–6 Molybdenum Alloy Castings and Casting Alloy for Surgical Implants, ASTM International, West Conshohocken, PA, USA.

Baltatu, M.S., P. Vizureanu, A.V. Sandu, N.F. Suarez, M.V. Saceleanu and J.C.M. Rosca. 2021. New titanium alloys, promising materials for medical devices. Materials 14: 5934.

Beck, T.R. 1973. Electrochemistry of freshly-generated titanium surfaces. I. Scraped-rotating-disk experiments. Electrochem. Acta 18: 807–814.

Beder, O.E., J.K. Stevenson and T.W. Jones. 1957. A further investigation of the surgical application of titanium metal in dogs. Surgery 41: 1012–1015.

Bessho, K., K. Fujimura and T. Iizuka. 1995. Experimental long-term study of titanium ions eluted from pure titanium miniplates. J. Biomed. Mater. Res. 29: 901–904.

Bianco, P.D., P. Ducheyne and J.M. Cuckler. 1996. Local accumulation of titanium released from a titanium implant in the absence of wear. J. Biomed. Mater. Res. 31: 227–234.

Boehm, H.P. 1966. Functional groups on the surfaces of solids. Angew Chem. 5: 533–544.

Boehm, H.P. 1971. Acidic and basic properties of hydroxylated metal oxide surfaces. Discuss. Faraday Soc. 52: 264–289.

Bothe, R.T., L.E. Beaton and H.A. Davenport. 1940. Reaction of bone to multiple metallic implants. Surg. Gynec. Obsbtet. 71: 598–602.

Brånemark, R., L.O. Ohrnell, R. Skalak, L. Carlsson and P.I. Brånemark. 1998. Biomechanical characterization of osseointegration: An experimental *in vivo* investigation in the beagle dog. J. Orthop. Res. 16: 61–69.

Breeson, A.C., G. Sankar, G.K.L. Goh and R.G. Palgrave. 2017. Phase quantification by X-ray photoemission valence band analysis applied to mixed phase TiO_2 powders. Appl. Surf. Sci. 423: 205–209.

Bruneel, N. and J.A. Helsen. 1988. In vitro simulation of biocompatibility of Ti-Al-V. J. Biomed. Mater. Res. 22: 203–214.

Brunette, D.M., P. Tenvall, M. Textor and P. Thomsen. 2001. Titanium in Medicine: Springer, Berlin, Germany.

Brånemark, P.I., B.O. Hansson, R. Adell, U. Breine, J. Lindström, O. Hallén et al. 1977. Osseointegrated implants in the treatment of the edentulous jaw. Experience from a 10-year period. Scand. J. Plastic Reconstruct. Surg. Hand Surg. 11: Suppl 16, 1–132.

Chaves, J.M., O. Florêncio, P.S. Silva Jr., P.W.B. Marques and S.G. Schneider. 2014. An elastic relaxation associated to phase transformations and interstitial atoms in the Ti–35Nb–7Zr alloy. J. Alloy. Compd. 616: 420–425.

Chávez-Díaz, M.P., R. Luna-Sánchez, J. Vazquez-Arenas, L. Lartundo-Rojas, J.M. Hallen and R. Cabrera-Sierra. 2019. XPS and EIS studies to account for the passive behavior of the alloy Ti-6Al-4V in Hank's solution. J. Solid State Electrochem. 23: 3187–3196.

Chen, P., A. Nagai, Y. Tsutsumi, M. Ashida, H. Doi and T. Hanawa. 2016. Differences in the calcification of preosteoblast cultured on sputter-deposited titanium, zirconium, and gold. J. Biomed. Mater. Res. 104A: 639–651.

Clark, G.C.F. and D.F. Williams. 1982. The effects of proteins on metallic corrosion. J. Biomed. Mater. Res. 16: 125–134.

Correa, D.R.N., P.A.B. Kuroda, C.R. Grandini, L.A. Rocha, F.G.M. Oliveira, A.C. Alves et al. 2016. Tribocorrosion behavior of β-type Ti-15Zr-based alloys. Mater. Lett. 179: 118–121.

Correa, D.R.N., L.A. Rocha, T.A.G. Donato, K.S.J. Sousa, C.R. Grandini, C.R.M. Afonso et al. 2020. On the mechanical biocompatibility of Ti–15Zr–based alloys for potential use as load-bearing implants. J. Mater. Res. Technol. 9: 1241–1250.

Davies, J.E., B. Lowenberg and A. Shiga. 1990. The bone titanium interface in vitro. J. Biomed. Mater. Res. 24: 1289–1306.

Diebold, U. 2003. The surface science of titanium dioxide. Surf. Sci. Rep. 48: 53–229.

Eda, Y., T. Manaka, T. Hanawa, P. Chen, M. Ashida and K. Noda. 2022. X-ray photoelectron spectroscopy-based valence band spectra of passive films on titanium. Surf. Interface Anal. 54: 892–898.

Ektessabi, A.M., T. Otsuka, Y. Tsuboi, K. Yokoyama, T. Albrektsson, L. Sennerby and C. Johansson. 1994. Application of micro beam PIXE to detection of titanium ion release from dental and orthopaedic implants. Int. J. PIXE. 4. 81–91.

Ektessabi, A.M., T. Otsuka, Y. Tsuboi, Y. Horino, Y. Mokuno, K. Fujii et al. 1996. Preliminary experimental results on mapping of the elemental distribution of organic tissues surrounding titanium-alloy implants. Nucl. Instr. Meth. Phys. Res. B 109/110: 278–283.

Eliaz, N. 2019. Corrosion of metallic biomaterials: A Review. Materials 12: 407.

Esposito, M., J. Lausmaa, J.M. Hirsch and P. Thomsen. 1999. Surface analysis of failed oral titanium implants. J. Biomed. Mater. Res. 48: 559–568.

Fanning, J. C. 1996. Properties and processing of a new metastable beta titanium alloy for surgical implant applications. pp. 1800–1807. *In:* Blenkinsop, P.A., W.J. Evans and H. Flower [eds.]. Titanium '95: Science and Technology, The University Press, Cambridge, UK.

Frauchiger, L., M. Taborelli, B.O. Aronsson and P. Descouts. 1999. Ion adsorption on titanium surfaces exposed to a physiological solution. Appl. Surf. Sci. 143: 67–77.

Fujisawa, H., Y. Mori, A. Kogure, H. Tanaka, M. Kamimura, N. Masahashi et al. 2018. Effects of intramedullary nails composed of a new β-type Ti-Nb-Sn alloy with low Young's modulus on fracture healing in mouse tibiae. J. Biomed. Mater. Res. Appl. Biomater. 106B: 2841–2848.

Fukushima, A., G. Mayanagi, K. Nakajo, K. Sasaki and N. Takahashi. 2014. Microbiologically induced corrosive properties of the titanium surface. J. Dent. Res. 93: 525–529.

Gefen, A. 2002. Computational simulations of stress shielding and bone resorption around existing and computer-designed orthopaedic screws. Med. Bio. Eng. Comp. 40: 311–322.

Gittens, R., A. Scheideler, L. Rupp, F. Hyzy, S.L. Geis-Gerstorfer, J. Schwartz et al. 2014. A review on the wettability of dental implant surfaces II: Biological and clinical aspects. Acta Biomater. 10: 2907–2918.

Goriainov, V., R. Cook, J.M. Latham, D.G. Dunlop and R.O.C. Oreffo. 2014. Bone and metal: An orthopaedic perspective on osseointegration of metals. Acta Biomater. 10: 4043–4057.

Hanawa, T. and M. Ota. 1991. Calcium phosphate naturally formed on titanium in electrolyte solution. Biomaterials 12: 767–774.

Hanawa, T. and M. Ota. 1992. Characterization of surface film formed on titanium in electrolyte using XPS. Appl. Surf. Sci. 55: 269–276.

Hanawa, T., K. Asami and K. Asaoka. 1998. Repassivation of titanium and surface oxide film regenerated in simulated bioliquid. J. Biomed. Mater. Res. 40: 530–538.

Hanawa, T., Y. Kohyama, S. Hiromoto and A. Yamamoto. 2004. Effects of biological factors on the repassivation current of titanium. Mater. Trans. 45: 1635–1639.

Hanawa, T. 2019. Titanium-tissue interface reaction and its control with surface treatment. Front. Bioeng. Biotechnol. 7: 170.

Hanawa, T. 2022. Biocompatibility of titanium from the viewpoint of its surface. Sci. Technol. Adv. Mater. 23: 457–472.

Healy, K.E. and P. Ducheyne. 1992. The mechanisms of passive dissolution of titanium in a model physiological environment. J. Biomed. Mater. Res. 26: 319–338.

Heimann, R.B. and M. Niinomi. 2020. Chapter 2 types and properties of biomaterials. pp. 75–165. *In:* Heimann, R.B. and De Gruyter [eds.]. Materials for Medical Application, Berlin, Germany.

Hiji, A., T. Hanawa, M. Shimabukuro, P. Chen, M. Ashida and K. Ishikawa. 2021a. Initial formation kinetics of calcium phosphate on titanium in Hanks' solution characterized using XPS. Surf. Interface Anal. 53: 185–193.

Hiji, A., T. Hanawa, T. Yokoi, P. Chen, M. Ashida and M. Kawashita. 2021b. Time transient of calcium and phosphate ion adsorption by rutile crystal facets in Hanks' solution characterized by XPS. Langmuir 37: 3597–3604.

Hiromoto, S., T. Hanawa and K. Asami. 2004. Composition of surface oxide film of titanium with culturing murine fibroblasts L929. Biomaterials 25: 979–986.

Hodgson, A.W.E., Y. Mueller and F.D. Virtanen. 2002. Electrochemical characterisation of passive films on Ti alloys under simulated biological conditions. Electrochim. Acta 47: 1913–1923.

Iman, M.A. and C.M. Gilmore. 1983. Fatigue and microstructural oroperties of quenched Ti–6Al–4V. Metall. Trans. 14A: 233–240.

ISO 5832-2:2018. 2018. Implants for surgery, Metallic materials, Part 2: Unalloyed titanium. International Organization for Standardization, Geneva, Switzerland.

Itakura, Y., T. Tajima, S. Ohoke, J. Matsuzawa, H. Sudo and S. Yamamoto. 1989. Osteocompatibility of platinum-plated titanium assessed *in vitro*. Biomaterials 10: 489–493.

Kelly, E.J. 1982. Electrochemical behavior of titanium. Mod. Aspect Electrochem. 14: 319–424.

Kim, S.C., T. Hanawa, T. Manaka, H. Tsuchiya and S. Fujimoto. 2022. Band structures of passive films on titanium in simulated bioliquids determined by photoelectrochemical response: principle goverining the biocompatibility. Sci. Technol. Adv. Mater. 23: 322–331.

Kuroda, D., M. Niinomi, M. Morinaga, Y. Kato and T. Yashiro. 1988. Design and mechanical properties of new β type titanium alloys for implant materials. Mater. Sci. Eng. A 243: 244–249.

Lavrys, S., I. Pohrelyuk, H. Veselivska, A. Skrebtsov, J. Kononenko and Y. Marchenko. 2022. Corrosion behavior of near-alpha titanium alloy fabricated by additive manufacturing. Mater. Corros. 73: 2063–2070.

Leventhal, G.S. 1951. Titanium, a metal for surgery. J. Bone Joint Surg. Am. 33-A: 473–474.

Lide, D.R. [ed.]. 2006. CRC Handbook of Chemistry and Physics, 87th ed., CRC Press, Boca Raton, FL, USA.

Listgarten, M.A., D. Buser, S.G. Steinemann, K. Donath, N.P. Lang and H.P. Weber. 1992. Light and transmission electron microscopy of the intact interfaces between non-submerged titanium-coated epoxy resin implants and bone or gingiva. J. Dent. Res. 71: 364–371.

Lutjering, G. and A. Gysler. 1984. Fatigue–A Critical Review. pp. 2065–2083. Titanium–Science and Technology. Proc. 5th International Conference on Titanium.

Lutjering, G., A. Gysler and Wagner, L. 1988. Crack Propagation in Ti-Alloys. pp. 71–80. Proc. 6th World Conference on Titanium.

Manam, N.S., W.S.W. Harum, D.N.A. Shri, S.A.C. Ghani, T. Kurniawan and M.H. Ismail. 2017. Study of corrosion in biocompatible metals for implants: a review. J. Alloy Comp. 701: 698–715.

Materials Properties Handbook. 1994. Titanium Alloys. pp. 5–11. ASM International, Materials Park, OH, USA.

Meachin, G. and D.F. Williams. 1973. Change in non-osseous tissue adjacent to titanium implants. J. Biomed. Mater. Res. 7: 555–572.

Merritt, K. and S.A. Brown. Effect of proteins and pH on fretting corrosion and metal ion release. J. Biomed. Mater. Res. 22: 111–120.

Mishra, A., J. Davidson, R. Poggie, P. Kovacs and T. FitzGerald. 1996. Mechanical and tribological properties and biocompatibility of diffusion hardened Ti-13Nb-13Zr –a new titanium alloy for surgical implants. pp. 96–113. *In*: Brown, S. and J. Lemons [eds.]. ASTM STP1272, Medical Applications of Titanium and Its Alloys: The Material and Biological Issues. ASTM International, West Conshohocken, PA, USA.

Miura, I. and K. Ida [eds.]. 1988. Titanium in Dentistry. Quintessence, Tokyo, Japan.

Mu, Y., T. Kobayashi, M. Sumita, A. Yamamoto and T. Hanawa. 2000. Metal ion release from titanium with active oxygen species generated by rat macrophages *in vitro*. J. Biomed. Mater. Res. 49: 238–243.

Mu, Y., T. Kobayashi, K. Tsuji, M. Sumita and T. Hanawa. 2002. Causes of titanium release from plate and screws implanted in rabbits. J. Mater. Sci. Mater. Med. 13: 583–588.

Murai, K., F. Takeshita, Y. Ayukawa, T. Kiyoshima, T. Suetsugu and T. Tanaka. 1996. Light and electron microscopic studies of bone-titanium interface in the tibiae of young and mature rats. J. Biomed. Mater. Res. 30: 523–533.

Nakagawa, M., S. Matsuya, T. Shiraishi and M. Ohta. 1999. Effect of fluoride concentration and pH on corrosion behavior of titanium for dental use. J. Dent. Res. 78: 1568–1572.

Nakayama, Y., T. Yamamuro, Y. Kotoura and M. Oka. 1989. *In vivo* measurement of anodic polarization of orthopaedic implant alloys: comparative study of *in vivo* and *in vitro* experiments. Biomaterials 10: 420–424.

Nakayama, Y., T. Yamamuro, P. Kumar, K. Shimizu, Y. Kotoura, M. Oka et al. 1990. Anodic polarization measurements of orthopaedic implant alloys in bovine serum albumin. J. Appl. Biomater. 1: 307–313.

Niinomi, M., T. Kobayashi, I. Inagaki and A.W. Thompson. 1990. The effect of deformation-induced transformation on the fracture toughness of commercial titanium alloys. Metall. Mater. Trans. A 21: 1733–1744.

Niinomi, M., T. Kobayashi and A. Shimokawa. 1993. Fatigue crack propagation in Ti-6Al-4V alloys containing retained metastable β phase titanium. pp. 1835–1842. *In:* Froes, F.H. and I. Caplan [eds.]. Titanium '92, Science and Technology, Proceedings of 7th World Conference on Titanium. Minerals, Metals and Materials Society, Pittsburgh, PA, USA.

Niinomi, M. 2002. Recent metallic materials for biomedical applications. Metall. Mater. Trans. A 33: 477–486.
Niinomi, M. 2019. Design and development of metallic biomaterials with biological and mechanical biocompatibility. J. Biomed. Mater. Res. 107A: 944–954.
Okada, M., E.S. Hara, A. Yabe, K. Okada, Y. Shibata, Y. Torii et al. 2020. Titanium as an instant adhesive for biological soft tissue. Adv. Mater. Interfaces 7: 1902089.
Okazaki, Y. 2001. A New Ti–15Zr–4Nb–4Ta alloy for medical applications. Current Opinion Solid State Mater. Sci. 5: 45–53.
Olver, J.W. and J.W. Ross. 1963. On the standard potential of the titanium(III)-titanium(II) couple. J Am. Chem. Soc. 85: 2565–2566.
Ouchi, C. 1994. Development and application of new titanium alloys SP-700. pp. 37–44. *In*: Fujishiro, S., D. Eylon and T. Kishi [eds.]. Metallurgy and Technology of Practical Titanium Alloys, Minerals, Metals and Materials Society, Pittsburg, PA, USA.
Palmquist, A., O.M. Omar, M. Esposito, J. Lausmaa and P. Thomsen. 2010. Titanium oral implants: surface characteristics, interface biology and clinical outcome. J. Royal Soc. Interface 7: S515–S527.
Pan, J., H. Liao, C. Leygraf, D. Thierry and J. Li. 1998. Variation of oxide films on titanium induced by osteoblast-like cell culture and the influence of an H_2O_2 pretreatment. J. Biomed. Mater. Res. 40: 244–256.
Parfitt, G.D. 1976. The surface of titanium dioxide. Prog. Surf. Membr. Sci. 11: 181–226.
Park, J.Y. and J.E. Davies. 2000. Red blood cell and platelet interactions with titanium implant surfaces. Clinic. Oral Implant. Res. 11: 530–539.
Pillar, R.M. and G.C. Weatherly. 1982. Development in Implant Alloys. pp. 371–473. Williams, D.F. [ed.]. Clinical Reviews in Biocompatibility, Vol. 1: CRC Press, Boca Raton, FL, USA.
Pourbaix, M. 1966. Atras of Electrochemical Equilibria. pp. 213–222. Pergamon, Oxford, UK.
Rao, V.B. and C.R. Houska. 1979. Kinetics of the phase-transformation in a Ti–15Mo–5Zr–3Al alloy as studied by X-ray-diffraction. Metall. Trans. A 10: 355–358.
Revie, R.W. and H.H. Uhlig. 2008. Corrosion and Corrosion Control: An Introduction to Corrosion Science and Engineering, 4th ed. Wiley, Berlin, Germany.
Rupp, F., L. Liang, J. Geis-Gerstorfer, L. Scheideler and F. Hüttig. 2018. Surface characteristics of dental implants: a review. Dent. Mater. 34: 40–57.
Ryhanen, J., E. Niemi, W. Serlo, E. Niemela, P. Sandvik, H. Pernu et al. 1997. Biocompatibility of nickel-titanium shape memory metal and its corrosion behaviour in human cell cultures. J. Biomed. Mater. Res. 35: 451–457.
Salvi, G.E., D.D. Bosshardt, N.P. Lang, I. Abrahamsson, T. Berglundh, J. Lindhe et al. 2015. Temporal sequence of hard and soft tissue healing around titanium dental implants. Periodontology 68: 135–152.
Sanderson, L., W. Ryan and P.G. Turner. 1992. Complications of metalwork removal injury. Injury 23: 29–30.
Seo, D.I. and J.B. Lee. 2023. Localized corrosion and repassivation behaviors of additively manufactured titanium alloys in simulated biomedical solutions. Npj Mater. Degradation 7: 44.
Serro, A.P., A.C. Fernandes, B. Saramago, J. Lima and M.A. Barbosa. 1997. Apatite desorption on titanium surfaces—The role of albumin adsorption. Biomaterials 18: 963–968.
Shah, F.A., P. Thomsen and A. Palmquist. 2018. A review of the impact of implant biomaterials on osteocytes. J. Dent. Res. 97: 977–986.
Shah, F.A., P. Thomsen and A. Palmquist. 2019. Osseointegration and current interpretations of bone-implant interface. Acta Biomater. 84: 1–15.
Silverman, D.C. 1982. Application of EMF-pH diagrams to corrosion prediction. Corrosion 38: 541–549.
Singh, A.P., N. Kodan and B.R. Mehta. 2016. Enhancing the photoelectrochemical properties of titanium dioxide by thermal treatment in oxygen deficient environment. Appl. Surf. Sci. 372: 63–69.
Speck, K.M. and A.C. Fraker. 1980. Anodic polarization behavior of Ti-Ni and Ti-6Al-4V in simulated physiological solutions. J. Dent. Res. 59: 1590–1595.
Sundell, G., C. Dahlin, M. Andersson and M. Thuvander. 2017. The bone-implant interface of dental implants in humans on the atomic scale. Acta Biomater. 48: 445–450.
Sundgren, J.E., P. Bodö, B. Ivarsson and I. Lundström. 1986a. Adsorption of fibrinogen on titanium and gold surfaces studied by esca and ellipsometry. J. Colloid Interface Sci. 113: 530–543.

Sundgren, J.E., P. Bodö and I. Lundstrom. 1986b. Auger electron spectroscopic studies of the interface between human tissue and implants of titanium and stainless steel. J. Colloid Interface Sci. 110: 9–20.

Tanaka, Y., K. Kurashima, H. Saito, A. Nagai, Y. Tsutsumi, H. Doi, Nomura, N. and T. Hanawa. 2009. *In vitro* short term platelet adhesion on various metals. J. Artf. Org. 12: 182–186.

Tang, L. and Eaton, J.W. 1993. Fibrinogen mediates acute inflammatory responses to biomaterials. J. Exp. Med. 178: 2147–2156.

Tengvall, P., I. Lundström, L. Sjöqvist, H. Elwing and L.M. Bjursten. 1989. Titanium-hydrogen peroxide interaction: model studies of the influence of the inflammatory response on titanium implants. Biomaterials 10: 166–175.

Thomsen, P., C. Larsson, L.E. Ericson, L. Sennerby, J. Lausmaa and B. Kasemo. 1997. Structure of the interface between rabbit cortical bone and implants of gold, zirconium and titanium. J. Mater. Sci. Mater. Med. 8: 653–665.

Trindade, R., T. Albrektsson, S. Galli, Z. Prgomet, P. Tengvall and A. Wennerberg. 2016. Osseointegration and foreign body reaction: Titanium implants activate the immune system and suppress bone resorption during the first 4 weeks after implantation. Clinic. Implant Dent. Related Res. 20: 82–91.

Tsutsumi, Y., D. Nishimura, H. Doi, N. Nomura and T. Hanawa. 2009. Calcium phosphate formation on titanium and zirconium and its application to medical devices. Mater. Sci. Eng. C 29: 1702–1708.

Tsutsumi, Y., T. Nishisaka, H. Doi, M. Ashida, P. Chen and T. Hanawa. 2015. Reaction of calcium and phosphate ions with titanium, zirconium, niobium, and tantalum. Surf. Interface Anal. 47: 1148–1154.

Wang, K. 1996. The use of titanium for medical applications in the USA. Mat. Sci. Eng. A 213: 134–137.

Wang, K., L. Gustavson and J. Dumbleton. 1993. Low modulus, high strength, biocompatible titanium alloy for medical implants. pp. 2697–2704. *In*: Froes, F.H. and H.L. Caplan [eds.]. Titanium '92: Science and Technology, TMS, Warrenda, PA, USA.

Wang, L., H. Yu, K. Wang, H. Xu, S. Wang and D. Sun. 2016. Local fine structural insight into mechanism of electrochemical passivation of titanium. ACS Appl. Mater. Interfaces 8: 18608–18619.

Wang, Y., M. Okada, S.C. Xie, Y.Y. Jiao, E.S. Hara, H. Yanagimoto et al. 2021. Immediate soft-tissue adhesion and the mechanical properties of the Ti-6Al-4V alloy after long-term acid treatment. J. Mater. Chem. B 9: 8348–8354.

Waterstrat, R.M., N.W. Rupp and O. Franklin. 1978. Production of a cast titanium-base partial denture. J. Dent. Res. 57: Special Issue, 254.

Westall, J. and H. Hohl. 1980. A comparison of electrostatic models for the oxide/solution interface. Adv. Colloid Interface Sci. 12: 265–294.

Williams, D.F. 1982a. Titanium and Titanium Alloys. pp. 10–44. *In*: William, D.F. [ed.]. Biocompatibility of Clinical Implant Materials, CRC Press, Boca Raton, FL, USA.

Williams, D.F. 1982b. Biological Effects of Titanium. pp. 170–177. *In*: William, D.F. [ed.]. Systematic Aspects of Biocompatibility, CRC Press, Boca Raton, FL, USA.

Williams, R. [ed.]. 2011. Surface Modification of Biomaterials: Woodhead Publishing, Sawston, UK.

Williams, R.L., S.A. Brown and K. Merritt. 1988. Electrochemical studies on the influence of proteins on the corrosion of implant alloys. Biomaterials 9: 181–186.

Woodman, J.L., J.J. Jacobs, J.O. Galante and R.M. Urban. 1984. Metal ion release from titanium-based prosthetic segmental replacements of long bones in baboons: a long-term study. J. Orthop. Res. 1: 421–430.

Yabe, A., M. Okada, E.S. Hara, Y. Torii and T. Matsumoto. 2021. Self-adhering implantable device of titanium: Enhanced soft-tissue adhesion by sandblast pretreatment. Colloid Surf. B 211: 112283.

Yilmaz, E., A. Gökçe, F. Findik and H.Ö. and H.Ö Gulsoy. 2018. Assessment of Ti–16Nb–xZr alloys produced via PIM for implant applications. J. Therm. Anal. Calorim. 134: 7–14.

Zardiackas, L.D., D.W. Mitchell and J.A. Disegi. 1996. Characterization of Ti-15Mo beta titanium alloy for orthopaedic implant applications. pp. 60–75. *In*: Browns, S.A. and J.E. Lemons [eds.]. Medical Applications of Titanium and Its Alloys, ASTM, West Conshohoken, PA, USA.

Chapter 7

Cobalt-Based Alloys

7.1 Introduction

Co-based alloys are materials with excellent mechanical properties such as strength and toughness, castability, corrosion resistance, and wear resistance. It also has better corrosion resistance than stainless steel, and better wear resistance than stainless steel, CP Ti, and Ti alloys. However, its plastic workability is generally lower than those of stainless steel, CP Ti, and Ti alloys. For medical applications, there are a cast Co–Cr–Mo alloy known as Vitallium, wrought Co–Cr–W–Ni alloy and a Co–Ni–Cr–Mo alloy with the brand name MP-35N, etc. Cast Co–Cr–Mo alloys have excellent pitting corrosion resistance and crevice corrosion resistance, and in particular have the best wear resistance among metallic biomaterials, so they are used for the femoral heads of artificial hip joints. It is also used as a denture base due to its excellent castability. Wrought Co-based alloys are designed to eliminate casting defects in cast Co–Cr–Mo alloys, and the strength and elongation obtained through solution heat treatment and cold working are equivalent to those of stainless steel. In addition, its corrosion resistance is inferior to cast Co–Cr–Mo alloy, but superior to stainless steel. For this reason, they are used as devices consisting of plates or wires such as guide wires, clips, orthodontic wires, and catheters. Because of better corrosion resistance than stainless steel and better wear resistance than Ti alloys, most sliding parts such as head of artificial hip joint are made of Co–Cr–Mo alloys, and it is difficult to replace them with other alloys at present. The composition and mechanical properties of typical Co-based alloys are summarized in Table 7.1 and Table 7.2. Comprehensive handbook on Co-based alloys (ASM Handbook Vol. 2 2023) should be used as reference.

7.2 History of Cobalt-Based Alloy

The history of the development of Co-based alloys begins in the 1900s. Stellite (Co–Cr alloy or Co–Cr–W alloy) developed by Haynes has established itself as an indispensable wear-resistant alloy for cutter blades, machine tools, etc. In the 1930s, Vitallium (Co–Cr–Mo alloy) was developed as a dental alloy (Morral 1966). The first application for orthopedics was in 1937 when Paterson developed an artificial joint made of Vitallium. In the 1940s, HS21 Co–Cr–Mo alloy was developed

Table 7.1. Composition, ASTM specification, brand name, and composition of major Co-based alloys.

Alloy sytem	ASTM specification	General bland name	Composition (mass%)
Co-Cr-Mo	F75	Vitallium HS21	27.0–30.0 Cr, 5.0–7.0 Mo < 0.5 Ni, < 0.75 Fe, < 0.35 C, < 1.0 Mn, < 1.0 Si, < 0.25 N
Co-Cr-W-Ni	F90	HS25	19.0–21.0 Cr, 14.0–16.0 W, 9.0–11.0 Ni 0.05–0.15 C, 1.0–2.0 Mn < 3.0 Fe, < 0.4 Si
Co-Ni-Cr-Mo-Ti	F562	MP35N	33.0–37.0 Ni, 19.0–21.0 Cr, 9.0–10.5 Mo < 1.0 Ti, < 1.0 Fe, < 0.15 Mn, < 0.15 Si, < 0.025 C
Co-Cr-Ni-Mo-Fe	F1058 grade1	Elgiloy	39.0–41.0 Co, 19.0–21.0 Cr, 14.0–16.0 Ni, 6.0–8.0 Mo, 1.5–2.5 Mn < 1.20 Si, < 0.15 C, < 0.1 Be, Balance Fe

Table 7.2. Mechanical properties of Co-base alloys for medical use (Data form ASTM).

ASTM	Young's modulus E/GPa	Yield strength σ_y/MPa	Tensile strength σ_{UTS}/MPa
F75	210	448–517	655–889
F799	210	896–1200	1399–1586
F90*1	210	1606	1896
F562*2	232	1500	1795
F1058 grade1*3	190	1240–1450	1860–2275

*1 Property of 44% cold worked material.
*2 Property of cold worked and aged material.
*3 Values change due to the diameter of wire.

as an improved Vitallium casting alloy for industrial applications. Therafter, much research has been carried out on its practical application as a heat-resistant material for turbochargers and gas turbine materials, and various heat-resistant Co-based alloys have been developed (Smith et al. 1991). After the advent of inexpensive and high-performance Ni-based superalloys from the 1950s to the 1970s, research and development into industrial Co-based alloys completely slumped. On the other hand, research on improving the mechanical properties of artificial joint materials, especially research on optimal heat treatment conditions for alloys with existing compositions (Cohen 1978, Dobbs and Robertson 1983, Montero-Ocampo 1999), and basic research on carbide precipitation (Clemow and Daniell 1979, Kilner et al. 1982, Taylor and Waterhouse 1983) have been developed mainly by artificial joint manufacturers in North America and Europe. Recently, Co–Cr–Al–Si alloys have been developed for medical use (Odaira et al. 2022). In the 1980s, it was pointed out that osteolysis caused by ultra high molecular weight polyethylene (UHMWPE) wear debris was the cause of the loosening of artificial hip joints that were made of a combination of a UHMWPE socket and a Co–Cr–Mo alloy head (Chan 1996). Since then, metal-on-metal artificial joints, in which the articular surfaces are made of a combination of Co–Cr–Mo alloys with excellent wear resistance, have been reconsidered. In addition, in the late 1990s, artificial hip joint surgery using resurfacing of the femoral head was applied clinically, and here again, the new metal-on-metal joint movement surface using Co–Cr–Mo alloy attracted attention. However, the occurrence of metallosis is considered a problem (Cipriano et al. 2008). On the other hand, metallosis occurs not only in metal-on-metal total hip arthroplasty (THA) but also in non-metallic THA, and it has a very wide and nonspecific clinical presentation (Oliveira 2015). Recently, medical-use Co–Cr–Mo alloys have attracted attention as stent materials due to their high elastic modulus and high density.

7.3 Cobalt-Based Alloys for Medical Devices

Because Co–Cr–Mo alloy has excellent strength, corrosion resistance, and wear resistance, it has established itself as an indispensable metallic biomaterial in orthopedics, cardiovascular surgery/internal medicine, and dentistry, as shown in Table 7.1. Various Co–Cr–Mo alloys have been standardized to meet the required properties depending on alloy composition and thermo-mechanical treatment. For example, although C-containing Co–Cr–Mo alloys exhibit superior wear resistance compared to other metallic biomaterials (see Subsection 5.8.3 and Fig. 5.13), they are hard and difficult to work, so they are used as cast. Co–Cr–Mo alloys with reduced C content have improved workability, while rought Co–Cr–Mo alloy having high strength and high elastic modulus through work and heat treatment can be used as wire and rods.

In the field of orthopedics, Co–Cr–Mo cast alloys (ASTM F75-23 2023), such as Vitallium, are used for sliding parts of artificial hip joints and knee joint. In particular, artificial knee joints have complex shapes, and manufacturing by investment casting is essential. By increasing the C content of this alloy, Cr- and Mo-rich carbides precipitate at dendrite interfaces and grain boundaries, contributing to the strengthening and wear resistance of this alloy. However, since the crystal grains become coarse during the cooling process, it is necessary to refine the grains in order to improve the strength. The grains of F75 and F799 are refined by hot working (ASTM F799-19 2019). The main constituent phase of F799 is the γ phase with a face-centered cubic (fcc), which is different from ε phase (hcp) of F75. The yield strength and tensile strength of F799 alloy are approximately twice as high as those of F75. ASTM F799 has recently been widely used as a spinal fixation rod. HS25 and L-605 used for wire, which were developed to improve the workability of Co–Cr–Mo alloys, are alloys with reduced C content and the addition of W and Ni (ASTM F90-23 2023). This alloy can be cold-working to a maximum of 44%, and the strength after working is more than twice that of F75.

In cardiological treatment, MP35N Co–Ni–Cr–Mo alloy (ASTM F562-22 2022) is used as stents. This alloy has excellent strength, ductility, and corrosion resistance, and has a tensile strength of over 1600 MPa. L-605 and MP35N exhibit high elastic modulus among Co-based alloys, so they are superior as stents. A Co–Cr–Ni–Mo–Fe alloy called Eligiloy (ASTM F1058-16 2017) is used for artificial heart springs and aneurysm clips. Although the elastic modulus of this alloy is lower than other

Co-based alloys, it can be worked into wire and foils, and its strength is also improved by aging treatment.

In the dental field, Co–Cr–Mo alloys called Vitallium and Ticonium (ISO 22674 2022) are used for removable partial dentures, crowns, and bridges. The mechanical property of the alloy is required as at least 2% of elongation to fracture, 500 MPa of yield strength, and 150 GPa of Young's modulus (Table 7.2). The Co–Cr–Mo alloy used for metal-porcelain restorations does not contain C, unlike Vitallium. Therefore, it cannot be strengthened with carbides, while Ga, W, Nb, Ru, etc., are added to improve workability and castability. Mo is a solid solution strengthening element and effective in reducing the coefficient of thermal expansion.

7.4 Mechanical Property of Cobalt-Based Alloys

Pure Co allotropically transforms from the γ phase (fcc), which is stable at high temperatures, to the ε phase (hcp), which is stable at low temperatures. Schematic diagrams of fcc and hcp structures are shown in Fig. 7.1 (Nishiyama 2012). This allotropic transformation is accompanied by a thermal history; during cooling, allotropic transformation occurs from γ phase to ε phase at 563 K (martensitic transformation starting temperature; M_s), and upon heating, it restores to γ phase again at 703 K (austenitic transformation starting temperature; A_s). This allotropic transformation occurs by shear deformation without atomic diffusion, i.e., by martensitic transformation. A schematic diagram of the transformation is also shown in Fig. 7.1.

The martensitic transformation temperature increases or decreases with alloying. Fig. 7.2 shows the effects of alloying elements on transformation of Co from hcp crystal to fcc crystal. The vertical axis shows the solid solution limit (maximum solid solution concentration: mol%) in Co, and the horizontal axis shows the temperature at which the transformation temperature from hcp to fcc changes with the addition amount of 1 mol%. This indicates that elements that lower this transformation

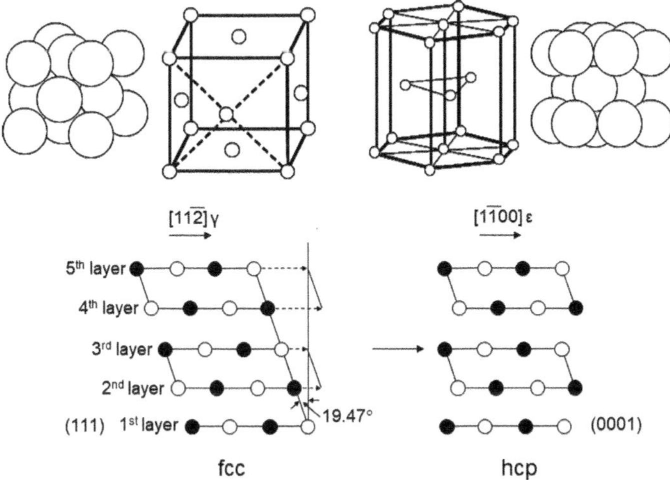

Fig. 7.1. Face-centered cubic lattice (fcc) and hexagonal close-packing lattice (hcp), and the transformation mechanism from fcc to hcp (Reproduced from the data of a reference (Nishiyama 2012).).

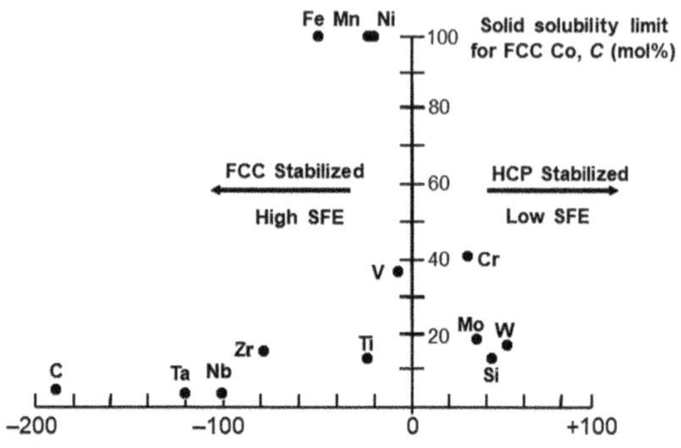

Fig. 7.2. Effect of additional elements on hcp→fcc phase transformation temperature (M_s) of Co. The vertical axis shows the solid solubility limit of the additional element and the horizontal axis shows the temperature at which 1% of the additional element changes to M_s. The higher the temperature from 0 to minus, the more stable the fcc crystal is. On the contrary, as the temperature increases from zero to positive, the hcp crystal becomes more stable. (Provided form Dr. Akihiko Chiba, Tohoku University).

temperature from hcp to fcc stabilize the γ phase, and conversely, elements that raise it have the effect of stabilizing the ε phase. Alloying elements such as Fe, Mn, Ni, and C stabilize the γ phase, while Cr, Mo, W, and Si stabilize the ε phase. If the γ phase exists as a metastable phase even at room temperature due to alloying, it transforms to the ε phase by strain-induced martensitic transformation during cold working. This strain-induced martensitic transformation is the main cause of decreasing the cold rolling, cold forging, and press workability of Co-based alloys composed of the metastable γ phase (Smis et al. 1987).

During the plastic deformation of Co–20Cr–15W–10Ni alloy (ASTM F90), the area fraction of the ε-phase in the as-received alloy is higher than that in the alloy heat-treated at 873 K (600 °C) for 14.4 ks in the low-to-middle strain region (≤ 50%), whereas the ε-phase of the heat-treated alloy is higher than that of the as-received alloy at the fracture point. During plastic deformation, the ε-phase is preferentially formed at the twin boundaries of the heat-treated alloy rather than at the grain boundaries. The thin ε-phase layer formed due to the alloy heat treatment acts as the origin of deformation twinning, which decreases the stress concentration at the grain boundaries (Ueki et al. 2018). In Co–27Cr–6Mo alloys heat-treated at 673–1373 K, lower elongation is observed after heat treatment at 1073 K due to formation of carbide precipitates. In contrast, when low-temperature heat treatment is applied at 673–873 K, both the ultimate tensile strength and elongation synchronously improve compared with the solution-treated alloy by the strain-induced martensitic transformation of the γ(fcc)-phase to ε(hcp)-phase during plastic deformation. Stacking faults (thin ε-phase) are observed to collide. This Co–Cr–Mo alloy effectively improves the performance and mechanical safety of spinal fixation implants, which often fracture because of fatigue cracking (Ueki et al. 2019). The dissolution of π-phase precipitates and the formation of Co_3Mo_2Si-type precipitates during reverse transformation promote the formation of fine γ-phase grains at the precipitate/ε-phase matrix interface, because the formation and dissolution of these precipitates affect the γ-phase stability of the matrix (Ueki et al. 2020).

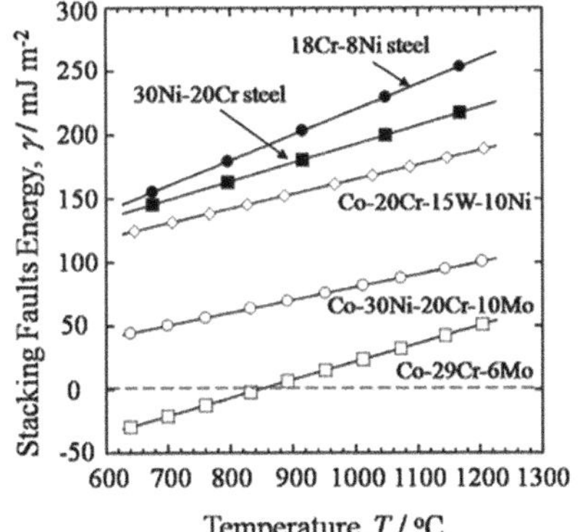

Fig. 7.3. Stacking fault energies of Co-based alloys calculated using Thermo-Calc database (Reprinted with permission from Springer Nature, Yamanaka et al. 2009. Metall. Mater, Trans. 40A: 1980–2009.).

Various types of Co-based alloys for medical devices are classified into cast materials and wrought materials depending on their plastic workability. Wrought materials are further classified into rod, plate, sheet, and wire, and this classification is determined by the difficulty of plastic workability of the Co-based alloy. The plastic workability of Co-based alloys, not only for medical applications, is greatly affected by the magnitude of stacking fault energy (SFE) (Allain et al. 2004). The temperature dependence of SFE of the medical Co-based alloy is shown in Fig. 7.3 (Nakayama et al. 1980). This figure shows the calculation results for the SFE in the neighborhood of the deformation temperature of the hot-compression test. For comparison, the values of SFE are also presented for the Co–39Ni–20Cr–10Mo alloy (SPRON510), in which the γ phase is stabilized by Ni addition, the type 304 austenitic stainless steel (Fe–18Cr–8Ni) (an example of a low-SFE alloy), and the 800H high-nickel steel (Fe-30Ni-20Cr). The various medical Co-based alloys shown in Table 7.1 are classified into the following three types based on their SFE values.

Large SFE

The SFE of Co–Cr–Ni–W alloys, represented by L-605 standardized as ASTM F90 (Taegue et al. 2004), is comparable to those of other metallic biomaterials, such as austenitic stainless steels. The γ phase exists stably up to room temperature, and deformation-induced martensitic transformation hardly occurs, so it has excellent plastic workability at room temperature and exhibits precipitation hardening by ageing. It has been put into practical use as a heat-resistant alloy (Chiba et al. 1999, Asgari et al. 2004), and has recently attracted attention as an alloy for stents due to its high elasticity and high density, which makes it highly visible in X-ray imaging.

Medium SFE

The Co–Ni–Cr–Mo alloy represented by MP35N, standardized as ASTM F562, exhibits high elasticity and high strength. When the amount of Ni increases, deformation-induced martensitic transformation is suppressed and plastic deformation such as cold rolling becomes possible. After cold working, the strength is increased by strain aging in the temperature range of 500 to 700°C (Chiba et al. 1999, 2001, Asgari et al. 2004). Elgiloy, which is known as a material for medical plates and wires such as guide wires, clips, and orthodontic wires, falls into this category.

Small SFE

So-called low Ni-containing Co–Cr–Mo alloys, such as Vitallium standardized as ASTM F75 in Table 7.1, as well as F799 and F1537, are classified into this category. In the case of Co–29Cr–6Mo alloy, at room temperature, about 20% of the high-temperature phase (γ phase) remains in addition to the non-thermal martensite (ε phase) formed during cooling (Lee et al. 2006, López and Saldivar-Garcia 2008, Chiba et al. 2009). By adding a small amount of N (approximately 0.1 to 0.2%), almost 100% of the γ phase remains as a metastable phase at room temperature. Because it inhibits plastic deformation such as rolling process, the F75 series Co-based alloy is essentially unsuitable for application as a wrought material. Artificial hip joint stems, femoral heads, and artificial knee joints are manufactured by precision casting.

Co–Cr–Mo alloy implants manufactured by additive manufacturing (AM) process osseointegrate and that the addition of a low amount of Zr to the bulk Co–Cr–Mo alloy further improves the bone anchorage (Stenlund et al. 2015). The spatial distribution of microstructures of a Co–Cr–Mo alloy rod fabricated by electron beam melting (EBM) method is observed along built direction. The topside of the rod is rich in γ-fcc phase and consists of fine grains with high local distortion density. The bottom part has an ε-hcp single phase and consists of relatively coarser grains with low local distortion density. The middle part of the rod consists of the mixture of both phases. On the other hand, a large number of precipitates including the main $M_{23}X_6$ phase and minor phases (η-phase and π-phase), are observed (Wei et al. 2018). On the other hand, the selective laser melting (SLM) process is applied to a Co–29Cr–6Mo alloy. Although the mechanical anisotropy is confirmed in the SLM builds due to the unique microstructure, the yield strength, ultimate tensile strength, and elongation are higher than those of the as-cast alloy and satisfied the type 5 criteria in ISO (ISO22674 2022). A significant microstructural inhomogeneity in EBM fabricated Co–Cr–Mo alloy along building direction is revealed, and post-production heat treatment regime homogenizes microstructures and enhances mechanical properties (Wei et al. 2019). A high cooling rate during post-heat treatment is effective in reducing grain and precipitate sizes, resulting in improved ductility and fatigue life (Cho et al. 2021). Additive manufacturing processes have opened new possibilities, allowing the production of complex components and individually tailored to the patient. In dentistry, SLM is the most popular of all powder bed fusion technologies (Konieczny et al. 2020).

7.5 Corrosion Resistance of Cobalt-Based Alloys

The reason why Co–Cr–Mo alloys exhibit excellent corrosion resistance is that, like stainless steel and CP Ti, a dense passive oxide film is formed on the alloy surface to protect the substrate metal. Co–Cr–Mo alloy exhibits better corrosion resistance than stainless steel because it contains a higher concentration of Cr than stainless steel.

Co–Cr alloys also exhibit excellent corrosion resistance in the absence of pitting and crevice corrosion. Figure 7.4 shows anodic polarization curves of variety of Co–Cr alloys (Tsutsumi et al. 2016). Shapes of the polarization curves are almost similar without pitting corrosion. Figure 7.5 shows change in corrosion rate after polishing of type 316L stainless steel, CP Ti, Ni-Ti alloy, pure Zr, and ASTM F90 Co–Cr–Mo alloy in 0.9%NaCl solution at 37°C. Decrease of corrosion rate with time in the Co-based alloy is relatively large. The corrosion of Co–Cr–Mo alloys in neutral or acid solutions was proceeded by selective dissolution of the Co (Sorp and Holm 1977). In addition, Co dissolves preferentially from a Co–Cr–W alloy in alkaline solution at 300°C (McIntyre et al. 1979). The low-Ni Co-based alloys are expected to show as high corrosion resistance. On the other hand, the passive current density of the Co–29Cr–6Mo alloy with a forging ratio of 50% is slightly lower than that with a forging ratio of 88% in the saline. The refining of grains by further forging causes the increase in the passive current density of the low-Ni Co–Cr–Mo alloy (Hiromoto et al. 2005).

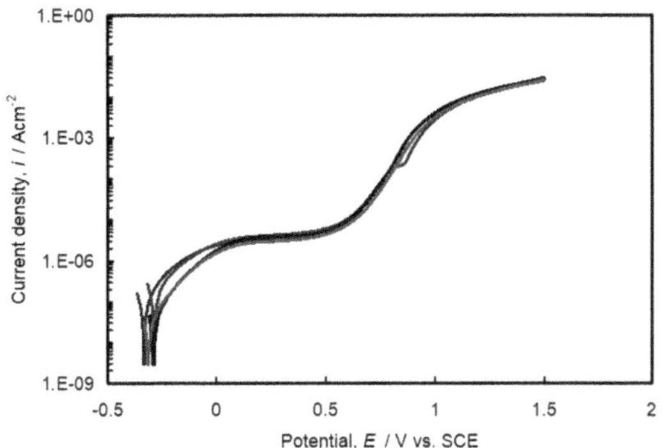

Fig. 7.4. Anodic polarization curves of Co–27–5Mo (ASTM F75), Co–20Cr–15W–10Ni (ASTM F90), Co–29Cr–6Mo, Co–33Cr–5Mo–0.34N, and Co–33Cr–9W–0.34N alloys in saline at 37°C (Provided by Dr. Yusuke Tsutsumi, National Institute for Materials Science). Anodic polarization curves of Co-based alloys are almost overlapped and no distinct difference is observed.

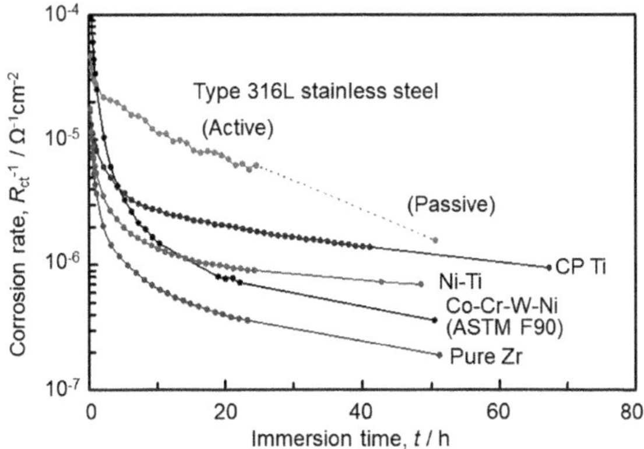

Fig. 7.5. Change in corrosion rate after polishing of type 316L stainless steel, CP Ti, Ni-Ti alloy, pure Zr, and ASTM F90 Co–Cr alloy in 0.9%NaCl solution at 37°C (Provided by Dr. Yusuke Tsutsumi, National Institute for Materials Science). Decrease of corrosion rate in the Co-based alloy is relatively large.

Dissolution of the SLM built Co–29Cr–6Mo alloy is smaller than that of the as-cast alloy; therefore, the SLM process for the Co–29Cr–6Mo alloy is a promising candidate for fabricating dental devices (Takaichi et al. 2013). Electrochemical properties of additively manufactured Co-based alloys are not significantly different than those of wrought low-C Co-based alloys (Mace et al. 2022). The potentiodynamic polarization tests have shown the lowest current density of the Co–Cr alloy in 0.9% NaCl, while the highest one was measured in phosphate buffered saline. Co–Cr alloys were passivated in all solutions, and the protective scale formed on Co–Cr alloy in 0.9% NaCl solution possesses the superior corrosion resistance according to electrochemical impedance sepectroscopy results (Ma and Niu 2019). The post-build heat treatments of Co–Cr–Mo alloy at temperatures that eliminate the melt pool boundaries are effective in reducing anisotropic corrosion behavior, and the lowest possible temperature is suitable for reducing the amount of released metal ions (Kajima et al. 2020).

7.6 Passive Film on Cobalt-Based Alloys

The surface oxide film of the Co–Cr–Mo alloy consists of cobalt oxide and chromium oxide of Co and Cr (Smith et al. 1991). The surface oxide film of a Co–Cr–Mo alloy is characterized as containing oxides of Co and Cr without Mo, and the film on another Co–Cr–Mo alloy, polished mechanically in de-ionised water, consists of oxide species of Co, Cr and Mo and has a thickness of about 2–3 nm (Hanawa et al. 2001). This surface film contains a large amount of OH^-– the oxide which is hydrated or oxyhydroxidised. Co is dissolved from a Co–Cr–Mo alloy during immersion in Hanks' solution and in a cell culture medium, as well as during incubation in a cell culture (Hanawa et al. 2001). After dissolution, the surface oxide consists of chromium oxide (Cr^{3+}) which contains molybdenum oxide (Mo^{4+}, Mo^{5+} and Mo^{6+}), as shown in Fig. 7.6. Calcium phosphate is also formed on the top surface. However, the alloys release Co ions in aqueous solution to stabilize the passive film, so Co ions are repeatedly released under wear conditions. The surface oxide film on Co–Ni–Cr–Mo alloy (MP35N) consists of oxides of Cr, Co, Ni and Mo containing a large amount of OH^-. During immersion in Hanks' solution, Co and Ni dissolve from the oxide and the composition changed as Cr^{3+} oxide containing a small amount of Co, Ni and Mo oxides. Also in Co–Ni–Cr–Mo alloy, preferential dissolution of Co and calcium phosphate formation occur (Nagai et al. 2012).

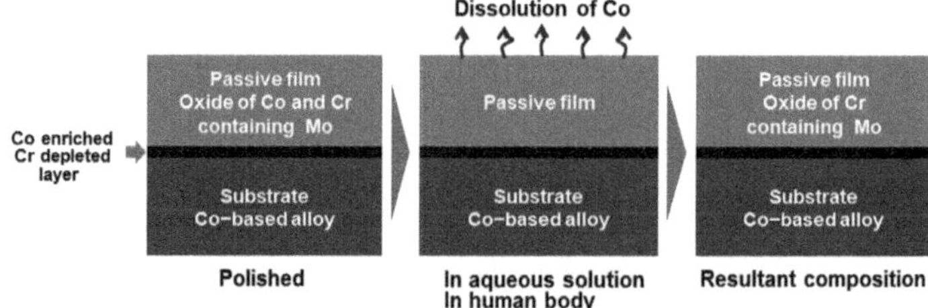

Fig. 7.6. Co ions are released from initial passive film in aqueous solutions or human body and the resultant passive film is chromium oxide containing small amount of Mo (Reprinted with permission from Francis Taylor open access, Hanawa. 2022. Sci. Technol. Adv. Mater. 23: 457–472.). Under wear condition, Co ions will be repeatedly released by the formation and destruction of the passive film.

7.7 Metallosis by Cobalt-Chromium Alloy

Co–Cr–Mo alloys can experience metallosis due to the Co release. A 56-yr-old female with metal neuropathy and a Co–Cr–Mo alloy hip prosthesis developed metallosis. Co and Cr levels in her blood decreased after exchange arthroplasty, and her symptoms improved. Elements containing Co or Cr can cause axonopathy (Ikeda et al. 2010). Cases with pseudotumors typically indicate poorly functioning implants and have significantly higher median metal ion concentrations: median Co levels are found to range from 6.9 to 29.7 μg/L (Czekaj et al. 2016). Co–Cr–Mo alloy debris are associated with persistent, dose-dependent peri-spine inflammation (Hallab et al. 2012).

The primary cause of the aforementioned metallosis is the release of Co ion. Co ions are released from the passive film on the alloys as decribed above. During release of Co ions, Cr, Mo, W, and Ni are enriched in the passive film, whereas Co is depleted, in accordance with their oxidation and reduction potentials. Therefore, under wear conditions, Co ions are released repeatedly (Maruyama et al. 2005, Hanawa et al. 2005), and the amount of Co ions released may be substantial. Therefore, the clinically observed metallosis above is due to the release of Co ions by friction wear in the human body.

7.8 Low-Nickel-Containing Cobalt-Chromium Alloy

The allergy problem of Ni is also a problem in Co-based alloys. Thus, Ni-free Co–Cr–Mo alloys are required. The Co–Cr–Mo alloy contains a small amount of Ni and this may preferentially dissolve under wear conditions. However, since the plastic workability of the Co–Cr–Mo alloy decreases in the absence of Ni, it is necessary to add strength and ductility to the Ni-free Co–Cr–Mo alloy by grain refinement. An Ni-free Co–(16-29)Cr–6Mo alloy with a grain size controlled by various forging ratios has been developed (Kurosu et al. 2007, Lee et al. 2007) that is named COBARION®. This alloy series are used for partial denture base and allergy-free accessories. Mechanical properties of Co–29Cr–6Mo alloy are improved with 0.01%Zr (Lee et al. 2007). The addition of Zr to Co–29Cr–6Mo–1N alloy decreases the release of Ni ion from the alloy, because the additional element forms a compound with Ni and Ni is fixed in the alloy (Kurosu et al. 2007). The Zr addition to the Co–29Cr–6Mo powders enhances the sintering of the compacts and suppresses the Co release from the compacts. In the metal injection molding (MIM) process, a small addition of Zr (less than 0.5 mass%) to the Co–29Cr–6Mo alloy is effective for densification during sintering and suppression of the Co release from the compacts (Murakami et al. 2010). The addition of 0.15%Zr to Co–29Cr–6Mo alloy improves its cytocompatibility (Numata et al. 2007). Co–28Cr–6Mo–0.23C–0.17N alloy cylindrical rods were fabricated by EBM with cylindrical axes along the build direction (Sun et al. 2015). The as-EBM-built rods consisting of both ε phase and γ phase can be transformed into single ε-hcp phase by the aging treatment at 800 °C for 24 h. The grain size increases along the build height at first, then decreases gradually to the position where the phase transitioned from γ-fcc to ε-hcp in the as-EBM-built rod. The decrease in stacking fault energy with increasing temperature keeps the dislocations expanding and increases the apparent activation energy.

7.9 Future Prospect

L-605 and MP35N, which are increasingly being used as stents, require large amounts of Ni to be added to the Co-based alloy in order to provide plastic workability. However, it has been reported that Ni is a typical element that causes allergies and carcinogenicity, and its use is strongly restricted in Europe by EU directives (BS EN 1811:1999, BS EN 12472:2020). Therefore, the use of alloys with Ni added poses a safety problem. Considering Ni allergy, there are safety issues with the current Co–Cr–Mo alloy standards for forging. Research and development on making Ni-free Co–Cr–Mo alloys for medical use is an important future research and development topic. On the other hand, mechanical property and corrosion resistance of Co-based alloys could be much improved by AM process. In order to expand the application to medical devices, further research to promote these and elucidation of the mechanism is necessary.

References

Allain, S., Chateau, J.P., Bouaziz, O., Migot, S. and N. Guelton. 2004. Correlations between the calculated stacking fault energy and the plasticity mechanisms in Fe–Mn–C alloys. Mater. Sci. Eng. A 387-389: 158–162.

Asgari, S., E. El-Danaf, E. Shaji, S.R. Kalidindi and R.D. Doherty. 1998. The secondary hardening phenomenon in strain-hardened MP35N alloy. Acta Mater. 46: 5795–5806.

Asgari, S. 2004. anoumalous plastic behavior of fine-grained MP35N alloy during room temperature tensile testing. J. Mater. Process. Technol. 155: 1905–1911.

ASM Handbook, Vol. 2. 2023. Properties and selection: Nonferrous allos and special-purpose alloys, ASM International, Materials Park, OH, USA.

ASTM F75-23. 2023. Standard Specification for Cobalt–28 Chromium–6 Molybdenum Alloy Castings and Casting Alloy for Surgical Implants, American Society for Testing and Materials, West Conshohocken, PA, USA.

ASTM F90-23. 2023. Standard Specification for Wrought Cobalt–20Chromium–15Tungsten–10Nickel Alloy for Surgical Implant Applications, American Society for Testing and Materials, West Conshohocken, PA, USA, 2023.

ASTM F1058-16. 2017. Standard Specification for Wrought 40 Cobalt–20 Chromium–16 Iron–15Nickel–7Molybdenum Alloy Wire and Strip for Surgical Implant Applications, American Society for Testing and Materials, West Conshohocken, PA, USA.

ASTM F562-22. 2022. Standard Specification for Wrought 35Cobalt–35Nickel–20Chromium–10Molybdenum Alloy for Surgical Implant Applications, American Society for Testing and Materials, West Conshohocken, PA, USA.

ASTM F799-19. 2019. Standard Specification for Cobalt–28 Chromium–6 Molybdenum Alloy Forgings for Surgical Implants, American Society for Testing and Materials, West Conshohocken, PA, USA.

BS EN 12472:2020. Method for the simulation of accelerated wear and corrosion for the detection of nickel release from coated items. European Standard.

Chan, F.W., J.D. Bobyn, J.B. Medley, J.J. Krygier, S. Yue and M. Tanzer. 1996. Engineering issues and wear performance of metal on metal hip implants. Clin. Orthop. 333: 96–107.

Chiba, A., X.G. Li and M.S. Kim. 1999. High work-hardening rate and deformation twinning of Co–Ni based super alloy at elevated temperatures. Phil. Mag. A79: 1533–1554.

Chiba, A. and M.S. Kim. 2001. Suzuki segregation and dislocation locking in supersaturated Co–Ni–based alloy. Mater. Trans. 42: 2112–2117.

Chiba, A. 2005. Co-Cr-Mo alloys. J. Jpn. Soc. Biomater. 23: 107–113.

Chiba, A., S.H. Lee, H. Matsumoto and M. Nakamura. 2009. Construction of processing map for biomedical Co–28Cr–6Mo–0.16N alloy by studying its hot deformation behavior using compression tests. Mater. Sci. Eng. A 513–514: 286–293.

Cho, H.H.W., A. Takaichi, Y. Kajima, H.L. Htat, N. Kittikundecha, T. Hanawa. 2021. Effect of post-heat treatment cooling conditions on microstructures and fatigue properties of cobalt chromium molybdenum alloy fabricated through selective laser melting. Metals 11: 1005.

Cipriano, C.A., P.S. Issack, B. Beksac, A.G. Della Valle, T.P. Sculco and E.A. Salvati. 2008. Metallosis after metal-on-polyethylene total hip arthroplasty. Am. J. Orthop. 37: E18–E25.

Clemow, A.J.T. and B.L. Daniell. 1979. Solution treatment behavior of Co–Cr–Mo alloy. J. Biomed. Mater. Res. 13: 265–279.

Cohen, J., R.F. Mose and J. Wulff. 1978. Recommended heat treatment and alloy additions for cast Co–Cr surgical implants. J. Biomed. Mater. Res. 12: 935–937.

Czekaj, J., M. Ehlinger, M. Rahme and F. Bonnomet. 2016. Metallosis and cobalt–chrome intoxication after hip resurfacing arthroplasty. Orthop. Sci. 21: 389–394.

Dobbs, H.S. and J.L.M. Robertson. 1983. Heat treatment of cast Co–Cr–Mo for orthopaedic implant use. J. Mater. Sci. 18: 391–401.

EN 1911:1999. 1999. Reference test method for release of nickel from products intended to come into direct and prolonged contact with the skin. European Standard.

Hallab, N.J., F.W. Frank Chan and M.L. Harper. 2012. Quantifying subtle but persistent peri-spine inflammation *in vivo* to submicron cobalt–chromium alloy particles. Eur. Spine J. 21: 2649–2658.

Hanawa, T., S. Hiromoto and K. Asami. 2001. Characterization of the surface oxide film of a Co–Cr–Mo alloy after being located in quasi-biological environments using XPS. Appl. Surf. Sci. 183: 68–75.

Hanawa, T., K. Nakazawa, K. Kano, S. Hiromoto, Y. Suzuki and A. Chiba. 2005. Friction-wear properties of nitrogen-ion-implanted nickel-free Co–Cr–Mo alloy. Mater Trans. 46: 1593–1596.

Hanawa, T. 2022. Biocompatibility of titanium from the viewpoint of its surface. Sci. Technol. Adv. Mater. 23: 457–472.

Hiromoto, S., E. Onodera, A. Chiba, K. Asami and T. Hanawa. 2005. Microstructure and corrosion behaviour in biological environments of the newforged low-Ni Co–Cr–Mo alloys. Biomaterials 26: 4912–4923.

ISO 22674:2022. 2022. Dentistry — Metallic materials for fixed and removable restorations and appliances. International Organization for Standardization, Geneva, Switzerland.

Ikeda, T., K. Takahashi, T. Kabata, D. Sakagoshi, K. Tomita and M. Yamada. 2010. Polyneuropathy caused by cobalt–chromium metallosis after total hip replacement. Muscle Nerve. 42: 140–143.

Kajima Y., A. Takaichi, N. Kittikundecha, H.L. Htat, H.H.W. Cho, Y. Tsutsumi et al. 2020. Dent. Mater. 37: e98–e108.

Kilner, T., R.M. Pilliar, G.C. Weatherly and C. Allibert. 1982. Phase identification and incipient melting in a cast Co–Cr surgical implant alloy. J. Biomed. Mater. Res. 16: 63–79.

Konieczny, B., A. Szczesio-Wlodarczyk, J. Sokolowski and K. Bociong. 2020. Challenges of Co–Cr alloy additive manufacturing methods in dentistry—the current state of knowledge (systematic review). Materials 13: 3524.

Kurosu, S., N. Nomura and A. Chiba. 2007. Microstructure and mechanical properties of Co–29Cr–Mo alloy aged at 1023K. Mater. Trans. 48: 1517–1522.

Lee, S.H., E. Takahashi, N. Nomura and A. Chiba. 2006. Effect of carbon addition on microstructure and mechanical properties of a wrought Co–Cr–Mo implant alloy. Mater. Trans. 47: 287–290.

Lee, S.H., N. Nomura and A. Chiba. 2007. Effect of Fe addition on microstructures and mechanical properties of Ni- and C-free Co–Cr–Mo alloys. Mater. Trans. 48: 2207–2211.

López, H.F. and A.J. Saldivar-Garcia: Martensitic transformation in a cast Co–Cr–Mo–C alloy. Metall. Mater. Trans. 39A: 8–18.

Ma, L. and J. Niu. 2019. A comparison of corrosion behaviors of additive manufacturing cobalt-chromium alloy in different solutions. Metall. Res. Technol. 116: 311.

Mace, A., P. Khullar, C. Bouknight and J.L. Gilbert. 2022. Corrosion properties of low carbon CoCrMo and additively manufactured CoCr alloys for dental applications. Dent. Mater. 38: 1184–1193.

Maruyama, N., H. Kawasaki, A. Yamamoto, S. Hiromoto, H. Imai and T. Hanawa. 2005. Friction-wear properties of nickel-free Co–Cr–Mo alloy in a simulated body fluid. Mater. Trans. 46: 1588–1592.

McIntyre, N.S., E.V. Murphy and D.G. Zetaruk. 1979. X-Ray photoelectron spectroscopic study of the aqueous oxidation of stellite-6 alloy. Surf. Interface Anal. 1: 105–110.

Montero-Ocampo, C., M. Talavera and H. Lopez. 1999. Effect of alloy preheating on the mechanical properties of as-cast Co–Cr–Mo–C alloys. Metall. Mater. Trans. 30A: 611–620.

Morral, F.R. 1966. Cobalt alloys as implants in humans. J. Mater. 1: 384–421.

Murakami, M., N. Nomura, H. Doi, Y. Tsutsumi, H. Nakamura, A. Chiba and T. Hanawa. 2010. Microstructures of Zr–added Co–Cr–Mo alloy compacts fabricated with a metal injection molding process and their metal release in 1 mass% lactic acid. Mater. Trans. 51: 1281–1287.

Nagai, A., Y. Tsutsumi, Y. Suzuki, K. Katayama, T. Hanawa and K. Yamashita. 2012. Characterization of air-formed surface oxide film on a Co–Ni–Cr–Mo alloy (MP35N) and its change in Hanks' solution. Appl. Surf. Sci. 258: 5490–5498.

Nishiyama, Z. 2012. Martensitic Transformation: Academic Press, Cambridge, MA, USA.

Numata, Y., B. Syuto, N. Nomura and A. Chiba. 2007. Cytocompatibility for Co–Cr–Mo alloy with a small amount of zirconium or carbon. J. Jpn. Inst. Metal. 71: 578–585.

Odaira, T., S. Xu, K. Hirata, X. Xu, T. Omori, K. Ueki et al. 2022. Flexible and tough superelastic Co–Cr alloys for biomedical applications. Adv. Mater. 34: 2202305.

Oliveira, C.A., I.S. Candelária, P.B. Oliveira, A. Figueiredo and F. Caseiro-Alves. 2015. Metallosis: A diagnosis not only in patients with metal-on-metal prostheses. Eur. J. Radiol. Open 2: 3–6.

Sims, C.T., N.S. Stoloff and Hagel, W.C. 1987. Cast intermetallic alloys and composites based on them by combined centrifugal casting—SHS process. pp. 135–162. *In*: Sims, C.T., N.S. Stoloff and W.C. Hagel [eds.]. Superalloys II: High-Temperature Materials for Aerospace and Industrial Power, John Wiley & Sons, New York, USA.

Smith, D.C., R.M. Pilliar, J.B. Metson and N.S. McIntyre. 1991. Dental implant materials. II. Preparative procedures and surface spectroscopic studies. J. Biomed. Mater. Res. 25: 1069–1084.

Sorp, S. and R. Holm. 1977. ESCA investigation of the oxide layers on some Cr containing alloys. Surf. Sci. 68: 10–19.

Stenlund, P., S. Kurosu, Y. Koizumi, F. Suska, H. Matsumoto, A. Chiba et al. 2015. Osseointegration Enhancement by Zr doping of Co-Cr-Mo implants fabricated by electron beam melting. Addit. Manuf. 6: 6–15.

Sun, S.H., Y. Koizumi, S. Kurosu, Y.P. Li and A. Chiba. 2015. Phase and grain size inhomogeneity and their influences on creep behavior of Co–Cr–Mo alloy additive manufactured by electron beam melting. Acta Mater. 86: 305–318.

Takaichi, A., Suyalatu, N. Nakamoto, N. Joko, N. Nomura, Y. Tsutsumi et al. 2013. Microstructures and mechanical properties of Co–29Cr–6Mo alloy fabricated by selective laser melting process for dental applications. J. Mech. Behav. Biomed. Mater. 21: 67–76.

Taylor, R.N.J. and R.B. Waterhouse. 1983. A study of the ageing behaviour of a cobalt based implant alloy. J. Mater. Sci. 18: 3265–3280.

Teague, J., E. Cerreta and M. Stout. 2004. Tensile properties and microstructure of Haynes 25 alloy after aging at elevated temperatures for extended times. Metall. Mater. Trans. 35A: 2767–2781.

Tsustumi, Y., H. Doi, N. Nomura, M. Ashida, P. Chen, A. Kawasaki et al. 2016. Surface composition and corrosion resistance of Co–Cr alloys containing high chromium, Mater. Trans. 57: 2033–2040.

Ueki, K., K. Ueda, M. Nakai, T. Nakano and T. Narushima. 2018. Microstructural changes during plastic deformation and corrosion properties of biomedical Co-20Cr-15W-10Ni alloy heat-treated at 873 K. Metall. Mater. Trans. A 49: 2393–2404.

Ueki, K., M. Abe, K. Ueda, M. Nakai, T. Nakano and T. Narushima. 2019. Synchronous improvement in strength and ductility of biomedical Co–Cr–Mo alloys by unique low-temperature heat treatment. Mater. Sci. Eng. A 739: 53–61.

Ueki, K., M. Kasamatsu, K. Ueda, Y. Koizumi, D. Wei, A. Chiba et al. 2020. Precipitation during γ-ε phase transformation in biomedical Co-Cr-Mo alloys fabricated by electron beam melting. Metals 10: 71.

Wei, D., Y. Koizumi, A. Chiba, K. Ueki, K. Ueda, T. Narushima et al. 2018. Heterogeneous microstructures and corrosion resistance of biomedical Co-Cr-Mo alloy fabricated by electron beam melting (EBM). Additive Manufact. 24: 103–114.

Wei, D., A. Anniyear, Y. Koizumi, K. Aoyagi, N. Nagasako, H. Kato et al. 2019. On microstructural homogenization and mechanical properties optimization of biomedical Co-Cr-Mo alloy additively manufactured by using electron beam melting. Addit. Manuf. 28: 215–227.

Yamanaka, K., M. Mori, S. Kurosu, H. Matsumoto and A. Chiba. 2009. Ultrafine grain refinement of biomedical Co-29Cr-6Mo alloy during conventional hot-compression deformation. Metall. Mater, Trans. A 40: 1980–2009.

CHAPTER 8

Stainless Steels

8.1 Introduction

Stainless steel, also known as inox, corrosion-resistant steel (CRES), or rustless steel, is an alloy of Fe that is resistant to rusting and corrosion. It contains at least 10.5%Cr and sometimes Ni, and may also contain other elements, such as C, to obtain the desired properties (Davis 1994). The corrosion resistance of stainless steel results from the Cr, which forms a passive film that can protect the material and self-heal in the presence of oxygen. Stainless steel was industrialized in 1912–1913. It was discovered that in order to obtain corrosion resistance, it was necessary to add a certain amount of Cr to a low-C steel, and the results of academic research by many predecessors contribute to industrial production of stainless steels. Even thereafter, stainless steel has been improved many times and is still being developed today. Performance of stainless steel has improved significantly continuously, and even for products with the same specifications, the performance is significantly different from what it was several decades ago. Comprehensive outline and details of stainless steel is referred from handbook (ASM Handbook 2023). Stainless steel is an essential material for the bodies of medical devices, treatment instruments, and surgical instruments. In addition, type 316L stainless steel is mainly used as an implant material. Although its corrosion resistance is inferior to Ti materials and Co-based alloys, its elongation to fracture and tortional resistance is large, making it an indispensable material for ligation wires.

8.2 Category

Different types of stainless steel are labeled with American Iron and Steel Institute (AISI) three-digit numbers (ASM International 2000). The ISO standard lists the chemical compositions of stainless steels of the specifications in existing ISO, ASTM, EN, JIS, and GB standards in a useful interchange table (ISO 15510:2014). Stainless steel is not corroded under an oxygen-containing atmosphere, but is locally corroded and sometimes forms pits in chloride solutions such as body fluids. Ni, Mo, Cu, Ti, Nb, N, etc., are added to stainless steels to improve their corrosion resistance, heat resistance, strength, and workability. The metallurgical structure, strength, and corrosion resistance of stainless steels depend on the concentrations of Ni and Cr.

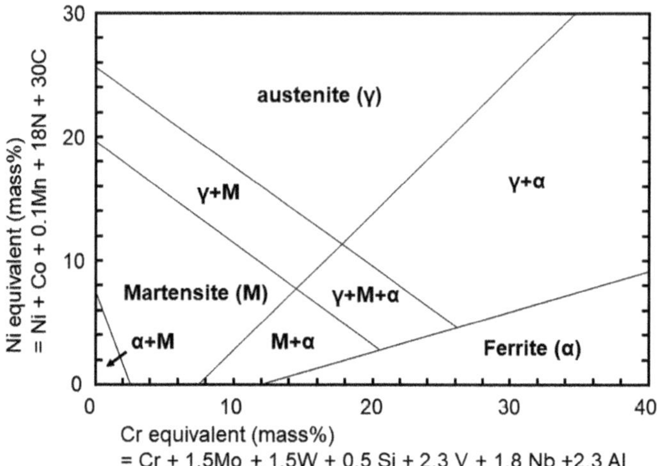

Fig. 8.1. Schaeffler diagram. The crystal phase of stainless steel is determined by the Cr equivalent and Ni equivalent of the additional elements.

Stainless steels are basically categorised as ferritic (Fe–Cr system), martensitic (Fe–Cr system), austenitic (Fe–Cr–Ni system), austenitic-ferritic (duplex), and precipitation hardening, according to their crystal phase, as shown by Schaeffler diagram (Pickering 1978, Schneider 1960) (Fig. 8.1). To improve the corrosion resistance of stainless steels, mainly three techniques are employed: the decrease of C content, the increase of Cr content, and the addition of Mo. The categories of popular stainless steel series are summarized in Fig. 8.2. Austenitic-type stainless steels have outstanding corrosion resistance, but do not have great strength. Therefore, austenitic stainless steels are strengthened by working and heat treatment and hardened with the addition of N. In addition, the addition of Mo improves their corrosion resistance, because their passive film becomes more stable. Properties of ferritic, martensitic, and autenitic stainless are compared in Table 8.1. In AISI numbering, the 200 series represents the Fe–Cr–Ni– Mn alloy system, the 300 series represents the Fe–Cr–Ni alloy system, the 400 series represents the Fe–Cr system, and the 600 series represents precipitation hardening type.

8.3 Stainless Steels for Medical Devices

The majority of stainless steels used for the stems of artificial hip joints and bone fixators are replaced by Ti alloys due to their lower corrosion resistance. However, stainless steel is still utilized for retrievable internal bone fixators and sternal and bone fixation wires due to its superior torsional property and elongation to fracture. Table 8.2 shows the types of stainless steel and their main medical uses. Stainless steel is used not only for implants but also for medical instruments such as injection needles, scissors, scalpels, and clips.

For implant materials, type 316L austenitic stainless steel is always used. Adding 2.0–3.0 mass% of Mo, increasing Ni from 8.0–10.0 mass% to 12.0–15.0 mass%, and decreasing C to less than 0.030 % increases its corrosion resistance (Hanawa 2019).

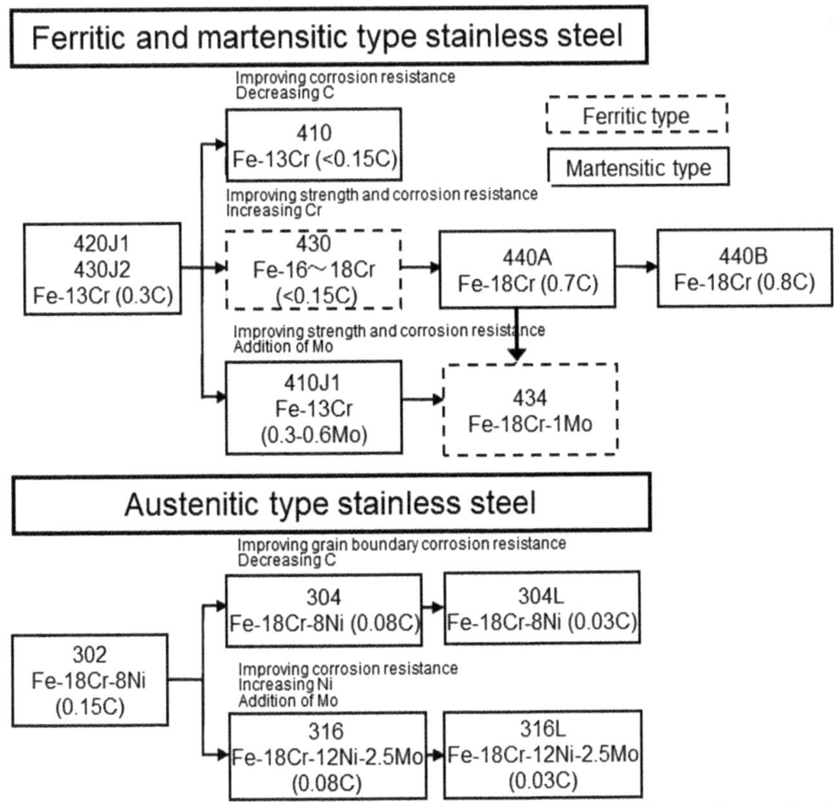

Fig. 8.2. Development progress of stainless steels and the categories of popular stainless steel series. To improve the corrosion resistance of stainless steels, mainly three techniques are employed: the decrease of C content, the increase of Cr content, and the addition of Mo.

Table 8.1. Comparison of representative properties among ferritic, martensitic, and austenitic stainless steels.

Property		Ferritic	Martensitic	Austenitic
Composition range (mass%)		Cr: 11.5–32 Mo: ~ 2.5 Ti: ~ 1 Nb: ~ 1 Cu: ~ 0.8	Cr: 11.5–18 Ni: ~ 0.6 Mo: ~ 0.75 C: ~ 0.75	Cr: 15–26 Ni: 3.5–28 Mo: ~ 7 Cu: ~ 3 Si: ~ 5 N: ~ 0.4
Corrosion resistance		Fair to Excellent	Fair to Good	Good to Excellent
Mechanical property	Strength	Fair	Good to Excellent	Fair to Good
	Toughness	Fair to Good	Poor to Good	Excellent
Heat resistance	Strength	Fair	Good to Excellent	Good to Excellent
	Oxidation resistance	Fair to excellent	Fair to Good	Good to Excellent
Applicability	Weldabilty	Fair to Good	Poor to Good	Excellent
	Workability	Good to Excellent	Poor to Fair	Good to Excellent

Table 8.2. Types, compositions, and application of representative stainless steels for medical devices (Data from ASTM).

Type	Composition (mass%)			Application example
	Cr	Ni	Other elements	
Austenitic system				
Type 304	18–20	8.0–10.5		Needle
Type 304L	18–22	9–13	< 0.030C	
Type 316	16–18	10–14	2–3Mo, < 0.08C	Tweezers; Scissors; Drill
Type 316L	16–18	12–15	2–3Mo, < 0.030C	Implant
Type 301	16–18	6–8		Handle, Drill
ASTM F1314	20.50–23.50	11.50–13.50	0.20–0.40N, 2.000–3.00Mo, 0.10–0.30Nb, 0.10–0.30V	Implant
ASTM F1586	19.5–22.0	9.0–11.0	0.25–0.50N, 2.0–3.0Mo, 0.25–0.80Nb	Implant
ASTM F2229	19.00–23.00	< 0.05	0.85–1.10N, 0.50–1.50Mo	Implant (Ni–free stainless steel)
XM–19	22.0	12.5	2.50Mo, 0.3N, 0.2V	Implant
Ortron 90	21.50	9.00	4.00Mn, 2.60Mo, 0.39N, 0.30Nb	Implant
Martensitic system				
Type 420J1	12.00–14.00	–	0.16–0.25C	Tweezers; Forceps; Sonde; Suture Hook; Drill; Scissors; Knife
Type 420J2	12.00–14.00	–	0.26–0.40C	
Feritic system				
Type 430F	16.00–18/00	–		Handle; Screw; Nut
Precipitation hardening system				
Type 630	15.00–17.50	3.00–5.00	3.00–5.00Cu, 0.15–0.45Nb	Clip; Staple
Type 631	16.00–18.00	6.50–7.75	0.75–1.50Al	
COP–1	19–21	19–21	19–21Co, 3.5–4.5Mo	Implant

"L" means "low carbon content". The composition and mechanical property of type 316L stainless steel are summarised in Tables 8.3. The presence of Mo reduces both the nucleation number and size of metastable pits. This is due to the bonding strength of the passive film to the substrate metal and the elimination of active pitting sites caused by the formation of molybdates or molybdenum oxyhyroxides (Ilevbare and Burstein 2001). In the case of type 316L stainless steel, solution treatment is carried out, followed by rapid cooling (such as water cooling), after the products have been

Table 8.3. Composition and mechanical property of type 316L stainless steel solution treated and annealed.

Composition (mass%)								
C	P	S	Si	Mn	Cr	Ni	Mo	Fe
< 0.03	< 0.045	< 0.03	< 1.0	< 2.00	16.0–18.0	12.0–15.0	2.0–3.0	Bal.
Tensile strength (MPa)			Offset yield strength (MPa)			Elongation (%)		
> 480			> 175			> 40		

heated to 1010–1150°C. This heat treatment causes the disappearnce of precipitates, as well as the release of strains which were induced during rolling. The release of strain energy causes recrystallization of the structures. Metallic biomaterials must possess essential prerequisite properties such as corrosion resistance, strength, toughness, and ductility. As explained above, these properties can be achieved through chemical composition, heat treatment, and working such as forging and rolling.

8.4 History of Stainless Steels for Medical Devices

Metals have great strength and are easy to form, so they have been used in medicine to maintain the structure of the human body by fixing them since ancient times. As for Fe-based materials, stainless steel, which is relatively safe, has been introduced after Ni-plated steel and V steel. The first stainless steel used for implants was type 302 alloy. Thereafter in 1926, type 316 alloy, which had better corrosion resistance in chloride solutions, began to be used. To further improve corrosion resistance in chloride solutions, type 316L alloy was developed in 1950 by reducing the C content of type 316 alloy to less than 0.03%, and this is still the mainstay for implants. Subsequently, N-containing austenitic stainless steel was developed that had superior corrosion resistance and mechanical properties compared to type 316L stainless steel. In the late 1990s, research and development of so-called Ni-free austenitic stainless steels, which do not contain Ni causing metal allergies, became active. Early Ni-free austenitic stainless steels contained a large amount of N as a substitute for Ni, as well as a large amount of Mn (Niinomi 2001). In the 2000s, various N-containing austenitic stainless steels were registered in ASTM standards for biological use. For example, high Mn, high N, and Ni-free stainless steels were standardized (ASTM F2229-21:2021) (Table 8.4). Since then, research and development of a manufacturing process for Ni- and Mn-free N-containing austenitic stainless steel has been progressing (Sumita et al. 2004).

8.5 Mechanical Property of Stainless Steels for Medical Devices

Figure 8.3 shows the standard tensile strength and minimum elongation to fracture of stainless steels registered with ASTM for use in implants and type 316L stainless steel. Ni in Fe–Cr–Ni series, which tends to cause metal allergies, is replaced with Mn, an element that stabilizes the austenite phase, developing the Fe–Cr–Mn series. In the Fe–Cr–Mn system, 0.5 mass% or more of N is added to stabilize the austenite phase. Austenitic stainless steel is not heat treatable, but it can be strengthened and hardened

Table 8.4. Chemical composition of ASTM registered biomedical stainless steels and type 316L stainless steel (Data from ASTM).

Alloys	C	Mn	P	S	Si	Cr	Ni	Mo	N	Cu	Nb	V	Fe
F138–08 Wrought F139–08 Wrought F1350–08 Wrought F2257–03 Wrought Fe–18Cr–14Ni–2.5Mo	< 0.030	< 2.00	< 0.025	< 0.010	< 0.75	17.00–19.00	13.00–15.00	2.25–3.00	< 0.10	< 0.50			Bal.
F745–07 Cast Fe–18Cr–12.5Ni–2.5Mo	< 0.06	< 2.0	< 0.045	< 0.030	< 1.0	16.50–19.00	11.00–14.50	2.00–3.00	< 0.20	< 0.50			Bal.
F1314–07 Wrought Fe–22Cr–13Ni–5Mn–2.5Mo	< 0.030	4.00–6.00	< 0.025	< 0.010	< 0.75	20.50–23.50	11.50–13.50	2.00–3.00	0.20–0.40	< 0.50	0.10–0.30	0.10–0.30	Bal.
F1586–08 Wrought Fe–21Cr–10Ni–3Mn–2.5Mo	< 0.08	2.00–4.25	< 0.025	< 0.01	< 0.75	19.5–22.0	9.0–11.0	2.00–3.00	0.25–0.50	< 0.25	0.25–0.80		Bal.
F2229–07 Wrought Fe–23Mn–21Cr–1Mo	< 0.080	21.00–24.00	< 0.03	< 0.01	< 0.75	19.00–23.00	< 0.05	0.50–1.50	0.85–1.10	< 0.25			Bal.
F2581–07 Wrought Fe–11Mn–17Cr–3Mo	0.15–0.25	9.50–12.50	< 0.02	< 0.01	0.20–0.60	16.50–18.00	< 0.05	2.70–3.70	0.45–0.55	< 0.25			Bal.
Type 316L	< 0.03	< 2.00	< 0.045	< 0.03	< 1.00	16.0–18.0	12.0–15.0	2.0–3.0					Bal.

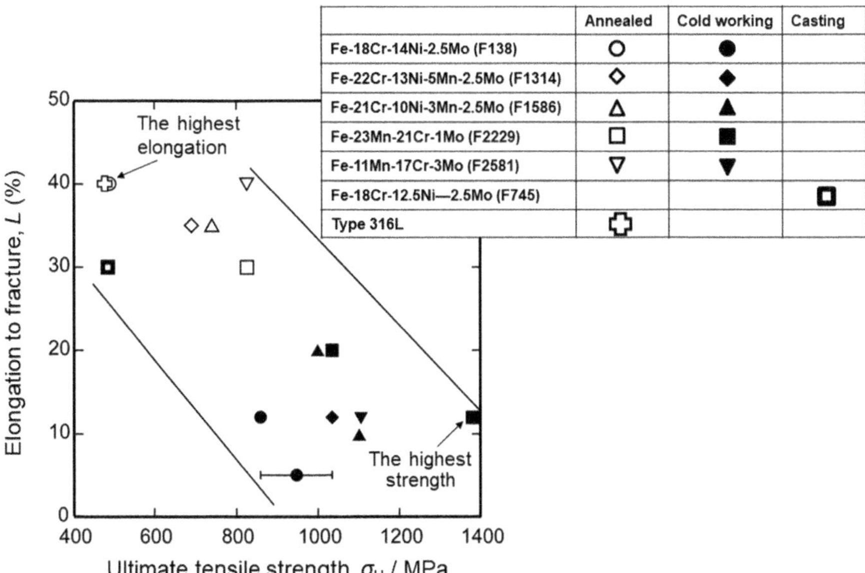

Fig. 8.3. Tensile strength and elongation at break of ASTM registered stainless steel and type 316L steel (Provided by Dr. Takayuki Narushima, Tohoku University).

by cold working (ASM Handbook 2023). The hardening of austenitic stainless steels due to cold working is related to the formation of stress-induced martensite. The more unstable the austenite phase is, the greater the increase in strength and hardness is. Taking advantage of this property, materials such as type 304 stainless steel are used as materials for injection needles. However, the formation of martensite due to cooling after cold working or heat treatment is undesirable from the viewpoint of MRI contrastability and ductility when applied as an implant.

The strength of austenitic stainless steel depends on alloying elements and grain size, and the following formula for its 0.2% offset yield stress was proposed (Pickling 1978).

$$0.2\%\ \text{offset yield stress (MPa)} = 15.4\times(4.4 + 23[\mathrm{C}] + 1.3[\mathrm{Si}] + 0.24[\mathrm{Cr}] + 0.94[\mathrm{Mo}] + 1.2[\mathrm{V}] + 0.29[\mathrm{W}] + 2.6[\mathrm{Nb}] + 1.7[\mathrm{To}] + 0.82[\mathrm{Al}] + 32[\mathrm{N}] + 0.16[\delta\ \text{ferritic pahse amount (vol\%)}] + 0.46[d(\mathrm{mm})]^{-1/2}) \quad (8.1)$$

The element concentration is expressed in mass%, and d is the crystal grain size. Composition-dependent formulas for tensile strength and area reduction rate is induced by equation (8.1).

Although austenitic stainless steel has problems with localized corrosion such as pitting corrosion, intergranular corrosion, and stress corrosion cracking, it basically has excellent corrosion resistance, excellent ductility, and nonmagnetic properties at room temperature. Although it has been replaced by Ti alloys, there is still great demand for implants that take advantage of its excellent ductility.

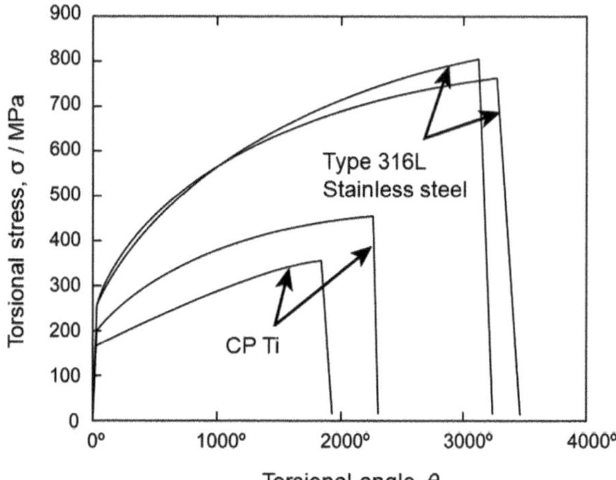

Fig. 8.4. Torsion test results for type 316L stainless steel and CP Ti sternal wires. CP Ti wires fracture with half rotation angle of type 316L stainless steels.

Figure 8.4 shows the torsion test results for commercially available sternal wires made of type 316L stainless steel and CP Ti. Stainless steel wire has a larger rotation angle to fracture and torsional strength than CP Ti wire. For this reason, austenitic stainless steel is used as a wire that is used in a ligated state.

In addition to austenitic stainless steel, there are ferritic and martensitic stainless steels. Martensitic stainless steel contains 11.5 to 18 mass% Cr and is used after being hardened and tempered. By quenching, a martensitic structure with high strength and hardness is obtained. In particular, type 440A and type 440B alloys, which contain 0.65 to 0.95 mass%C and 16 to 17 mass%Cr, are usually used in surgical scalpels.

8.6 Magnetism

Magnetic attachments used in dental prostheses that use the attractive force of magnets for retention force use Sm–Co alloys and Ne–Fe–B alloys as magnets in the dentures, and they are attracted to stainless steels implanted in tooth by the magnetic force of the magnets. Ferritic magnetic stainless steels (type 444, type XM27, and type 447J1) with excellent corrosion resistance is used for the side yoke and the yoke that covers the magnet. Austenitic stainless steel is paramagnetic, while when plastic strain is applied through cold working, stress-induced martensite is formed and it may become ferromagnetic. Figure 8.5 shows the change in magnetic permeability with cold rolling reduction for type 316 and type 304 stainless steels (Stainless Steel Handbook 1995c). Magnetic permeability increases as the rolling reduction increases, and this increase is remarkable in type 304 stainless steel, which has a low austenitic phase stability. As mentioned above, due to its excellent ductility, stainless steel is being considered for application in wires and ultrafine wires used in the human body (Narushima et al. 2005). Changes in magnetic properties due to cold rolling and cold drawing are being considered. The temperature at which 50% of

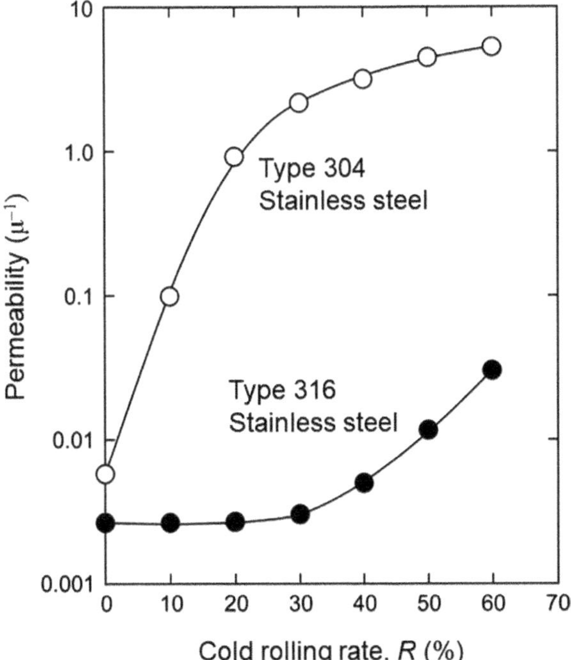

Fig. 8.5. Effect of cold rolling rate on magnetic permeability (Reprinted with permission from Japan Stainless Steel Association, *Stainless Steel Handbook, 3rd ed.* 1995, 569.).

crystals becomes martensite when a true strain of 0.30 is applied by cold working as M_{d30}, and expressed it as a function of alloy composition using the following equation (Angle 1954).

$$M_{d30}(°C) = 413 - 462[C+N] - 9.2[Si] - 8.1[Mn] - 13.7[Cr] - 9.5[Ni] - 18.5[Mo] \quad \text{(mass\%)} \tag{8.2}$$

Addition of C and N is effective for preventing stress-induced martensite formation, but martensite may be formed by cooling after heat treatment. The martensitic transformation temperature (Ms) of austenitic stainless steel is expressed by the following formula. Martensitic stainless steel contains 11.5 to 18% Cr and is used after being hardened and tempered. By quenching, a martensitic structure with high strength and hardness is obtained. In particular, type 440A and type 440B stainless steels, which contain 0.65 to 0.95% C and 16 to 17% Cr, are used for surgical scalpels.

$$M_s(°C) = 502 - 810[C] - 1230[N] - 13[Mn] - 30[Ni] - 12[Cr] - 54[Cu] - 46[Mo] \quad \text{(mass\%)} \tag{8.3}$$

8.7 Corrosion Resistance

Anodic polarization of stainless steel in saline has been investigated for a long time (Schmid and Hackerman 1961). In the human body, the presence of inorganic ions, cells, and proteins, the production of active oxygen by phagocytes, and low equilibrium oxygen partial pressure affect the surface reactions of metals. Chloride ions cause pitting corrosion in stainless steel. When cells adhere to a stainless steel surface, the area near the interface between the cells and the material is thought to become a site of crevice corrosion (see Subsection 2.11.3 and Figs. 2.11B and Fig. 2.22). Low equilibrium oxygen partial pressure inhibits the regeneration of the passive film and reduces the corrosion resistance of stainless steel. Stainless steel has a lower Cr content compared to Co–Cr–Mo alloys, which may reduce its corrosion resistance in biological environments.

In biological environments, type 316L stainless steel typically exhibits pitting corrosion due to anodic polarization, as shown in Figs. 3.10 and 6.11. Severe crevice corrosion of spinal rods is observed in the human body (Akazawa et al. 2005) (Fig. 5.10). In addition, severe pitting corrosion is observed on sternal wires implanted for over 30 years (Tomizawa et al. 2006) (Fig. 5.9). Non-metallic inclusions in stainless steel are known to be harmful and become the nucleus for pitting corrosion (Stainless Steel Handbook 1995b). Manganese sulfide (MnS) inclusions are particularly harmful for pittingcorrosion. Consequently, the corrosion resistance of type 316L stainless steel is considerably less than that of Ti and Ti alloys.

The corrosion resistance of stainless steel in the human body is due to the passive film that forms on its surface in an aqueous environment. The passive film formed on the stainless steel surface is several-nm thick and has an amorphous structure containing bound water enriched with Cr. Figure 8.6 shows the anodic polarization curve of type 304 stainless steel in 1 N-H_2SO_4 solution in comparison with Fe, Cr, and Ni (Fujimoto et al. 2001, Stainless Steel Handbook 1995a, Shibata and Okamoto 1972). It can be seen that Cr is greatly involved in the appearance of the passive region in stainless steel. All stainless steels registered with ASTM for medical use (Table 8.4) are austenitic, and the main alloying elements are Cr, Ni, Mo, Mn, and nitrogen. Although Cr is a ferrite phase stabilizing element, it promotes passivation and is effective in improving corrosion resistance in acids and pitting corrosion resistance. Ni is a stabilizing element for austenite phase that stabilizes the passive film and improves corrosion resistance in non-oxidizing solutions, but Ni may exhibit toxicity such as metal allergy. Mo not only contributes to the stability of the passive film but also improves pitting corrosion resistance in chloride solutions. Pitting corrosion is a typical localized corrosion in the presence of chloride ions, such as in the human body, and the simultaneous addition of 30% or more Cr and 3% or more Mo is effective.

The passive film on stainless steel has a two-layer structure, with the outer layer consisting of hydroxide and the inner layer consisting of oxide (Tsuchiya et al. 2004, Fujimoto et al. 2007). Trivalent chromium ions (Cr^{3+}) are concentrated in the inner layer oxide, and the stainless steel base and coating are thought to be bonded through oxide ions (OH^-). It is believed that this inner layer oxide is primarily responsible for the corrosion resistance of the passive film. The passive film is a non-stoichiometric

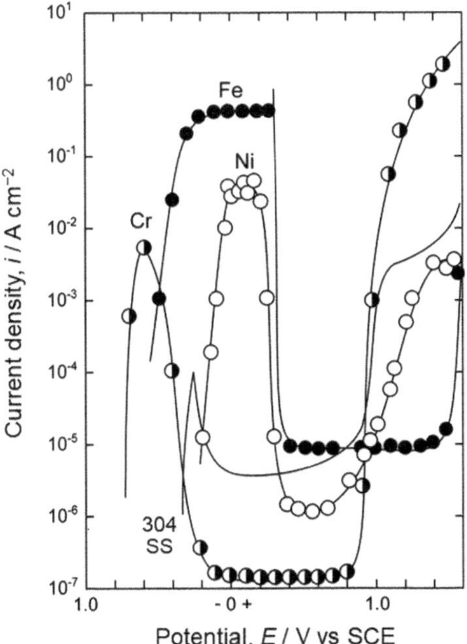

Fig. 8.6. Anodic polarization curves of type 304 stainless steel (SS) and its component metals (Fe, Cr, and Ni) in 1-N H_2SO_4 at 298 K (Reprinted with permission from Japan Stainless Steel Association, *Stainless Steel Handbook, 3rd ed.* 1995, 253.). Cr is the most effective element to appear in the passive state of the stainless steel.

compound and does not have a well-defined crystal structure. The higher the amount of Cr, the more it exhibits amorphous properties.

In austenitic stainless steel, carbide $Cr_{23}C_6$ precipitates at the grain boundaries due to short-time heating at 673 to 1073 K followed by slow cooling. A Cr-depleted zone is generated in the adjacent area, making intergranular corrosion more likely (Fig. 8.7). Therefore, reducing carbon content is effective in improving intergranular corrosion resistance (see Subsection 2.11.5). The phenomenon of increased intergranular corrosion is called "sensitization". Intergranular corrosion resistance can be improved by adding Nb and Ti and forming these carbides within the grains.

N is an effective additive element in stainless steel from the following viewpoints (Osozawa 1998).

I. Substitution of nickel as an austenite phase stabilizing element.
II. Improvement of strength.
III. Improvement of resistance to localized corrosion such as pitting corrosion in chloride environments.

From the perspective of medical applications, it is hoped that N will replace Ni, which is expensive and has concerns about its toxicity. The mechanism of the improvement of local corrosion is that N becomes NH^{4+}, prevents the pH drop in the pit or crevice, concentrates at the metal substrate-passive film interface and on the active surface, and forms dense oxide-nitride in the passive film. It has been reported

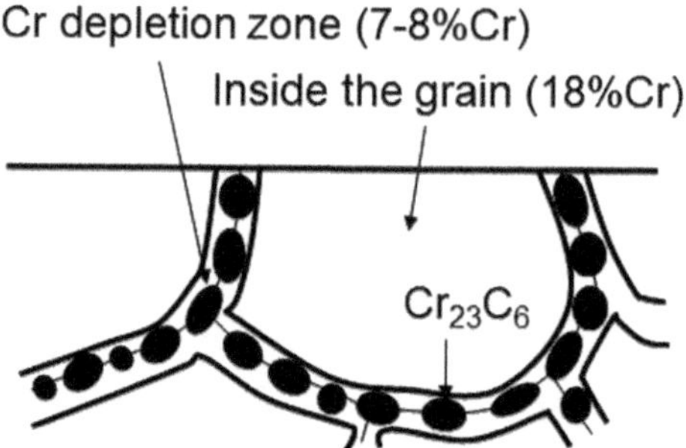

Fig. 8.7. Grain boundaries of sensitized type 304 stainless steel by the formation of carbide in the Cr depletion zone.

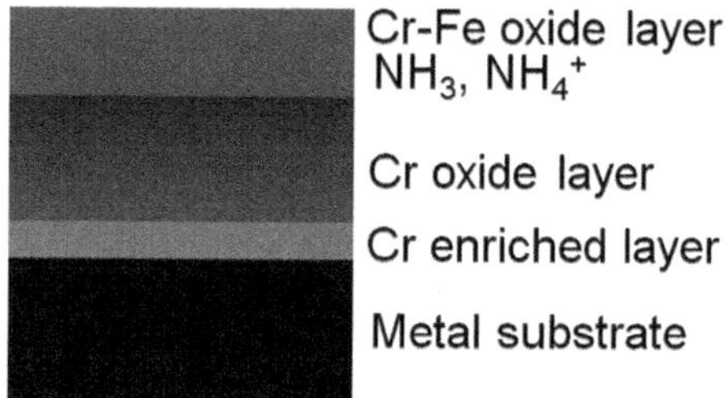

Fig. 8.8. Structure of surface oxide layer of high N stainless steel.

that NO^{3-} forms, dissolves as NO^{3-}, and acts as an inhibitor (Matsushima et al. 1998). The schematic model of the surface oxide layer on high N stainless steel is shown in Fig. 8.8. The pitting resistance equivalent (PRE) of stainless steel is expressed by equation (8.4) using the main active ingredients Cr, Mo, and N concentrations (Osozawa 1998).

$$\mathrm{PRE} = [\mathrm{Cr}] + 3.3[\mathrm{Mo}] + n[\mathrm{N}]\ (\mathrm{mass\%}) \tag{8.4}$$

Element concentrations are expressed in mass%. n is believed to be approximately 10 to 30, with reports of n being 20 (Uggowitzer et al. 1996) and 25 (Manzel et al. 1996). Although Mn is an element that stabilizes the austenite phase, it may reduce the corrosion resistance of stainless steel. Since high-N and high-Mn austenitic stainless steel is important as a biomaterial, equation (8.4) has also been reported, in which n in equation (8.5) is set to 30 and the negative effect of Mn is taken into account (Rndelli et al. 1995).

$$\mathrm{PRE_{Mn}} = [\mathrm{Cr}] + 3.3[\mathrm{Mo}] + 30[\mathrm{N}] - [\mathrm{Mn}]\ (\mathrm{mass\%}) \tag{8.5}$$

$\mathrm{PRE_{Mn}} > 45$ is required for localized corrosion resistance.

Stress corrosion cracking, which is considered to be a weak point of austenitic stainless steel, is caused by a combination of three factors: environmental factors, stress factors, and material factors. Defects formed by partial destruction of the passive film due to stress induces localized corrosion such as pitting corrosion or intergranular corrosion in the presence of chloride ions.

8.8 Improvement of Corrosion Resistance by Additive Manufacturing

The relationship between the microstructure of building objects by additive manufacturing (AM) and corrosion has been reported based on a number of research papers. Stainless steel materials manufactured by AM differs from wrought and cast materials in terms of solute segregation, defects at the atomic level and nm level such as dislocations, defects at the μm and mm levels such as holes and cracks, and residual stress. The AM process has a significant effect on corrosion resistance. Specifically, the pitting potential of type 316L stainless steel formed by selective laser melting (SLM) in a 0.6-M NaCl aqueous solution is much higher than that of wrought material (Sander et al. 2018). In austenitic stainless steel, rapid cooling in the AM process improves pitting corrosion resistance by suppressing the formation of MnS inclusions, but the behavior of erosion and intergranular corrosion is still controversial (Haghdadi et al. 2021). By analyzing the corrosion behavior of stainless steel due to differences in AM process conditions, steel types, and environments, the main factors that affect the corrosion behavior of stainless steel formed by the AM process are extracted. In SLM-built type 316L stainless steel, scan speed, laser power, and laser energy density influence grain size and void formation, which are important parameters for corrosion. In addition, the post-built heat treatment influences passive film composition and stability and repassivation potential. In type 316L stainless steel fabricated by direct laser deposition (DLD), the effect of heat treatment on the Cr concentration in the passive film has been studied (Ko et al. 2021).

AM is a dynamic non-equilibrium process, and the microstructure of the built stainless steel is special, which changes the corrosion behavior. Changes in corrosion behavior are currently not well understood, and there are often contradictions and inconsistencies in the literature. The unique microstructure formed during the AM process influences corrosion, especially localized corrosion, such as pitting, erosion corrosion, intergranular corrosion, fatigue corrosion, and stress corrosion cracking (Laheh et al. 2021).

The following matters were clarified regarding the corrosion resistance behavior of type 316L steel built by the laser powder bet fusion (LPBF) process (Sun et al. 2019, Tsutsumi et al. 2021).

(1) LPBF modeling dramatically improves the local corrosion resistance of type 316L stainless steel in saline.

(2) The excellent local corrosion resistance of LPBF built specimens does not depend on exposed crystal faces and grain boundary density.

(3) The LPBF process suppresses metastable pitting corrosion and does not inhibit the repassivation process.

(4) The presence of only inclusions of approximately 100 nm or less in the LPBF built specimen contributes to the excellent corrosion resistance of the LPBF built specimen because the ultra-rapid cooling of ~ 10^7 K/s in the LPBF process suppresses the growth of inclusions.

The effects of crystal structure and solute segregation on the corrosion behaviors of alloys fabricated by AM have not yet been elucidated for any alloy system. The effects of residual stress, surface roughness, and ultrafine grain structure on the corrosion properties of alloys built by AM are future research topics. At present, there are almost no corrosion studies of stainless steel built objects using AM processes other than SLM and LDL. The parameters that control stainless steel corrosion are heat treatment conditions, building conditions (scan speed, laser power, etc.), and additive elements. Heat treatment is the most important factor that influences the corrosion behavior of stainless steel, not only in the AM process. No comparison of corrosion behavior between stainless steels of the same specification manufactured by different AM processes has been made. Research on the corrosion behavior of stainless steel manufactured by AM will likely increase in the future. In particular, it is important to elucidate the relationship between the unique metallurgical structure and corrosion behavior by the AM process, and it is necessary to continue efforts to improve corrosion resistance by controlling the microstructure and grain boundary density by the AM process.

8.9 Reaction with the Host Body

In the human body, the presence of inorganic ions, proteins, cells, the production of active oxygen by phagocytes, and low equilibrium oxygen partial pressure affect the surface reactions of metals. As mentioned above, chloride ions cause pitting corrosion in stainless steel. When cells adhere to the stainless steel surface, crevice corrosion may occur at the interface between the cells and the material (see Fig. 2.22). Low equilibrium oxygen partial pressure inhibits the reformation of the passive film and reduces the corrosion resistance of stainless steel. Stainless steel has a lower Cr content than Co–Cr–Mo alloys, so its corrosion resistance may decrease depending on the biological environment. According to an evaluation based on electrochemical measurements of type 316L stainless steel under a cell culture, the cells were found to release biomolecules as an extracellular matrix, causing corrosion to occur because the cells themselves act as barriers to the diffusion of dissolved oxygen (Hiromoto and Hanawa 2006a,b). When cathodically polarized in a similar environment, a decrease in oxygen reduction current was observed for both type 316L stainless steel and CP Ti, which is due to the fact that the cells themselves and the extracellular matrix act as diffusion barriers for dissolved oxygen and released metal ions, leading to corrosion behavior.

Auger electron spectroscopy (AES) of the surfaces of type 316L stainless steel pins and wires that had been implanted for 20 to 136 days near cortical bone and bone marrow revealed that Ca and P were incorporated into the passive film (Sundgren et al. 1986). The formation of calcium phosphate was also reported by X-ray photoelectron spectroscopy (XPS) when type 316L stainless steel was immersed for 7 d in Hanks' solution, which simulates the inorganic components of the extracellular matrix in the huma body (Hanawa et al. 2002). The surface reaction of type 316L stainless steel in cell culture has also been investigated, and the presence of mouse-derived fibroblast cells, L929, results in the formation of sulfides and sulfites on the surface of 316L stainless steel. These results suggest that calcium phosphate is formed on stainless steel surfaces as well as CP Ti, but its formation rate is extremely slow and does not lead to hard tissue compatibility like CP Ti, known as osseointegration. Conversely, this also has the advantage that adhesion to bone does not progress in areas where bone fixators are expected to be retrieved after healing.

8.10 Development of Nickel-Free High Nitrogen Stainless Steels

As already mentioned, the addition of N to stainless steel is effective in improving corrosion resistance and mechanical properties. In particular, it is known that while strengthening by cold working inevitably reduces ductility, adding N causes less reduction in ductility. Austenitic stainless steel that contains 0.3 mass% or more of N is recognized to be a high-N stainless steel. There are two methods for adding N: the melting method and the solid phase N absorption method. The melting methods include include electro slag remelting (ESR), pressurized electro slag remelting (PESR), and counter pressure casting (CPC). Solid N absorption treatment uses N_2 gas from the surface of ferritic stainless steel to diffuse N atoms into the material and transform it into austenite, and the reaction formula is expressed by the following equation.

$$1/2N_2(g) = N \text{ (mass\%, in austenite phase)} \tag{8.6}$$

If the N partial pressure and temperature are given, the N solubility can be determined by equation (8.6). Under the conditions of 1473 K and 1 atm N_2, the following formula (8.7) has been proposed as an estimation formula for nitrogen solubility using an activity coefficient that takes into account the second-order interaction coefficient.

$$[N](\text{mass\%})=0.9\exp(1.7\times(-1.65+9.9\times10^{-2}[Cr]-7.6\times10^{-4}[Cr]^2+3.4\times10^{-2}[Mn] -2.59\times10^{-5}[Mn]^2-5.0\times10^{-4}[Cr][Mn]))(\text{mass\%}) \tag{8.7}$$

Ni is a high-risk element from the viewpoint of allergic problems. Thus, Ni-free austenitic stainless steel is required. Schaeffler diagram can be used for the development of high-performance austenitic stainless steels (see Fig. 8.1). The y-axis corresponds to the Ni-equivalent for the elements which stabilise the austenitic microstructure; the x-axis corresponds to the Cr-equivalent for the elements which stabilise the ferritic microstructure. N, which is one of the austenitizing elements, is an important alloying element for austenitic stainless steels in terms of corrosion resistance and strength (Ornhagen et al. 1996). N dissolved in austenitic stainless steel acts to increase its strength and improve its resistance to pitting corrosion and crevice corrosion in solutions containing chloride ions. The mechanisms have been summarised as follows (Baba et al. 2002):

(1) N in solid solution is dissolved and produces NH_4^+, hence depressing oxidation inside a pit;

(2) Concentrated N at the passive film/alloy surface stabilises the film and prevents attack from anions (Cl^-);

(3) Nitrate ions are produced to improve resistance to pitting corrosion;

(4) N addition stabilises the austenitic phase; and

(5) N blocks kink and controls the increase of electric current for pit production.

Therefore, high-N austenitic stainless steels containing over 0.3mass%N are used. As an alternative, Ni-free austenitic stainless steel, having a high concentration of N and Mn instead of Ni and displaying high strength and corrosion resistance, has been developed (Sumita et al. 2004). Fe–(19-23)Cr–(21-24)Mn–(0.5-1.5)Mo–(0.85-1.1)N (BioDur® 108) in the United States (Gebau and Brown 2001), Fe–18Cr–18Mn–2Mo–0.9N in Germany (Menzel et al. 1996), and Fe–(15-18)Cr–(10-12)Mn–(3-6)Mo–0.9N in Switzerland (Uggowitzer et al. 1996) have been developed for medical use. These alloys are fabricated with ESR process where N is absorbed into the alloy during melting under a high-pressure N atmosphere. A new manufacturing process, where N is absorbed into ferritic stainless steel after forming at 1200 °C, has also been developed (Kuroda et al. 2003). Recently, Ni-free austenitic stainless steel has been developed using additive manufacturing (Cheng et al. 2022). N-containing and Ni-free stainless steels developed for medical use are summarized in Table 8.5. From the viewpoint of paramagnetism and corrosion resistance, it is necessary to stabilize the austenite phase. It is necessary to suppress the formation of ferrite, σ phase, and martensite during heat treatment and cold working, including the cooling

Table 8.5. Compositions, manufacturing processes, and mechanical properties of Ni-free stainless steel.

Composition (mass%)	Manufacturing process	Tensile strength; Elongation
Fe-(15-18)Cr-(10-12)Mn-(3-6)Mo-0.9N	PESR CPC	981-1110 MPa; 53-70 % (ST after forging)
Fe-18Cr-18Mn-2Mo-0.9N	PESR	600 MPa (Offset yield strength, ST); 2100 MPa (50% CW)
Fe-(19-23)Cr-(21-24)Mn-(0.5-1.5)Mo-(0.85-1.1)N	ESR	931 MPa; 49 % (ST) 2206 MPa, 3% (80%CW)
Fe-24Cr-1N	Solid phase nitrogen absorption method (1473K, 1atm, ~ 129.6ks)	800 MPa; 25 %
Fe-24Cr-2Mo-1N	Solid phase nitrogen absorption method (1473K, 1atm, ~ 129.6ks)	1000 MPa; 45%

PESR: Pressured electro-slug remelting; CPC: Counter pressure casting; ESR: Electro-slug remelting. ST: Solution treated; CW: Cold working process. For this purpose, it is effective to increase the Ni equivalent, and an equation (8.8) as a condition for a single austenite phase is expressed (Uggowitzer et al. 1996).

$$\text{Ni equivalent} \geqq \text{Cr equivalent (Cr equivalent)}-8 \quad (8.8)$$
$$\text{Ni equivalent} = [\text{Ni}] + [\text{Co}] + 0.1[\text{Mn}] - 0.01[\text{Mn}]^2 + 18[\text{N}] + 30[\text{C}] \text{ (mass\%)}$$
$$\text{Cr equivalent} = [\text{Cr}] + 1.5[\text{Mo}] + 1.5[\text{W}] + 0.5[\text{Si}] + 2.3[\text{V}] + 1.75[\text{Nb}] \text{ (mass\%)}$$

Regarding corrosion resistance, as can be seen from equations (8-7) and (8-8), the addition of Cr and Mo in addition to N is effective. In this way, it is preferable to add a large amount of N, not only to make the austenite a single phase and improve corrosion resistance, but also to suppress martensitic transformation during cold working (equation (8-8)). However, when the amount exceeds the solubility at the heat treatment temperature, Cr2N precipitates, rapidly decreasing the toughness and corrosion resistance. Taking these into consideration, approximately 1mass% of N is added to Ni-free stainless steel for medical use.

References

Angel, T. 1954. Formation of martensite in austenitic stainless steels. J. Iron Steel Inst. 177: 165–173.

ASM Handbook, Vol. 1. 2023. Properties and Selection: Irons, Steels, and High-Performance Alloys. ASM Internationa, Materials Park, OH, USA.

ASM International. 2000. Introduction to Stainless Steels. Alloy Digest Sourcebook: Stainless Steels. ASM International, Materials Park, OH, USA.

ASTM Volume 13.01. 2012. Medical and Surgical Materials and Devices (I): E667 F2477, American Socity for Testing and Materials, West Conshohocken, PA, USA.

ASTM F2229-21. 2021. Standard Specification for Wrought, Nitrogen Strengthened 23 Manganese-21 Chromium-1 Molybdenum Low-Nickel Stainless Steel Alloy Bar and Wire for Surgical Implants, American Socity for Testing and Materials, West Conshohocken, PA, USA.

Akazawa, T., S. Minami, K. Takahashi, T. Kotani and T. Hanawa. 2005. Corrosion of spinal implants retrieved from patients with scoliosis. J. Orthop. Res. 10: 200–205.

Cheng, B., F. Wei, W.H. The, J.J. Lee, T.L. Meng, K.B. Lau et al. 2022. Ambient pressure fabrication of Ni-free high nitrogen austenitic stainless steel using laser powder bed fusion method. Addit. Manuf. 55: 102810.

Davis, Joseph R. [ed.]. 1994. Stainless Steels. ASM Specialty Handbook. ASM International, Materials Park, OH, USA.

Fujimoto, S., K. Tsujino and T. Shibata. 2001. Growth and properties of Cr-rich thick and porous oxide films on Type 304 stainless steel formed by square wave potential pulse polarisation. Electrochim. Acta 47: 543–551.

Fujimoto, S. and H. Tsuchiya. 2007. Semiconductor properties and protective role of passive films of iron base alloys. Corros. Sci. 49: 195–202.

Gebeau, R.C. and R.S. Brown. 2001. Biomedical implant alloy. Adv. Mater. Proc. 159: 46–48.

Haghdadi, N., M. Laleh, M. Moyle and S. Primig. 2021. Additive manufacturing of steels: a review of achievements and challenges. J. Mater. Sci. 56: 64–107.

Hanawa, T. 2019. Chapter 1 Overview of metals and applications. pp. 3–29. *In:* Niinomi, M. [ed.]. Metals for Medical Devices, 2nd ed., Elsevier, Berlin, Germany.

Hanawa, T., S. Hiromoto, A. Yamamoto, D. Kuroda and K. Asami. 2002. XPS characterization of the surface oxide film of 316L stainless samples that were located in quasi-biological environments. Mater. Trans. 43: 3088–3092.

Hiromoto, S. and T. Hanawa. 2006a. Electrochemical properties of 316L stainless steel with culturing L929 fibroblasts. J. Roy. Soc. Interface 3: 495–505.

Hiromoto, S. and T. Hanawa. 2006b. Corrosion of implant metals in the presence of cells. Corros. Rev. 24: 323.

ISO 15510:2014. 2014. Stainless steels—Chemical composition. International Organization for Standardization, Geneva, Switzerland.

Ilevbare, G.O. and G.T. Burstein. 2001. The role of alloyed molybdenum in the inhibition of pitting corrosion in stainless steels. Corros. Sci. 43: 485–513.

Kuroda, D., T. Hanawa, T. Hibaru, S. Kuroda, M. Kobayashi and T. Kobayashi. 2003. Characterization of the surface oxide film on an Fe–Cr–Mo–N system alloy in environments simulating the human body. Mater. Trans. 44: 414–420.

Laheh, M., A.E. Hughes, W. Xu, I. Gibson and M.Y. Tan. 2021. A critical review of corrosion characteristics of additively manufactured stainless steels. Int. Mater. Rev. 66: 563–599.

Menzel, J., W. Kirschner and G. Stein. 1996. High nitrogen containing Ni-free austenitic steels for medical applications. ISIJ Int. 36: 893–900.

Narushima, T., K. Suzuki, T. Murakami, C. Ouchi and Y. Iguchi. 2005. Fatigue properties of stainless steel wire ropes for electrodes in functional electrical stimulation systems. Mater. Trans. 46: 2083–2088.

Niinomi, M. 2001. Recent metallic materials for biomedical applications. Metall. Mater. Trans. A 32: 477–486.

Pickering, F.B. 1978. Physical Metallurgy and the Design of Steels. P.231. Applied Science Publisher, Essex, England, UK.

Rondelli, G., B. Vicentini and A. Cigada. 1995. Influence of nitrogen and manganese on localized corrosion behaviour of stainless steels in chloride environments. Mater. Corros. 46: 628–632.

Sander, G., J. Tan, P. Balan, O. Gharbi, D.R. Feenstra, L. Singer et al. 2018. Corrosion of additively manufactured alloys: A review. Corrosion 74: 1318–1350.

Schmid, G.M. and N. Hackerman. 1961. Anodic polarization of stainless steel in chloride solutions. J. Electrochem. Soc. 108: 741.

Schneider, H. 1960. Investment casting of high-hot strength 12% chrome steel. Foundry Trade J. 108: 562–563.

Shibata, S. and G. Okamoto. 1972. Effect of potential of etching treatment and passivation treatment on the stability of passive stainless steels. Boshoku Gijutu 21: 263–270.

Stainless Steel Handbook, Ver. 3. 1995a. p. 253. Japan Stainless Steel Association, Tokyo, Japan.

Stainless Steel Handbook, Ver. 3. 1995b. p. 358. Japan Stainless Steel Association, Tokyo, Japan.

Stainless Steel Handbook, Ver. 3. 1995c. p. 569. Japan Stainless Steel Association, Tokyo, Japan.

Sumita, M., T. Hanawa and S.H. Teoh. 2004. Development of nitrogen-containing nickel-free austenitic stainless steels for metallic biomaterials–Review. Mater. Sci. Eng. C24: 753–760.

Sun, S.H., T. Ishimoto, K. Hagihara, Y. Tsutsumi, T. Hanawa and T. Nakano. 2019. Excellent mechanical and corrosion properties of austenitic stainless steel with a unique crystallographic lamellar microstructure via selective laser melting. Scripta Mater. 159: 89–93.

Sundgren, J.E., P. Bodo and I. Lundstrom. 1986. Auger electron spectroscopic studies of the interface between human tissue and implants of titanium and stainless steel. J. Colloid Interface Sci. 110: 9–20.

Tsuchiya, H., S. Fujimoto and T. Shibata. 2004. Semiconductive properties of passive films formed on Fe-18cr in borate buffer solution. J. Electrochem. Soc. 151: B39–B44.

Tsutsumi, Y., T. Ishimoto, T. Oishi, T. Manaka, P. Chen, M. Ashida et al. 2021. Crystallographic texture- and grain boundary density-independent improvement of corrosion resistance in austenitic 316L stainless steel fabricated via laser powder bed fusion. Addit. Manuf. 45: 102066.

Uggowitzer, P.J., R. Magdowski and M.O. Speidel. 1996. Nickel free high nitrogen austenitic steels. ISIJ Int. 36: 901–908.

Chapter 9

Other Metals and Functional Alloys

9.1 Introduction

In previous chapters, CP Ti and Ti alloys, Co-based alloys, and stainless steels that are used as major metallic biomaterials are explained. In addition to these, there are many other metals that are not used in large quantities or are still under research and development, but are expected to be put to practical use in the future. In this chapter, noble metals and alloys, shape memory and superelastic alloy, Ta and Nb, biodegradable alloys, magnet alloy, Zr alloys, and high entropy alloys are explained. Research and development regarding these materials is also actively conducted, and many papers have been published. However, in this chapter, historical circumstances are emphasized and only representative papers are cited in a limited space. Noble metals, such as Au and Au alloys, precious alloys for metal-ceramic restorations, silver alloys, brazing metals, and Pt and Pt alloys are used for medical devices, especially in dentistry and cardiology. Shape-memory and superelastic Ni-Ti alloys have several medical applications that are used in guidewire, stents, orthodontic wires, and endodontic files. Research and development of shape memory and superelastic alloys made from Ti-based or precious metals is underway. As for biodegradable alloys, Mg-based alloys are being studied at the clinical level. Other biodegradable metals being studied include pure Fe and Zn alloys. Magnet alloy is used for magnetic attachment in dentistry and for diagnosis instruments. Ta and Nb are essential additive elements for Ti alloys, and Ta is used for repairing bone defects and peripheral nerves. Zr alloys have improved wear resistance due to the formation of zirconia on their surfaces through high-temperature oxidation, and have been put into practical use as heads of artificial joints. In addition, Zr alloys with low magnetic susceptibility is being studied as a material that can reduce magnetic resonance imaging (MRI) artifact volume. High-entropy alloys are being actively researched around the world as materials that exhibit unique properties due to their unique structures, and research into medical alloys has also begun. This chapter provides an overview of these metals.

9.2 Noble Metals and Their Alloys

9.2.1 Outline

Noble metals are chemically inert or inactive especially toward oxygen and difficult to form into compounds. Noble metals are also classified as precious metals that is defined as the less common and valuable metals often used to make coins or jewelry. Therefore, from the viewpoint of chemical property, noble metal is much more proper to use in this chapter. Noble metals and their alloys used in medicine include Au, which is used as markers for imaging stents, Pt and Ir, which are used as embolic coils, and Au, Ag, and Pd alloys, which are used in dentistry. Noble metals such as Ag, Pt, Pd, and Cu are used as constituent elements of these alloys. In addition, an Au alloy (Au-Cu-Al) that exhibits shape memory and super-elasticity has been developed (Goo et al. 2023). For more information on dental alloys, refer to the classic textbooks on dental materials (Anusavice 2003, Powers and Sakaguchi 2006). In this chapter, noble metals and their alloys used for medical devices are explained.

9.2.2 Noble Metals

The eight elements, Au, Ag, Ir, Os, Pd, Pt, Rh, and Ru are generally called noble metals. They have excellent chemical stability and exhibit extremely good corrosion resistance. There is a textbook (Su 2012) on noble metals. Apart from price and rarity, noble metals that are less likely to corrode or oxidize are electrochemically stable. Hg and Cu, which have higher standard electrode potential than hydrogen, are sometimes added to noble metals. Au and Ag have long been used as solvent metals for noble metal alloys because they are soft and ductile. White metal elements are categorized to Pd group (Pd, Rh, and Ru) and Pt group (Pt, Ir, and Os), both of which are harder and less ductile than Au and Ag. These are mainly used as additive elements in noble metal alloys. However, Pd and Pt have high ductility and are also used as solvent metals for noble metal alloys. Although Pd has high corrosion resistance, it is suspected that it may cause metal allergy (Kielhorn et al. 2002).

As summarized in Table 9.1, noble metal alloys for biomedical use can be broadly classified into alloys whose main components are Au, Pd, Ag, and Pt, and most of them are used in dentistry. Many of these noble metal alloys maintain the properties required for metallic biomaterials as summarized below, and each alloy is designed to exhibit properties appropriate for its use.

I. Excellent corrosion resistance.
II. Chemically stable and inert in the human body.
III. No toxicity to the human body.
IV. Radiopaque and excellent imaging properties.
V. Sufficient mechanical properties according to the application.
VI. Excellent workability and castability.

Au is an extremely soft and ductile metal. However, the occlusal pressure of molars is comparable to the person's weight, and it is insufficient in strength to be used as a dental metallic material or as a substitute for teeth. Generally, it is used in

Table 9.1. Main noble metal alloys and categorization with basic components.

Category	Type	Composition	Purpose
Au alloy	Dental casting Au alloy	Au-Ag-Cu-Zn Au-Ag-Cu-Pt-Pd-Zn	Dental restorations and prostheses
	Metal-ceramic prostheses	Au-Pt-Pd-Sn-In-Zn Au-Pd-Sn-In-Zn Au-Pd-Ag-Sn-In-Zn	Dental metal-ceramic prostheses
	Brazing alloy	Au-Ag-Cu-Zn	Dental solder
Ag Alloy	Dental Ag alloy	Ag-Pd-Cu-Au	Dental restorations and prostheses
	Dental amalgam	Ag-Sn-Cu-Hg	Dental restorations
Pd alloy	Metal-ceramic prostheses	Pd-Ag-Sn-In-Zn Pd-Cu-Sn-In-Zn	Dental metal-ceramic prostheses
Pt and Pt alloy	Pt Pt alloy	Pt, Pt-Ir	Embolic wire Electrode
	Fe-Pt magnet alloy	Fe-Pt-Nb	Magnet for medical devices

the oral cavity as a dental casting alloy with improved mechanical properties and a lower melting point (Knosp et al. 2003). Au foil which was used as a dental filling material is now rarely used. Although limited to small cavities, Au foil restoration that uses forge welding (hammer welding; blacksmith welding) takes advantage of the property of Au foil to easily adhere through forge welding and the work hardening of Au foil. The Au content is usually expressed as weight percent concentration (wt%) or mass percent concentration (mass%), while Au purity (F) and carat (K) are also used. Au purity (F) corresponds to the mass of Au contained in 1000 g of Au alloy, and carat (K) corresponds to the mass of Au contained in 24 g of Au alloy. Therefore, pure Au is 24 K.

9.2.3 Dental Casting Gold Alloys

Dental casting alloys are specified by ANSI/ADA (Table 9.2) (ANSI/ADA Specification 1997). Dental casting alloys are required to have both mechanical properties and excellent castability depending on the application, while maintaining the excellent corrosion resistance and chemical stability of noble metals. The main alloying elements are selected to contribute to improving mechanical properties and decreasing the melting point. Table 9.3 summarizes representative additive elements and their effects to alloys.

Ag and Cu are the main elements that form the basic composition of Au alloys. Cu forms a complete solid solution with Au, and solid solution hardening improves hardness, yield strength, and ultimate tensile strength. When approximately 10 mass% or more of Cu is added, it undergoes solid-phase transformation into a regular lattice of Au_3Cu or AuCu at temperatures below 680 K, so improvement in mechanical properties due to age hardening can be expected. Cu greatly contributes to decreasing the melting point, but when added in large amounts, it causes the Au alloy to turn red and deteriorate its corrosion resistance. Ag is also completely dissolved in Au, while

Table 9.2. Classification of casting metals for full-metal and metal-ceramic prostheses and partial dentures.

Metal type	All-metal prostheses	Metal-ceramic prostheses	Partial denture flameworks
High noble (HN)	Au-Ag-Pd Au-Pd-Cu-Ag HN metal-ceramic alloys	Pure Au (99.7 wt%) Au-Pt-Pd Au-Pd-Ag (5–12 wt%Ag) Au-Pd-Ag (> 12 wt%Ag) Au-Pd	Au-Ag-Cu-Pd
Noble (N)	Ag-Pd-Au-Cu Ag-Pd Noble metal-ceramic alloys	Pd-Au Pd-Au-Ag Pd-Cu-Ga Pd-Ga-Ag	–
Predominantly base metal (PB)	CP Ti Ti-Al-V Ni-Cr-Mo Co-Cr-W Cu-Al	CP Ti Ti-Al-V Ni-Cr-Mo-Be Ni-Cr-Mo Co-Cr-Mo Co-Cr-W	CP-Ti Ti-Al-V Ni-Cr-Mo Co-Cr-Mo Co-Cr-W

Table 9.3. Effect of additional elements in noble metal alloys.

Additional element	Effect	
	Positive	Negative
Ag	Decreases reddish	Decreases corrosion resistance
Cu	Decreases melting point Improves mechanical property	Decreases corrosion resistance Reddish
Pt	Improves mechanical property and elastic modulus	Increases melting point Increases segregation
Pd	Improves mechanical property and elastic modulus	Increases melting point Decreases corrosion resistance
Zn	Inhibits oxidation	Decreases corrosion resistance
Ir	Grain refinement	–

the addition of Ag does not change the mechanical properties because of the identical atomic size (see Subsection 2.5.2 and Fig. 2.13). Ag shows the effect of reducing the Au content and preventing redness caused by Cu addition.

Pt and Pd are elements that are harder than Au and have a higher elastic modulus. These are added to Au alloys for large prosthetic devices because it contributes to improving the elasticity of Au alloys, and at the same time improves yield strength and strength. Like Ag, it has the effect of preventing redness due to the addition of Cu, but it cannot be added in large amounts to Au alloys for casting because it significantly increases the melting point. These elements have similar effects on Au alloys, while Pt is used in combination with Pd because it tends to segregate and is expensive. There are Zn and Ir as trace additive elements. Zn is added to noble metal alloys for casting as a deoxidizer. Ir has an extremely high melting point and does not melt easily. By adding a small amount of fine Ir powder to an Au alloy, the Ir becomes a crystal nucleus, which promotes crystal refinement and contributes to suppressing segregation, improving corrosion resistance and mechanical properties (see Subsection 2.5.2).

Dental casting Au alloys are categorized into four types based on yield stress and elongation to fracture: type I, type II, type III, and type IV (ANSI/ADA 2006).[1] The type-classified Au alloys are Au–Ag–Cu–Pt–Pd–Zn alloys whose main components are Au, Ag, and Cu. As can be seen from the composition of Au alloys by type listed in Table 9.4, Cu and Ag increases and Au decreases in the order from type I to IV. Pt and Pd are mainly added to types III and IV. As mentioned in the above, Cu is added to decrease the melting point and improve hardness and strength, while Pt and Pd are added mainly to improve strength and elasticity, and exhibit mechanical properties depending on the application. The greater the amount of Cu added, the lower the melting point, while the greater the amount of Pt or Pd added, the higher the melting point. Therefore, the composition is such that the sum of these does not exceed 10 mass%, and the liquidus temperature of each type of Au alloy is specified to be 1323K (1050°C) or lower. Table 9.5 lists the mechanical properties and main uses of Au alloys by type. Types I-IV Au alloys are defined as soft, medium-hard, hard, and ultra-hard, respectively, and as the amount of Cu added increases, hardness, yield strength, and tensile strength increase, but conversely, elongation to fracture decreases. There are no heat treatment regulations for type I and type II, while type III and type IV can be hardened by heat treatment (regular age hardening) using a regular lattice of Au_3Cu or AuCu, and are used for large prosthetic appliances that require strength.

The inlay shown in Fig. 4.19 requires marginal sealing properties rather than strength, so Type I Au alloy, which is soft and has high elongation, is used. Type II and III Au alloys are used for crowns that must withstand occlusal pressure (Fig. 4.19), and type III Au alloys are used for bridges where occlusal pressure is applied as bending strength (Fig. 4.20). Metal denture bases of large prosthetic devices and clasps that require elasticity (Fig. 4.21) are exposed to even greater stress, so Type IV Au alloys are used and, if necessary, hardened heat treated. Au alloys by type exhibit high corrosion resistance according to Tamman's law of resistance limit

Table 9.4. Composition of dental casting alloys by type.

Type	**Composition (mass%)**					
	Au	**Ag**	**Cu**	**Pt**	**Pd**	**Zn**
I	80.2–95.8	2.4 – 12.0	1.6 – 6.2	0 – 1.0	0 – 3.6	0 – 1.2
II	73.0 – 83.0	6.9 – 14.5	5.8 – 10.5	0 – 4.2	0 – 5.6	0 – 1.4
III	71.0 – 79.8	5.2 – 13.4	7.1 – 12.6	0 – 7.5	0 – 6.5	0 – 2.0
VI	62.4 – 71.9	8.0 – 17.4	8.6 – 15.4	0.2 – 8.2	0 – 10.1	0 – 2.7

[1] These types correspond to types 1 to 4 in Table 4.2 specified by ISO (ISO 22674 2022).

Table 9.5. Mechanical property of dental casting alloys by type.

Type	Property	Heat treatment	Offset yield strength (MPa)	Elongation to fracture (%)	Main purpose
I	Soft	Softening	80 – 180	> 18	Inlay
II	Medium hard	Softening	180 – 240	> 12	Crown
III	Hard	Softening	240	> 12	Crown Bridge
VI	Super hard	Softening	300	> 10	Denture base Clasp Large scale prostheses
		Hardening	450	> 3	

Liquidus temperature is less than 1323 K (1050°C).

because they form single-phase solid solutions containing 50 at% or more of noble metals (Au and Pt group elements).

9.2.4 Dental Wrought Alloys

Wrought alloys are used in two ways in dental prostheses. First, they can be brazed to a previously cast restorations. An example is a wrought wire clasp on a removable partial denture framework (Fig. 4.20). Second, they can be embedded into a cast framework by "casting to" the alloy, as a precision attachment is "cast to" the retainer of crown, bridge, or partial denture. Composition of typed wrought dental alloys are listed in Table 9.6.

Table 9.6. Composition of typical wrought dental alloys.

Alloy	Composition (wt%)					
	Au	Ag	Cu	Pd	Pt	Others
Pt–Au–Pd	27	–	–	27	45	
Au–Pt–Pd	60	–	–	15	24	Ir: 1.0
Au–Pt–Cu–Ag	60	8.5	10	5.5	16	
Au–Pt–Ag–Cu	63	14	9	–	14	
Au–Ag–Cu–Pd	63	18.5	12	5	–	Zn: 1.5
Pd–Ag–Cu	–	39	16	43	1	

9.2.5 Noble Metal Alloys for Metal-Ceramic Restorations

Porcelain-fused-to-metal is a method of multiple additive layers of porcelain to a cast metal surface to obtain a color tone and texture similar to natural teeth (Fig. 9.1). A cross section of the metal-ceramic crown is shown in Fig. 9.1. Generally, an opaque porcelain that firmly adhered to the metal is used as a base, a dentine porcelain that gives off the color of dentin, and a highly transparent enamel porcelain that is fired on top of that. In this way, alloys for fusing porcelain are called alloys for metal-ceramics, and are available in noble metal and non-noble metal types. Porcelain has

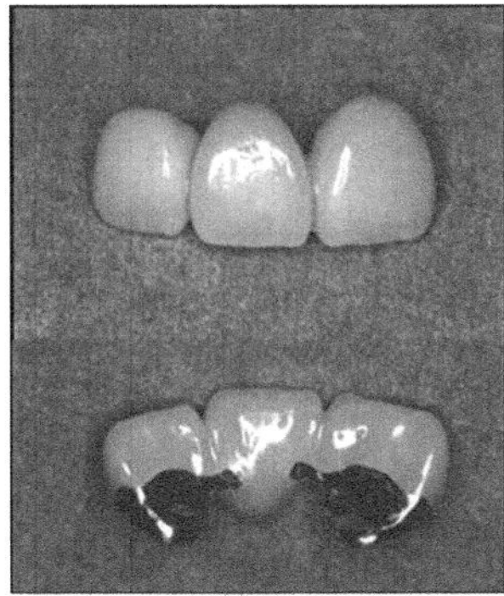

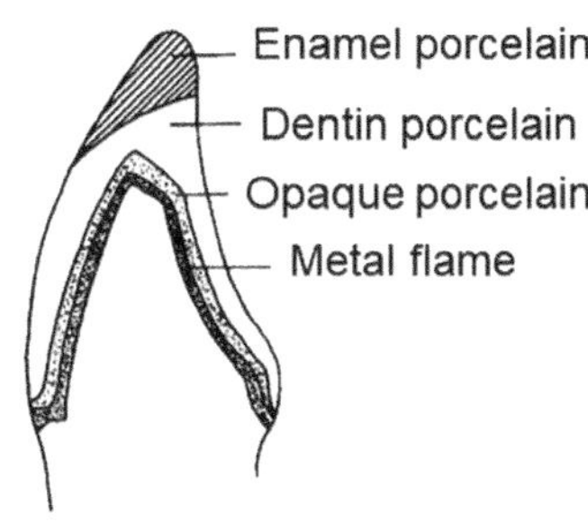

Fig. 9.1. Appearance and cross-sectional view of a metal-ceramic restoration (Provided by Yukyo Takada, Tohoku University). Porcelain layers are formed by repeated powder painting and sintering.

a higher modulus of elasticity and a lower coefficient of thermal expansion than metals. During heating and cooling by fusing, if there is a large difference in thermal expansion, thermal residual stress will generate at the interface between the metal and the porcelain. In order to prevent porcelain from peeling off easily, it is important to have a modulus of elasticity and coefficient of thermal expansion similar to those of porcelain.

Noble metal alloys for metal-ceramic restorations are classified into Au alloys and Pd alloys. The former are a high carat Au–Pt–Pd system, a medium to low carat Au–Pd system, and an Ag-added Au–Pd–Ag system; the latter are a Pd–Ag system and a Pd–Cu system. In addition, Pd and Pt foils are also used for metal-ceramic crowns.

The composition and elastic modulus of precious alloys for metal-ceramic restorations are shown in Table 9.7 (O'Brien 2002). In high carat Au–Pt–Pd gold alloys containing 74-88 mass% Au, Pt and Pd are added to increase the hardness and yield strength of the alloy, and to raise the solidus temperature to 1323-1473K (1050–1200°C) in the addition of In and Sn to increase the bonding strength with the porcelain. In Au–Pd and Au–Pd–Ag alloys, which have a lower Au content, 22 to 45 mass% of Pd is added, and the solidus temperature is as high as 1473 to 1573 K (1200 to 1300°C), the elastic modulus is also higher than that of Au–Pt–Pd alloys. The coefficient of thermal expansion of these materials (14–15 × 10^{-6}/K) is close to that of dental porcelain (11.5–13.5 × 10^{-6}/K). Ag and Cu can cause greening or yellowing of porcelain. Therefore, in the case of Au–Pd–Ag alloys containing a large amount of Ag, discoloration prevention treatment is required.

Pd–Ag-based and Pd–Cu-based alloys contain 50 mass% or more of Pd, containing Ag and Cu as the main additive elements, respectively. Like Au alloys for metal-ceramic restorations, In, Sn, and Ga are added to increase bonding strength. Pd–Ag alloy has the highest elastic modulus among the noble metal alloys for metal-ceramic restorations. Both Pd alloys contain large amounts of Ag and Cu, so they require treatment to prevent discoloration.

All Au alloys for metal-ceramic restorations have superior corrosion resistance because they contain Au and Pt group elements in amounts equal to or higher than other types of Au alloys. Pd alloys for metal-ceramic restorations with the alloying

Table 9.7. Compositions of noble metal alloys for metal-ceramic prostheses.

Alloy system	Composition (mass%)								Elastic modulus (GPa)
	Au	Pt	Pd	Ag	Cu	Sn	In	Others	
Au – Pt – Pd	74 – 88	0 – 20	0 – 16	0 – 15	–	0 – 3	0 – 4	Zn < 2	90
Au – Pd	45 – 68	0 – 1	22 – 45	–	–	0 – 5	2 – 10	Zn < 4	124
Au – Pd – Ag	42 – 62	–	25 – 40	5 – 16	4 – 20	0 – 4	0 – 6	Zn < 3	110
Pd – Ag	0 – 6	0 – 1	50 – 75	1 – 40	–	0 – 9	0 – 8	Zn < 4 Ga < 6	138
Pd – Cu	0 – 2	0 – 1	66 – 81	–	4 – 20	0 – 8	0 – 8	Zn < 4 Ga:3 – 9	96

elements of Cu, Sn, and Ga have somewhat poor corrosion resistance and tend to dissolve a large amount of Pd ions (Pfeiffer and Schwickerath 1994, 1995).

9.2.6 Brazing Alloys

Brazing alloys (ISO 9333 2022) have a melting point of 373–423 K (100–150°C), which is a lower melting point than that of the base metal. Brazing alloys require the strong bonding with the base metal and the prevention of galvanic corrosion (Figs. 2.22 and 5.7). It is required to have a small potential difference with the base metal and a color tone similar to that of the base metal. Au brazing alloys are divided into those for metal-porcelain restorations and those for general Au alloys, and both are stipulated to contain at least 58.33 mass% Au and have a peel strength of at least 350 MPa. It is common to use Au brazing alloy that matches the carat of the base metal, and various grades from 20 to 14 K are commercially available. Typical compositions and melting temperatures of dental Au brazing alloys are 45.0–80.9Au, 8.1–35Ag, 6.8–20Cu, 2–3Sn, and 2–4Zn in mass%, and melting temperature is in the range of 691–871°C (Powers and Sakaguchi 2006).

9.2.7 Silver-Palladium Alloys

Main components of Ag-Pd-Cu-Au-Zn alloy are Ag, Pd, Cu, and Au. Cu is added to Ag to improve mechanical properties and lower the melting point, and Pd increases sulfidation resistance and suppresses discoloration. In order to obtain sufficient corrosion resistance and sulfidation resistance, it is necessary to add a large amount of Pd. However, since Pd significantly raises the melting point of the Ag alloy, these improvements can be achieved by combining it with Au, which does not contribute much to raising the melting point. There are casting and non-casting types. For casting, Au is 12 mass% or more, Pd is 20 mass% or more, and Ag is 40 mass% or more. On the other hand, for non-casting products, Au is 12 mass% or more, Pd is 25 mass% or more, and Ag is 40 mass% or more. Pd content is larger for non-casting products that do not require melting. Most Ag-Pd-Cu-Au alloys for casting are 12 mass% Au, while 20 mass% Au are also commercially available. Ag-Pd-Cu-Au-Zn alloys for casting can be hardened by heat treatment, and the mechanical properties of type III to IV Au alloys can be obtained as desired, as shown in Table 9.8.

Table 9.8. Mechanical property of Ag-Pd alloys and their main uses.

Heat treatment	Hardness (HV)	Tensile strength (MPa)	Elongation (%)	Main use
Softened	90 – 160	390 – 590	10 – 40	Inlay; Crown
Hardened	200 – 320	640 – 980	2 – 15	Bridge; Clasp; Denture base

Although Ag-Pd-Cu-Au-Zn alloys have very good corrosion resistance, while compared to Au alloys for dental casting, the amount of released ions is slightly higher and the color may turn brown.

9.2.8 Dental Amalgam

Dental amalgam (ISO 24234 2021) is made of intermetallic compound alloy (Ag_3Sn) powders and Hg, and can be roughly divided into conventional type (low Cu type) and high-Cu type depending on the Cu content. There are two types of high-Cu amalgam alloy: single composition type and mixed type. The shape of the powder can be divided into lathe-cut, spherical, and a mixture of both. Conventional amalgam alloy (Ag_3Sn) amalgamates with Hg to form an alloy consisting of γ phase (Ag_3Sn), γ_1 phase (Ag_2Hg_3), and γ_2 phase ($Sn_{7\text{-}8}Hg$). The γ_2 phase is brittle and deteriorates mechanical properties and corrosion resistance, leading to marginal fracture of amalgam restorations. On the other hand, in high Cu amalgam, since the content of Cu is high, Sn forms an η' phase (Cu_6Sn_5) phase, which is an intermetallic compound with Cu instead of Hg, γ phase, ε phase (Cu_3Sn), and γ_1 phase. It has a low creep value and is less likely to produce a brittle phase (γ_2 phase), making it less prone to marginal fracture. A large amount of Sn ions is released due to the dissolution of the γ_2 (Sn_8Hg) phase, and Sn and Cu ions are released due to the dissolution of the η' (Cu_6Sn_5) phase (Marek 1992).

9.2.9 Platinum and Platinum Alloys

Pt is a stronger and more elastic metal than Au and Ag. Pure Pt has high hardness, elongation, and excellent corrosion resistance, so pure Pt is used in embolization coils (see Subsection 4.4.3 and Fig. 4.16) and electrodes. Pt alloys contain small amounts of additive elements which are used for medical purposes (Cowley and Woodward 2011). Additive elements include W and Pd group elements such as Ir, Rh, and Ru, as shown in Table 9.9. The addition of these elements from 4 to 10 mass% improves strength even more than Pt without impairing elongation. Like Au, Pt is radio-opaque and has excellent imaging properties, so Pt, Pt–Ir alloys, Pt–W alloys, etc., are used *in vivo* as electrodes and embolic coils. Embolic coils are made by processing Pt or these Pt alloys into thin wires with a diameter of approximately 35 to 80 μm and winding them in a double helix (White et al. 2006).

Table 9.9. Mechanical property of Pt and Pt alloys.

Composition	Tensile strength (MPa)	Elongation to fracture (%)
Pt	147	37
Pt-5mass%Ru	412	34
Pt-5mass%Ir	274	-
Pt-10mass%Ir	382	-
Pt-5mass%Rh	206	-
Pt-10mass%Rh	314	35
Pt-4mass%W	500	25

9.3 Shape Memory and Superelastic Alloys

9.3.1 Martensitic Transformation

Martensitic transformation is an important phenomenon to understand shape memory and superelastic effects of metals. The martensitic transformation is a displacement-type diffusion-less transformation in which atomic arrays in a crystal work together to undergo shear deformation, and the relative positional relationships of the atoms are maintained before and after the transformation. The high-temperature phase is called the “parent phase” or “austenite phase,” and is hereinafter referred to as the “P phase”. The P phase is often a cubic crystal with high symmetry. The low-temperature phase is called the “martensite phase,,” or the “M phase”. The M phase is often a tetragonal, rhombohedral, or orthorhombic crystal with low symmetry. The transformation from M phase to P phase by heating is called “austenitic transformation” or “reverse martensitic transformation”. On the other hand, the transformation from P phase to M phase is called as “martensitic transformation”. In addition, the transformation start temperature is expressed as M_s, the transformation end temperature as M_f, the reverse start temperature as A_s, the transformation end temperature as A_f, and the test temperature as T.

In the deformation of shape memory alloys, it is necessary to understand martensitic variants and their reorientation. Consider that the P phase is a cubic crystal with a lattice constant a_0, and when it is cooled to $T < M_f$, it transforms into a tetragonal M phase with lattice constants a_1, a_0, c ($a_1 > a_0 > c$), as shown in Fig. 9.2. Here, if one of the three a_0 axes in the cubic crystal shrinks to become the c-axis, and the remaining two axes expand to become the a_1-axis, there are three ways of transformation, depending on the number of c-axes. All are equivalent, but since there are differences in the direction of strain, those with different crystal orientations are called variants. Each variant is twinned to each other. Figure 9.2 shows a schematic diagram of martensitic variants. Note that the type of variant changes depending on the crystal structure of the P phase and M phase and the lattice correspondence relationship between the two phases.

When work is done externally, the macroscopic shape changes, so each variant is combined and generated to cancel out each other's distortions as much as possible during metamorphosis so as not to change the external shape. This is

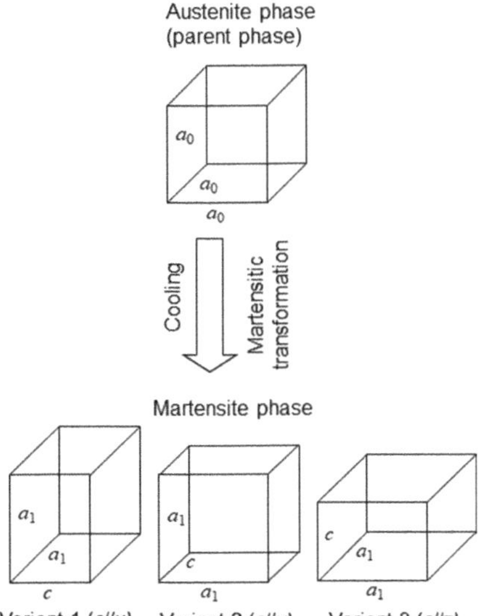

Fig. 9.2. Formation of variants by martensitic transformation (Provided by Dr. Hideki Hosoda, Tokyo Institute of Technology).

called self-accommodation of the martensitic variant, and for this reason, shape memory alloys do not undergo macroscopic external changes during transformation. However, microscopically, each variant causes unevenness, so when viewed under a microscope, a pattern called surface relief can be seen. The self-adjusted martensitic structure of the Ti–Nb–Al alloy in Fig. 9.3 is the state of the shape memory alloy before deformation.

There are many metals that undergo martensitic transformation. Normally, the volume change during transformation is large, and due to the restraint around the M phase, a large amount of lattice invariant deformation such as dislocations and twins is introduced during transformation, causing an irreversible change in the internal state. This is called "non-thermoelastic transformation". Although it is important in quenching and strengthening steel, it does not produce a shape memory effect. On the other hand, when the volume change is small and the lattice-invariant deformation is small, no irreversible defects are created inside the material, so the internal state does not change due to transformation-reverse transformation. Therefore, the formed martensite can grow reversibly by lowering the temperature or maintaining it at an isothermal temperature. This is called "thermoelastic transformation" and is necessary for the shape memory effect to occur.

Transformation may occur not only due to such cooling but also due to stress loading. This is called "stress-induced martensitic transformation", and the stress is called transformation-induced stress. Stress-induced martensitic transformation is essential for superelasticity and is very important. Transformation-induced stress increases in proportion to temperature rise. The reason for this is that the higher the temperature, the more stable the P phase becomes and the Gibbs energy difference between it and the *M* phase increases. For quantitative understanding, the Clausius-Clapeyron relation is applied to stress-induced transformation under uniaxial stress

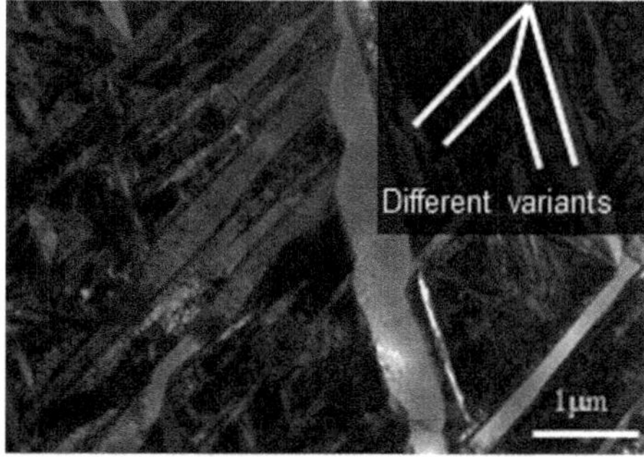

Fig. 9.3. Microstructure of Ti–Nb–Al (Provided by Dr. Hideki Hosoda, Tokyo Institute of Technology).

conditions. If temperature is T, transformation-induced stress is σ_{SIMT}, strain caused by transformation is ε_T, difference in enthalpy from P phase to M phase is ΔH, and difference in entropy is ΔS, then the following formula holds true:

$$\frac{d\sigma_{SIMT}}{dT} = -\frac{\Delta S}{\varepsilon_T} = -\frac{\Delta H}{\varepsilon_T T} \tag{9.1}$$

This allows the phase diagram of P and M phases to be expressed in terms of the relationship between temperature and stress, as shown in Fig. 9.4. The figure shows both cases where the slip deformation stress is (I) low and (II) high. The maximum temperature at which stress-induced transformation occurs is called M_d, and is the temperature at which the transformation-induced stress is equal to the stress for slip deformation or fracture stress. At high temperatures above M_d, no transformation occurs, and sliding deformation and destruction occur. If the sliding deformation stress is low, it corresponds to an annealing condition such as homogenization

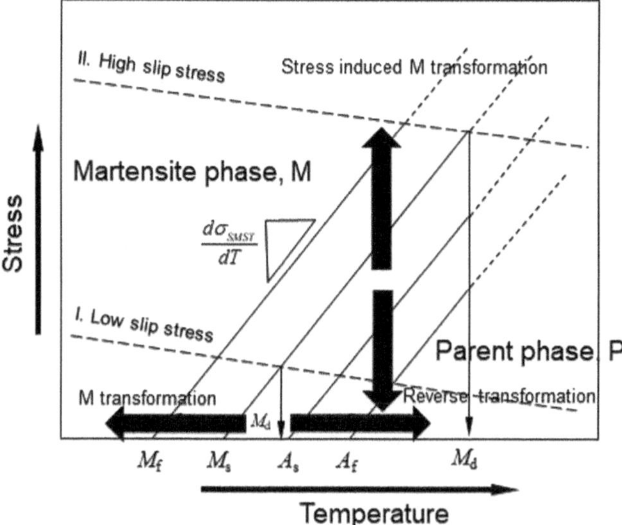

Fig. 9.4. Phase diagram of shape memory alloys according to temperature and stress (Provided by Dr. Hideki Hosoda, Tokyo Institute of Technology).

treatment, and if it is high, it corresponds to a case where the strength has been improved by processing heat treatment. When the sliding deformation stress is low, $M_d < A_s$, and at this temperature, the M phase is only unloaded and does not transform back to the P phase. On the other hand, when the sliding deformation stress is high, $A_f < M_d$, and at this temperature, the stress-induced M phase can reversely transform into the P phase simply by unloading. As will be explained later, this is superelasticity. In this way, as the strength of the material increases, M_d increases and superelasticity develops, so strengthening is very important in shape memory alloys.

9.3.2 Shape Memory and Superelasticity

The shape memory effect is a phenomenon in which a material that is deformed returns to its original shape when heated. It is called "shape memory" because it remembers its initial shape. Superelasticity is a phenomenon in which a strain of several percent that greatly exceeds the elastic limit returns only by unloading, and is called "superelasticity" because it returns as if it were an elastic deformation. Both are phenomena of shape recovery, but another important feature is that a nearly constant holding force can be obtained regardless of the amount of strain. Figure 9.5 shows the differences in the stress-strain diagrams of ordinary metals, shape memory alloys, and superelastic alloys.

Figure 9.6 shows the deformation mechanism in each temperature range, and Fig. 9.7 shows the corresponding stress-strain curve. Note that in actual shape memory alloys, plastic deformation due to slip is often introduced during deformation, so Fig. 9.7 shows a case where residual strain is also introduced. This shows the mechanism of shape memory effect. When cooled from P phase to below M_f under no stress, the M phase generated by cooling adjusts itself and there is no apparent deformation. Thereafter, let's assume that a uniaxial compressive stress is applied to this. When the phase transformation shown in Fig. 9.2 is assumed and the external stress is parallel to the a_0 axis of one of the original cubic crystals, the number of variants whose stress direction and c-axis are parallel increases, the potential energy decreases, so in the stress-loaded state, the variant that shrinks in the stress direction becomes energetically advantageous, and the unfavorable variant becomes more

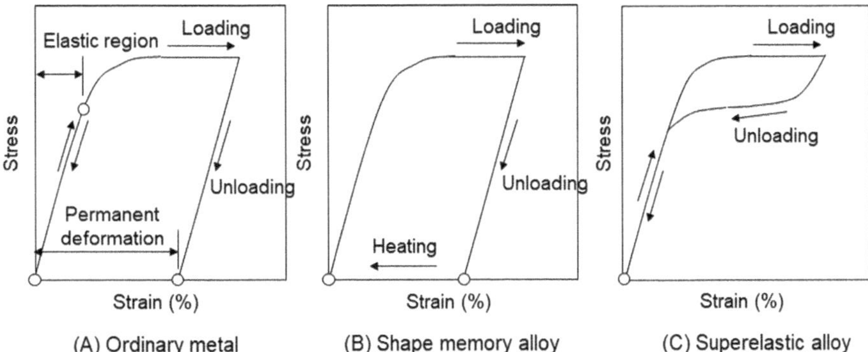

Fig. 9.5. Comparison of stress-strain curves of conventional metals (A), shape memory alloys (B), and superelastic alloys (C).

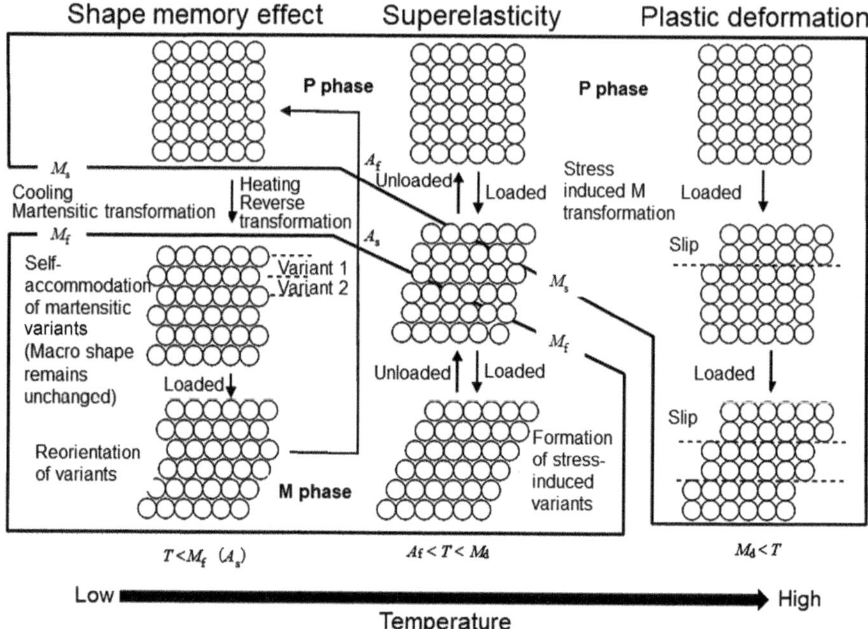

Fig. 9.6. Deformation mechanism of shape memory alloy at each temperature region (Provided by Dr. Hideki Hosoda, Tokyo Institute of Technology).

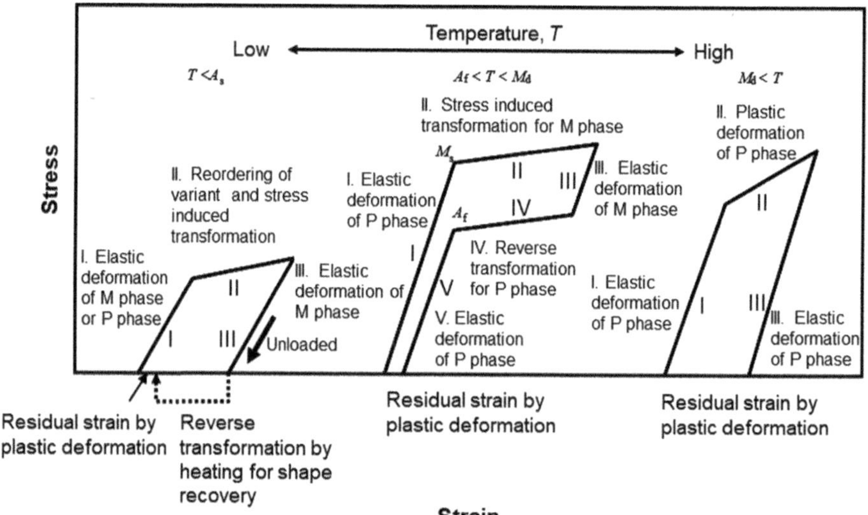

Fig. 9.7. Stress-strain curves of shape memory alloy in each temperature region (Provided by Dr. Hideki Hosoda, Tokyo Institute of Technology).

advantageous due to twin deformation. Rearrange and transform into variants. Figure 9.8 shows the changes in the lattice during variant rearrangement. Then, the stress is unloaded. Since any variant is equivalent to energy under stress-free conditions, the transformed variant is preserved and the deformation is also preserved. When the unloaded sample is heated above A_f, it transforms back to the original P phase and returns to its original shape. Even if it is cooled down to its original temperature, its shape will not change. The shape memory effect is obtained by this deformation-temperature cycle.

The shape memory effect also occurs in the temperature range of $M_s < T < A_s$ in the P phase. In this case, the M phase undergoes stress-induced transformation due to external force. Under stress, an advantageous variant is generated, resulting in the same variant state as when stress is applied in the case of $T < M_f$ above. After that, when heated above A_f, reverse transformation occurs and a shape memory effect is obtained. Note that after all, martensite forms the same variant due to external force; even if a larger stress is applied, the martensite cannot be deformed further by variant

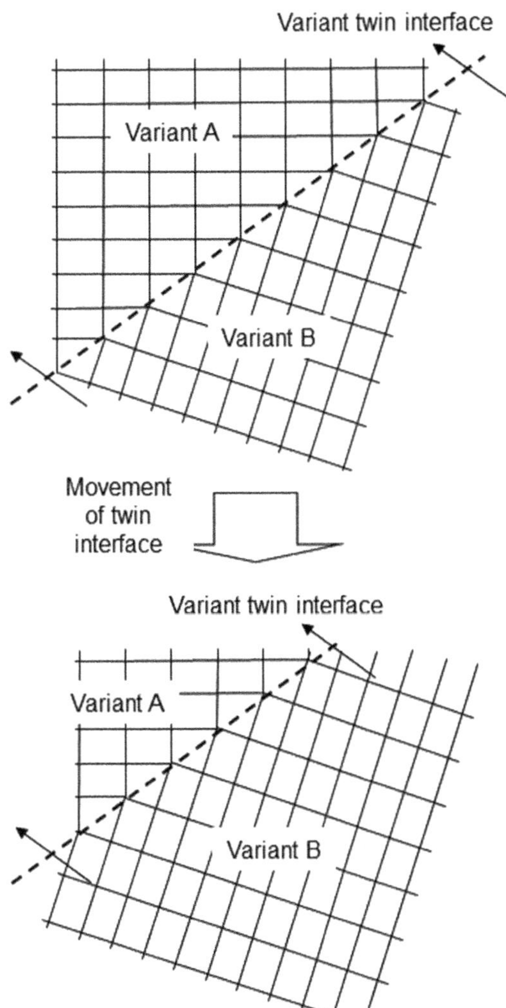

Fig. 9.8. Reorientation of martensite variants. Stress application → Movement of twin interface → Growth of variant B → Deformation (Provided by Dr. Hideki Hosoda, Tokyo Institute of Technology).

rearrangement, so deformation proceeds only by normal plastic deformation such as slip. In this way, there is a limit to the shape recovery strain of a shape memory alloy. The maximum shape recovery strain is the difference in lattice strain between the state in which all M phases are aligned in the same variant and the P phase.

When $A_s < T < A_f$, a stress-favorable variant is generated and deformed and unloaded, a portion undergoes reverse transformation and incomplete superelasticity is expressed, while the remaining M phase remains and a partial shape memory effect is also expressed. However, in the temperature range $A_f < T < M_d$, the stress-induced transformed M phase completely transforms back to the P phase simply by unloading. At this time, the strain caused by the difference in lattice strain is several percent strain, which far exceeds the elastic deformation, but it is called superelastic because it is completely recovered by unloading alone. Another feature of superelasticity is first order phase transformation due to stress. Since transformation and reverse transformation proceed with almost constant stress, the superelastic deformation stress remains almost constant regardless of strain. Young's modulus is clearly almost zero. Therefore, the superelastic wire for orthodontics can always produce a constant orthodontic force (see Fig. 4.23). Finally, when $M_d < T$, the stress required for stress-induced transformation is not reached and plastic deformation due to slip occurs like in normal metals, so no shape recovery behavior is observed.

To summarize the above, the deformation mechanism of shape memory alloys can be classified as follows depending on the test temperature and material transformation temperature. It is important to understand these relationships when using shape memory alloys.

(1) When $T < A_s$, shape memory effect

(2) When $A_s < T < A_f$, a mixture of incomplete superelasticity and shape memory effect

(3) If $A_f < T < M_d$, superelasticity

(4) If $M_d < T$, permanent deformation

Note that if the material's slip deformation stress is close to the martensitic variant's rearrangement stress or transformation-induced stress, slip will also be introduced during deformation and plastic deformation will remain. However, if the sliding deformation stress can be made high enough, almost no sliding deformation will be introduced and complete shape recovery will be obtained. Therefore, improving the sliding deformation stress, along with improving the superelastic temperature range, is important for the expression and stabilization of shape memory and superelastic properties, and such treatment is called shape memory treatment or superelastic treatment. In order to put shape memory alloys into practical use, in addition to developing materials with good properties, it is also essential to develop processing methods for these materials.

9.3.3 Nickel-Titanium Alloy

Ni–Ti alloys consisting of equal atomic amounts of Ni and Ti (49–51mol%Ni) show unique mechanical properties such as shape memory, superelasticity, and dumping.

Table 9.10. Mechanical property of Ni–Ti alloy.

Young's modulus (GPa)	80 – 100 (P phase)
Vickers hardness (HV)	180 – 200 (M phase); 200 – 400 (P phase)
Yield strength (MPa)	50 – 200 (M phase); 100 – 600 (P phase)
Ultimate tensile strength (MPa)	700 – 2000
Superelastic deformation stress (MPa)	100 – 600 (Loaded); 0 – 300 (Unloaded)
Elongation to fracture (%)	20 – 60

Mechanical property of Ni–Ti alloy is summarized in Table 9.10. Because of these unique properties, the Ni–Ti alloy is used for guide wires, stents, orthodontic arch wires, endodontic reamers and files (Hanawa 2019, Thompson 2000).

The range of composition for the Ni–Ti alloy displaying these properties is very narrow, nearly a 1:1 atomic ratio. This Ni–Ti alloy has a particular transformation temperature as a biomaterial, and an austenitic phase (P phase) at a higher temperature and a martensitic phase (M phase) at a lower temperature with a heat-elastic martensitic phase. When external stress is loaded onto the crystal, the crystal deforms by the twin deformation, not by slip deformation, and the relative configuration of the atoms is not changed. Therefore, when the temperature is again increased, the crystal returns to the original structure and original morphology. The twin compensates for 8% of the deformation in tensile strain. Slip will occur over this strain and it is then impossible to recover the original morphology. This transformation is caused by the change in temperature. However, superelasticity is caused by stress, not by a change in temperature, and is known as a stress-induced transformation. The transformation between the P phase and M phase is caused by stress: The P phase transforms to the M phase by stress and the M phase transforms to the P phase by the release of stress. The characteristics of the Ni–Ti alloy change according to the transformation temperature and the service temperature, with the transformation temperature being influenced by composition, impurity, and heat history. In particular, slight change of composition generates great change of transformation temperature.

The reason why only Ni–Ti alloy has been put into practical use is that this alloy is chemically and physically stable and can withstand long-term use, and that it has a shape memory treatment that improves slip deformation stress without inhibiting transformation. The working method for Ni–Ti alloy is described below (Frazin-Nia and Yoneyama 2009).

Low Temperature Treatment (Work Hardening)

After cold working with an area reduction rate of about 30%, heat treatment for several min to several tens of min at a temperature range of about 373 to 673 K reduces slip deformation stress due to work hardening mainly due to structurally stabilized high-density dislocations (see Subsection 2.5.2). This is the most important treatment in practice because it does not depend on the composition.

Aging Treatment (Precipitation Treatment)

This process mainly utilizes precipitation hardening due to Ti_3Ni_4, which is a metastable precipitate (see Subsection 2.5.2 and Fig. 2.14). The only precipitate that causes strengthening in the Ni–Ti binary system is the semi-coherent precipitate Ti_3Ni_4 that forms at 50.5 mol%Ni or more. The treatment method is to perform solid solution treatment at 973K or higher and aging treatment at 573–773K for about 10 min to 1 hr to achieve high-density precipitation of Ti_3Ni_4. This is very important as a superelastic processing method.

Medium Temperature Treatment (Grain Refinement)

After cold working, the material is held at a relatively high temperature of around 773 K for several min to several hr, and the method mainly utilizes grain refinement strengthening through recrystallization (see Subsection 2.5.2). Because it requires severe plastic deformation, it can only be used at close to stoichiometric compositions with good workability.

Training Treatment

Although slippery dislocations move due to cyclic deformation, they gradually become work hardened and the mobile dislocations become immobile. As a result, the apparent residual strain decreases with repeated deformation and the shape memory and superelastic properties become stable. This is called a training effect. Although it can be used for many shape memory alloys, it is not practically used because it takes time and effort.

Another option is solution hardening. Solid solution hardening is not used in Ni–Ti alloy because it requires the addition of a large amount of third element, which causes a large change in the transformation temperature and causes embrittlement.

9.3.4 Corrosion Resistance of Nickel-Titanium Alloy

The safety level of the Ni–Ti alloy is lower than that of CP Ti, but is the same as that of stainless steels and Co-based alloys, because the Ni–Ti alloy is covered by a surface oxide film consisting mainly of titanium oxide and nickel hydroxide. However, the Ni–Ti alloy contains about 50mol%Ni and its use in medicine is limited from the viewpoint of safety. Ni–Ti alloy is used as guidewires and self-expanding stents. However, 37.2% (45 of 121 cases) of Ni–Ti stents are fractured in 10.7 mon of service (Scheinert et al. 2005). Corrosion may be related to the fracture, while the main cause is fatigue. In the case of stent grafts of Ni–Ti, severe pitting and crevice corrosion appears between Ni–Ti alloy and a polymer as an artificial blood vessel (Heintz et al. 2001). The observed corrosion defects of pitting and irregular shape are precursors to material failure. They weaken the thin wire, resulting in stress cracks and eventual fracture of the stent wire when subjected to circulation pulses. In addition, the fatigue mechanism of Ni-Ti alloy is still unknown to use stents and endodontic files (Kang and Song 2015, Mahtabi et al. 2015). Therefore, Ni-free Ti-based superelastic alloys have been researched (Shinohara et al. 2015).

9.3.5 Nickel-Free Shape Memory and Superelastic Alloys

When a metal is implanted in the human body for a long time, the material dissolves slightly against the body fluid. For this reason, it is necessary to consider the allergy of the released metal. The problem of Ni–Ti alloy is that Ni, which is an allergic element, is contained. However, Ni–Ti alloys have no alternative material and have extremely few allergic cases, so they are currently widely used (Oshida and Miyazaki 1991). Since metal allergy is due to the release of metal ions, there is no problem if the corrosion resistance is improved and ion release is prevented by the surface oxide film. The reason why Ni allergy is not a problem in the Ni–Ti alloy is that a passive oxide film covers the surface. However, from the possibility that the film is destroyed and Ni released, toxic-element-free alloys are required, which can replace Ni–Ti alloy for further safety.

The normal martensite of CP Ti is hcp lattice and non-heated α', but it is generated with an appropriate composition, which is a diagonal crystal and passionate type α", and its shape memory and superelasticity are expressed. For this reason, Cr, Nb, Mo, Hf, Ta, etc., which reduces M_s as an additive element, has been developed (Suzuki 1984). By changing in composition of Ti–Nb–Ta–Zr alloy, shape memory effect appears (Niinomi et al. 2005). Also, Ti–Nb–Sn alloy, Ti–Nb–Cu alloy, Ti–Nb–Al alloy, Ti–Nb–Ta alloy, Ti–Mo–Ga alloy, Ti–Mo–Ge alloy, Ti–Mo–Al alloy, Ti–Ta alloy, Ti–Ta–Zr alloy, Ti–Sc–Mo alloy, Ti–Mo–Sn alloy, Ti–Mo–Ag–Sn alloy, Ti–7Cr–Al alloy, etc., have been developed (Niinomi 2003, Ikeda et al. 2004, Maeshima and Nishida 2004, Ikeda et al. 2005, Inamura et al. 2005, Kim et al. 2006). Many of these have good cold working ability with a cross-sectional reduction rate of 90% or more. For this reason, the texture increases under strong working, and the elastic strain is increased by the anisotropy of the transformation strain and the Young' modulus. For example, about 5% and 7% of elastic strain for Ti–Nb–Al alloy (Fukui et al. 2004) and Ti–Nb–Cu alloy (Horinouchi et al. 2007) appear, respectively, and these are comparable to the Ni–Ti alloy. Ti–Nb–Sn alloy, Ti–Mo–Sn alloy, Ti–Nb–Zr alloy, etc., are already commercialized. Ti–Nb–Al alloy shows the equivalent orthodontic effect to Ni–Ti alloy in animal experiments (Kanetaka et al. 2007).

9.4 Biodegradable Metals

9.4.1 Outline

The term "biodegradable metal (BM)" has been used worldwide to describe these new kinds of degradable metallic biomaterials for medical applications and there were many new findings reported over the last two decades. The degradation mechanisms of BMs and its environmental influencing factors, which include the degeneration of mechanical integrity, and the metabolism of the degradation products, are reviewed (Zheng et al. 2014). The definition of BMs can be given as follows: BMs are metals expected to corrode gradually *in vivo*, with an appropriate host response elicited by released corrosion products, then dissolve completely upon fulfilling the mission to assist with tissue healing with no implant residues. Therefore, the major component of BM should be essential metallic elements that can be metabolized by the human body, and demonstrate appropriate degradation rates and modes in the human body.

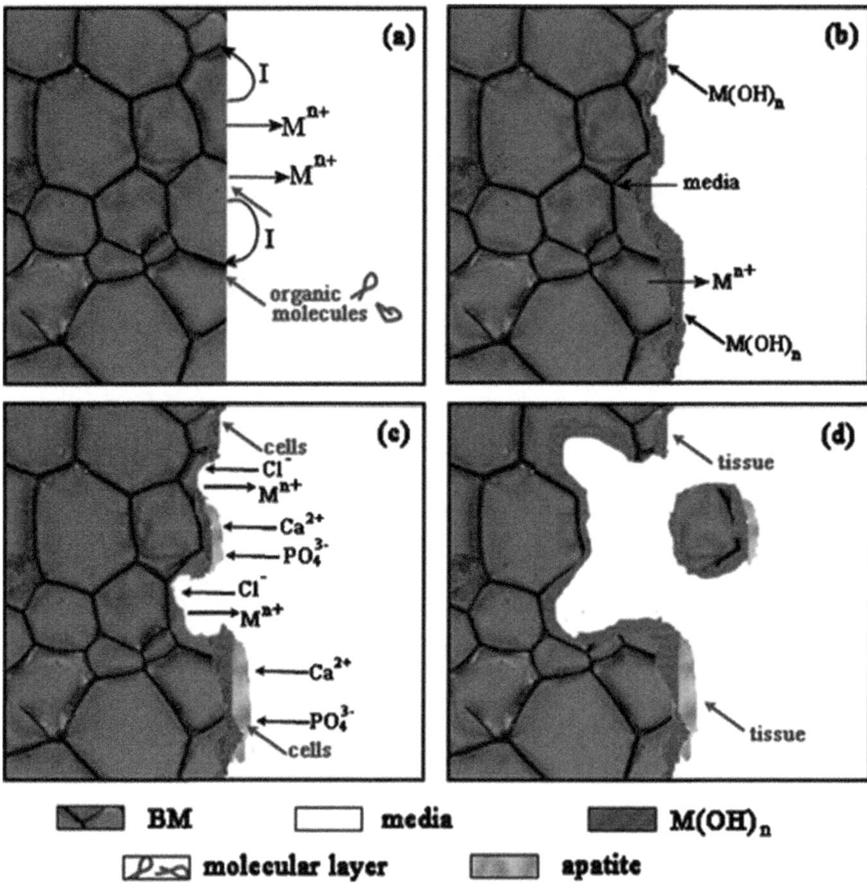

Fig. 9.9. Schematic diagram of the degradation mechanism of the biodegradable metal (BM) in a physiological environment. Immediately after contacting the body fluid, the BM is oxidized into metal cations following the anodic reaction. Simultaneously, the organic molecules, such as proteins, amino acids and lipids, will adsorb over the metal surface, thereby influencing the dissolution of BM (a) and (b). Chloride adsorption causes the breakdown of the M(OH)n protective layer and leads to pitting corrosion (c). Depending on the particle size, the fibrous tissue or macrophages might enclose these particle, which may be further degraded until the metallic phase is completely exhausted (d). (Reprinted with permission from Elsevier, Zheng et al. 2014. Mater. Sci. Eng. R 77: 1–34.).

In other words, BMs are metals and alloys expected to corrode gradually *in vivo*, with an appropriate host response elicited by released corrosion products, then dissolve completely upon fulfilling the mission to assist with tissue healing with no implant residues (Li et al. 2014). The degradation mechanism of the BM in a physiological environment is shown in Fig. 9.9.

9.4.2 Magnesium Alloys

The mechanical properties and degradation rate of cast and wrought Mg alloys in Hank's solution at 37°C are well reviewed (Zheng et al. 2014). The key to

manufacturing Mg-based alloys that are suitable as biodegradable orthopedic implants is adjusting their degradation rates and mechanical integrity in the physiological environment. Biodegradable Mg alloys have been widely investigated in the field of biomaterials because they can be gradually dissolved and absorbed by the human body. The use of Mg alloys as BMs for stents and bone fixators is expected. Mg has the smallest density of all commercially utilized metals, while pure Mg cannot be utilized as a structural material due to its low strength; therefore, at least one of the following element is added to form the alloy: Al, Zn, Mn, Zr, or rare-earth metals. The addition of rare-earth metals improves castability and pressure resistance. Clinical trials of stents consisting of Mg alloys (WE30) are underway (Peeters et al. 2005, Erbel et al. 2007). Mg alloys used as stents in Germany contain Al, Y, Ce, Nd and/or rare-earth metals. Controlling degradation and corrosion of Mg in the human body is difficult due to its extreme activity. In addition, hydrogen evolution occurs when it dissolves. Control of the degradation rate, so that it is safe for the human body, is a key factor for enabling the utilization of Mg alloys for medical devices. History of biodegradable Mg alloy is well reviewed (Witte 2010, Herber et al. 2021) and the corrosion and biocompatibility is summarized (Virtanen 2011). Mg alloys are expected to be applied in biomedical fields as BMs because Mg is a bioessential element even though it is corrosive in an aqueous environment.
Mg is dissolved with the following reaction:

$$Mg + 2H_2O \rightarrow Mg^{2+} + 2OH^- + H_2\uparrow. \quad (9.2)$$

Because the control of degradation, i.e., corrosion, of Mg in the human body is difficult due to the extreme activity of Mg, alloying is absolutely necessary to control the corrosion rate. In addition, hydrogen evolution occurs when Mg is dissolved and a gas cavity is formed during the implantation of Mg alloys (Witte et al. 2005). Control of the corrosion rate for safety in the human body is a key factor in the utilization of Mg alloys for medical devices. Efforts to achieve this purpose are currently underway (Heublein et al. 2003). Two types of schematic illustration of corrosion process of AZ31 alloy during exposure to 0.9% NaCl solution with different glucose contents are shown in Fig. 9.10 (Li et al. 2018).

It has been found that bare Mg alloy implants suffer from rapid corrosion. Therefore, surface coating is applied to improve the corrosion resistance and biocompatibility of Mg alloys. Electrodeposition of HA on Mg alloys have been studied (Guan and Brown 2001, Wen et al. 2009; Hiromoto and Tomozawa 2010, Kannan and Wallipa 2013). Also, calcium compounds are coated on Mg alloys (Wang et al. 2014). A composite coating of HA and stearic acid is developed on the substrate surface (Zhang et al. 2012). These composite coatings could provide effective protection and enhance the corrosion resistance of the Mg alloy.

Regarding biomedical applications, Mg has been used as a material for bone replacement since ancient times. However, in recent years, it has attracted attention as a stent for expanding stenosed sites such as blood vessels and esophagus (Li et al. 2022). As a bone fixation material, Mg has a high specific strength of approximately 120 kN m kg^{-1}, which is inferior to that of Ti alloy, approximately 220 kN m kg^{-1}, but it is possible to increase through alloy design. From the perspective of regenerative medicine, it is expected that Mg alloys will not ultimately remain in the body and will

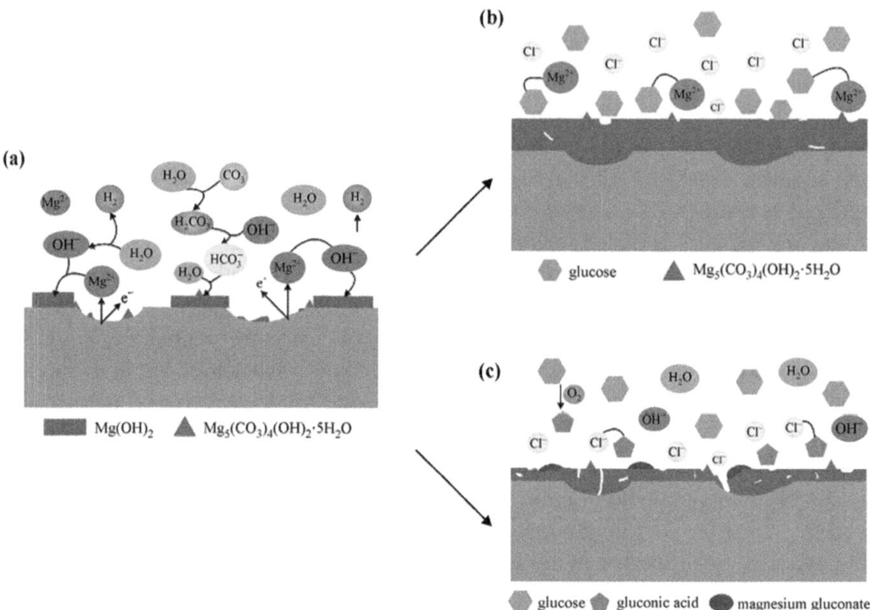

Fig. 9.10. Two types of schematic illustration of corrosion process of AZ31 alloy during exposure to 0.9%NaCl solution with different glucose contents: (a) initial corrosion of AZ31 alloy in neat 0.9%NaCl solution; (b) 0.9%NaCl solution containing 1.0 g/L glucose; (c) 0.9%NaCl solution containing 2.0 and 3.0 g/L glucose (Reprinted with permission from Frontiers Media S.A. open access, Li et al. 2018. Front. Mater. Sci. 12: 148–197.).

completely replace bones. However, the dissolution rate of Mg implants is generally as fast as 1/3 to 1/4 of the period required for bone regeneration. Moreover, it cannot withstand the stress loading required in bone fixation sites. It is also necessary to consider how to remove the hydrogen gas generated, so it has not yet been put into clinical application. However, when a porous body of Mg–9Al–1Zr alloy (AZ91) was implanted into the distal condyle of a rabbit femur, the Mg alloy completely dissolved after 3 mon and no abnormalities such as inflammatory reactions to the surrounding bone were observed, and it is expected to be used as a bone substitute material in the future (Witte et al. 2007).

In addition to bone replacement, Mg-based stents have been actively studied and developed as medical materials that take advantage of the small amount of implantation into the body (less than 10 mg for vascular stents) and their resistance to dissolution and corrosion. In addition, Mg is an essential element in the human body. With conventional type 316L stainless steel stents, the problem is that vascular endothelial cells invade the inner wall of the stent, passing endothelialization and restenosis of the blood vessel, making it difficult to replace the stent. Furthermore, while progress is being made in the development of drug eluting stent, the lack of proper endothelialization may be an obstacle to clinical application. In order to overcome these shortcomings, research on Mg alloy stents is being conducted (Erbel et al. 2007, Ikeo et al. 2021, Kawamura et al. 2023). A German medical device manufacturer is developing a stent using Mg–4Y–3RE (RE: rare earth metal) alloy (WE43).

9.4.3 Pure Iron and Zinc Alloy

Pure Fe is one of other candidates of BM (Mueller et al. 2006, Peuster et al. 2006, Hermawan et al. 2008). Degradation rate of pure ion in physiological solution is very low, so the acceleration of the degradation rate is the main subject to utilize pure Fe for medical implants. Fe–Mn–Pd alloy is designed to accelerate degradation rate (Schinhammer et al. 2010).

Zn alloys is also studied as BM and many compositions are proposed (Levy et al. 2017). Zn with a small amount of Zr showed finer grains, but brittle fracture mode and minor mechanical properties have been improved. Zn–0.05Zr alloy shows a yield strength of 104 MPa, ultimate tensile strength of 157 MPa, and elongation to fracture of 22% (Wątroba et al. 2018).

9.5 Magnet Alloys

Figure 9.11 shows the changes in magnetic force due to the development of magnet alloys. Magnetic attachments used in dental prostheses that use the attractive force of a magnet for retention force use Sm–Co alloy or Ne–Fe–B alloy as the magnet. Magnetic alloys are used in the strong magnetic field generators of advanced contrast imaging devices such as computed tomography (CT), MRI, and positron emission tomography (PET).

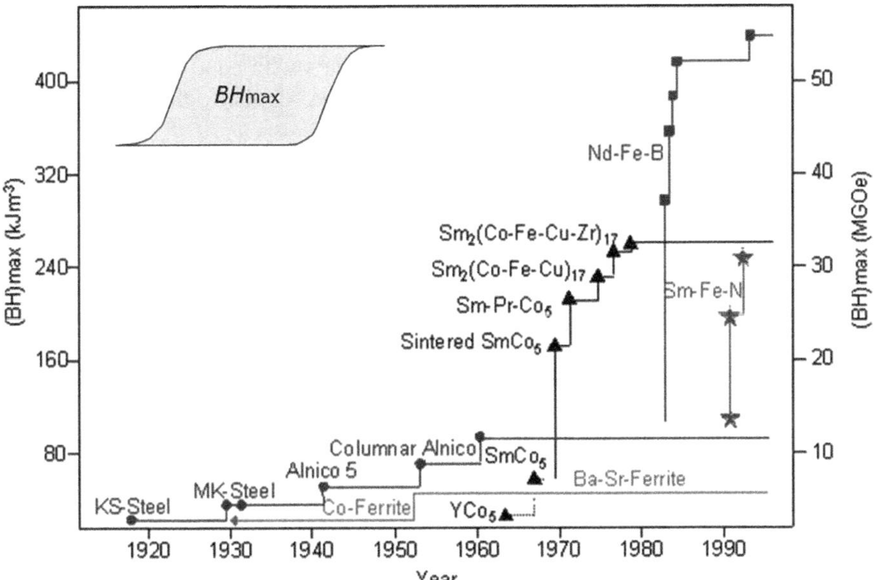

Fig. 9.11. The development of permanent magnets in the 20th Century. BH_{max} has improved exponentially, doubling every 12 years (https://www.birmingham.ac.uk/Documents/college-eps/metallurgy/research/Magnetic-Materials-Background/Magnetic-Materials-Background-1-History.pdf).

9.6 Tantalum and Niobium

Ta and Nb are transition metal elements of the same Group 5 on the periodic table, and both exhibit similar physical properties. Ta and Nb are elements with very low toxicity, and are expected to be used as bioinert materials. On the other hand, Ta has a density that is about twice as high as Nb and a melting point that is over 550°C higher, so caution must be required when casting and using it. Due to its high chemical stability, Ta is expected to be used as an implant device, and has limited use in the orthopedics and dentistry, such as in defected bone repair and as a marker for X-ray imaging. Ta and Nb are often used as constituent elements of Ti-based alloys. Since Ta and Nb exhibit a bcc structure, they are important elements, along with Mo, as β-phase stabilized elements.

Biological applications of Ta have been attempted for a long time. Ta was implanted in the body in 1938 and implanted into skull bone defects in 1943, and Ta foil was used to repair peripheral nerves (Pudenz 1943, Pobertson and Peacher 1943). Ta has low reactivity with soft tissues and can tolerate contact with brain substance and meninx due to excellent corrosion resistance (Weast and Astle 1981). The mechanical properties and corrosion resistance that Ta should exhibit as an implant are specified (ASTM F560 2022). The *in vivo* response of Ta is strongly dependent on its shape and size. Powders smaller than 50 μm are transported in the lymphatic system through phagocytosis by macrophages, whereas powders larger than that are immobilized and encapsulated with fibrous tissue (Venugopal and Luckley 1978). When thin-film, wire, rod, or sphere-shaped Ta is implanted into bone, osseointegration is observed, and direct contact with bone without soft tissue intervention is observed using an optical microscope, similar to that of CP Ti. This phenomenon indicates high compatibility with bone.

Since the late 1990s, porous Ta has been developed and used as bone prosthetic materials and bone contact parts of artificial joints (Bobyn et al. 1999, 2004, Mohandas et al. 2014). Figure 9.12 shows the three-dimensional microstructure of porous Ta material and an example of its application to an artificial hip joint cup (Bobyn et al. 2004). Porous Ta has various mechanical, chemical, and biological advantages, including:

I. The high density, which is a demerit of Ta, is solved by porous body, and at the same time, the apparent elastic modulus is reduced.
II. By using chemical vapor deposition/infiltration (CVD/CVI), the poor castability of high-melting point Ta is resolved and creation of a complex shape like a dodecahedron and connecting pores is obtained.
III. By using Ta, sufficient strength is achieved with a porosity of about 75–80% and a pore size of about 500 μm.
IV. New bone easily in-grows into the pores, and osseointegration is observed between the bone and the implant.
V. By making it porous, high shearing force due to the anchor effect of new bone is performed.
VI. In pores, remodeling occurs with the normal Haversian system in animals.

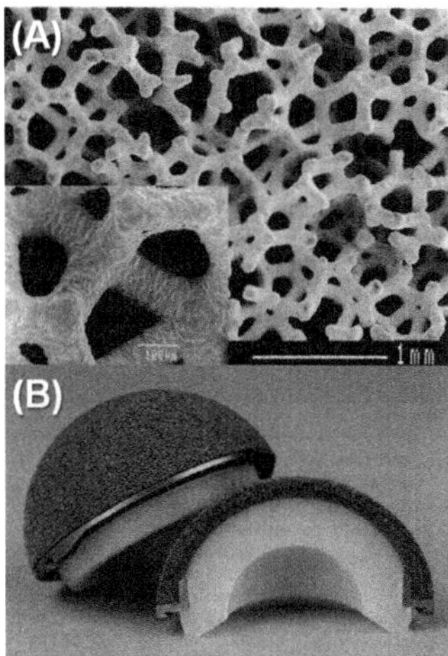

Fig. 9.12. (A) Microstructure of connected porous Ta for medical devices and (B) application example to artificial hip joint cup (Reprinted with permission from Wolters Kluwer, Bobyn et al. 2004. J. Bone Joint Surg. B81: 907–914.).

By taking these advantages of porous Ta material, applications to not only the cup of an artificial hip joint but also the tibial contact part of an artificial knee joint, screws of bone fixators, the bone contact/fixation part of custom-made artificial joints, and spinal fixation devices are expanding.

9.7 Zirconium Alloys

9.7.1 General Property

At room temperature, Zr exhibits hcp crystal structure, α phase, which changes to β phase, a bcc crystal structure, at 863°C, and exists in the β–phase until the melting point (Schnell and Albers 2006). The α–ω and ω-β phase transformations of Zr are discussed (Zhang et al. 2019). Among the numerous radioactive isotopes of Zr, 93Zr is among the most common. It is released as a product of 235U, mainly in nuclear plants and during nuclear weapons tests in the 1950s and 1960s. It has a very long half–life (1.53 million yr), its decay emits only low energy radiations, and it is not highly hazardous. Therefore, major demand of Zr alloys is coming from nuclear industry and they are conventionally used for protective tubes of nuclear fuel rods.

Zr is highly resistant to corrosion by alkalis, acids, salt water and other agents. The increase of the Nb and Ta amount in Zr alloy led to the improving of electrochemical behavior in fetal bovine serum (Branzoi et al. 2017). Zr and Zr-based alloys show pitting corrosion in the presence of chloride ions including in human body fluid, unlike Ti. Sn played an important role in determining the corrosion resistance of Zr in chloride environments (Tsutsumi et al. 2020). To increase localized corrosion resistance of Zr, an electrochemical treatment is attempted (Manaka et al. 2021).

The cathodic polarization curves of CP Ti and Zr in Hanks' solution and saline are shown in Fig. 9.13. The surface oxide film (passive film) on CP Ti is not completely oxidized and is relatively reactive; that on Zr is more passive and protective than that

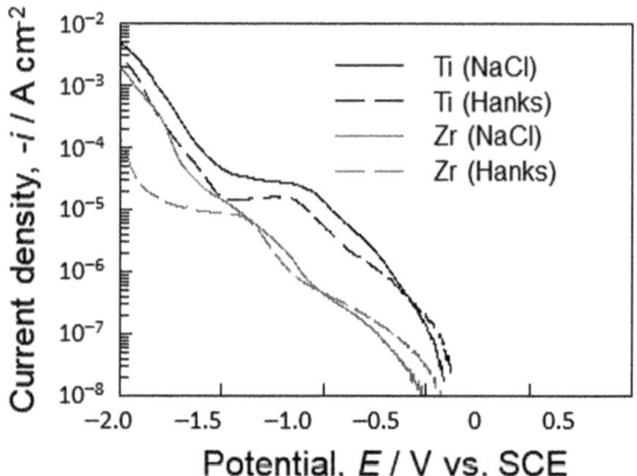

Fig. 9.13. Cathodic polarization curves of CP Ti and pure Zr in saline and Hanks' solution (Reprinted with permission from Elsevier, Tsutsumi et al. 2009. Mater. Sci. Eng. C 29: 1702–1708.). The passive film on Zr is more protective than that on Ti against cathodic polarization.

on Ti (Tsutsumi et al. 2009). Neither calcium nor phosphate stably exists alone on Ti, and calcium phosphate is naturally formed on it; calcium phosphate formed on CP Ti is stable and protective. On the other hand, calcium ion is never incorporated on Zr, while zirconium phosphate, which is easily formed on Zr, is highly stable and protective. Moreover, the surface oxide films on CP Ti, Nb, and Ta are not completely oxidized and are relatively reactive, while that on Zr is stably oxidized; that on Zr is more passive and protective than those on CP Ti, Nb, and Ta (Tsutsumi et al. 2015). CP Ti plays the most important role in forming calcium phosphate, while Zr inhibits the formation of calcium phosphate on Ti alloys. In this regard, calcium phosphate formation is inhibited in Hanks' solution when Zr is coated on CP Ti (Kobayashi et al. 2007) and bone formation is prevented in rat tibia (Takada et al. 2017). Therefore, the ability of calcium phosphate formation of CP Ti is weakened by the addition of Zr in Ti–Zr alloys (Hanawa et al. 1992). The stability of Zr is explained from the viewpoint of band gap of the passive film on it. The passive film on Zr consists of mainly ZrO_2 with hydroxyl groups. The band gap energies of ZrO_2 ceramics are 4.27–4.93 eV by theory and 5.78–6.1 eV by experiment that varies according to the crystal system (French et al. 1994). In the case of the passive film on Zr, the band gap energies are 3.01–3.47 eV in the outer hydroxide layer and 4.44–4.91 eV in the inner oxide layer (Kim et al. 2005). These values are much larger than those of TiO_2 and the passive film on CP Ti (see Fig. 6.21).

Zr is categorized in the safest element groups (Yamamoto et al. 1998). The proliferation, mitochondrial activity, cell morphology of MC3T3–E1 cells and GM7373 cells are good after 7 days incubation in direct contact with polished Zr. The biocompatibility range of the investigated metals is (the order increasing biocompatibility): Nb=Ta, CP Ti, Zr=Al=type 316L stainless steel=Mo (Eisenbarth et al. 2004). Zr shows excellent cell proliferation and varied ALP activity for SaOS2 cells (Zhang et al. 2017). Protein adsorption on Zircaloy has been investigated to apply biomedical devices. Adsorption of bovine serum albumin by Zircaloy-2 increases with deformation by cold rolling (Trivedi et al. 2015). Regarding the mineralization level, the mineral composition, and the alignment and order of the mineral particles, the maturity of the newly formed bone after 8 wk of implantation is already very high and the bone material quality obtained on Zr implants is at least as good as for Ti (Hoerth et al. 2014). On Zr and Zr alloys for medical and dental use, an excellent review paper has been published (Mehjabeen et al. 2018).

9.7.2 Application to Artificial Joints

Decreasing the wear of polyethylene cups is the predominant goal to succeed total hip replacement (THR) bearings. The wear of THR bearings with ceramicized ball heads depends more on the behavior of the polyethylene cups than on the treatment of the ball head surface. The risk of coating damage and of its consequences has to be taken into account in selecting this type of bearing (Piconi et al. 2017). The oxidation of Zr–2.5Nb alloy surface produces a relatively thick (7 μm), adherent, and abrasion–resistant ceramic surface layer. The coefficient of friction of bovine articular cartilage rubbed against oxidized Zr was lower than with Co–Cr alloy surfaces, and there is a trend toward less wear with oxidized Zr (Patel and Spector 1997). The oxide/metal interface is continuous, without pores or voids which might be detrimental to oxide adhesion. The ceramic like zirconia surface layer is highly adherent to the metal alloy and further supported the use of this novel alloy as a scratch–resistant counter-face for total joint replacement prostheses (Hernigou et al. 2007, Bourne et al. 2005, Sonntag et al. 2012, Bader et al. 2008). The Zr–2.5Nb alloy has a relatively low modulus of 100 GPa. The Zr alloy is combined with an all–plastic tibial component, replacing the metal tray and plastic insert used in other knee replacements. It is believed that this new knee could last for 20–25 yr (Hernigou et al. 2007, Bourne et al. 2005), substantially more than the 15–20 yr over which Co–Cr alloy and polyethylene implants (Spector et al. 2001). By the bearing surfaces of both the femoral and tibial components of retrieved total knee arthroplasty (TKA), oxidized Zr femoral bearing surfaces create less *in vivo* damage to both surfaces than those of Co–Cr alloy (Heyse et al. 2011).

The amounts of bacteria that adhered to the material are significantly lower for Oxinium® and Co–Cr–Mo than for CP Ti (Shida et al. 2013). Minimum level of roughness affecting initial bacterial adherence activity differs according to materials, and that even a surface roughness of below 30 nm R_a in Oxinium, Ti–6Al–4 V and type 316L stainless steel can promote bacterial adhesion. In addition, relative hydrophobic Co–Cr–Mo surfaces were less susceptible to bacterial adherence (Yoda et al. 2014).

9.7.3 Zirconium-Based Alloys

MRI artifact volume is proportional to the magnetic susceptibility difference between metal and surroundings as shown in Fig. 9.14 (Imai et al. 2013). Pure Zr shows low magnetic susceptibility as well as high corrosion resistance, but poor proof and tensile strengths. Therefore, Zr alloys strengthened with solid solution strengthening elements have been developed to decrease artifact volume of implant devices.

Zr–Nb alloys shows that the ω phase contributes to the decrease of the magnetic susceptibility, independently of the formation process of the ω phase (Nomura

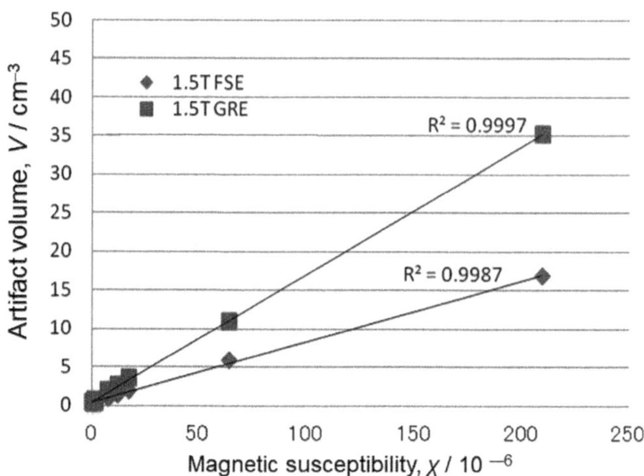

Fig. 9.14. Relationship between magnetic susceptibility and artifact volume of metals (Provided by Dr. Naoyuki Nomura, Tohoku University). Artifact volume of metals is proportional to the magnetic susceptibility of the metals.

et al. 2009). Relationship among the mechanical property, crystal structure and magnetic susceptibility is shown in Fig. 9.15. Cold–workable Zr–14Nb with low magnetic susceptibility could be a promising alloy for medical devices under MRI (Kondo et al. 2013). The mechanical properties of Zr–14Nb can be controlled by thermomechanical processing while keeping low magnetic susceptibility (Kondo et al. 2016). As a matter of fact, MRI artifact by Zr–14Nb alloy is sufficiently small (Kajima et al. 2020). The 0.2% offset yield strength and the ultimate tensile strength of the Pt and Pd-added Zr–20Nb alloys increase with the Pt and Pd concentrations. Pt and Pd solute in β–Zr is a substitutional element and contributes to the increase in the strength by solid solution hardening (Kondo et al. 2011).

In cast Zr–Mo alloys, the minimum value of the susceptibility is closely related to the appearance of the athermal ω phase in the β phase. The appearance of the α' and β phase leads to an increase in magnetic susceptibility (Suyalatu et al. 2010). Magnetic susceptibility is reflected in the phase constitution: the susceptibility shows a local minimum at Zr–(0.5–1)Mo with mostly α' phase and a minimum at Zr–3Mo with mostly β and ω phases. The ultimate tensile strength of α'–based Zr–Mo alloys is tailored from 674 to 970 MPa, and the corresponding elongation varied from 11.1% to 2.9% (Suyalatu et al. 2011). As shown in Fig. 9.16 (Nomura 2021), the best balance between mechanical property and magnetic susceptibility is Zr–0.5-1 mass%Mo. It is possible to produce a homogeneous large–scale ingot of Zr–1Mo with high elongation and low magnetic susceptibility (Ashida et al. 2015). A good balance of mechanical properties and low magnetic susceptibility in the Zr–1Mo alloy is obtained by cold swaging (Ashida et al. 2015). In addition, the Zr–1Mo alloy decreases MRI artifact as shown in Fig. 5.5. A low magnetic Zr–1Mo alloy is fabricated by a powder bed fusion (PBF) process using a fiber laser (Sun et al. 2017, 2020a,b). Additive manufacturing of Zr–1Mo alloy is performed to find optimal manufacturing conditions (Sun et al. 2020c, d, 2021a, b, Zhou et al. 2021).

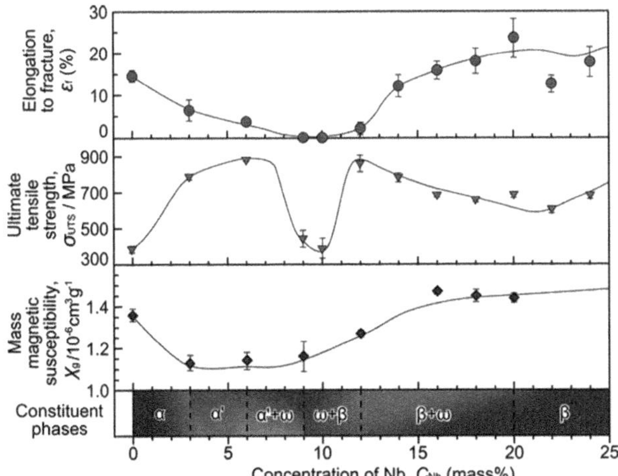

Fig. 9.15. Changes in mass magnetic susceptibility, ultimate tensile strength, and elongation to fracture of Zr-Nb alloy with Nb content and their crystal phases (Reprinted with permission from NOVA science publishers, *Advances in Materials Science Research, Vol.52* (Hanawa and Nomura: Chapter 4 Zirconium and zirconium alloys for biomedical use, 2022), 107–144.). ω phase decreases magnetic susceptibility, strength, and elongation.

A phase stability (B_o–M_d) map is constructed by performing theoretical calculations and was subsequently used to determine alloy compositions (Zr–14Nb–5Ta–1Mo and Zr–14Nb–10Ta–1Mo alloys). A higher strength of 796 MPa and an elongation of 15% are obtained for the Zr–14Nb–5Ta–1Mo alloy. Furthermore, the fabricated Zr–14Nb–5Ta–1Mo and Zr–14Nb–10Ta–1Mo alloys are characterized by low magnetic susceptibilities of 16.96×10^{-9} and 17.34×10^{-9} m^3 kg^{-1}, respectively, and Young's moduli of 61 GPa and 58 GPa, respectively. These alloys show a good balance of mechanical properties with low Young's moduli and magnetic susceptibility (Ashida et al. 2020).

Swaged Zr–Ag composites up to the reduction ratio of 96% for Zr–(4, 16, 36, 64)Ag and 86% for Zr–81Ag are successfully obtained. The magnetic susceptibility of the composites linearly decreases with the increasing volume fraction of Ag (Imai et al. 2017).

The microstructures, mechanical properties, corrosion behaviors, *in vitro* cytocompatibility and magnetic susceptibility of Zr–1X alloys with various alloying elements are systematically investigated. Among the experimental Zr–1X alloys, Zr–1Ru alloy possessing high strength coupled with good ductility, good *in vitro* cytocompatibility and low magnetic susceptibility may be a good candidate alloy for medical devices within a magnetic resonance imaging environment (Zhou et al. 2013). Zr–Ti–Nb alloys are also investigated (Mishchenko et al. 2020).

The tendency for the formation of a spontaneous oxide is greater for $Zr_{97.5}Nb_{1.5}Ti_{1.0}$, $Zr_{97.5}Nb_{1.5}Mo_{1.0}$, and $Zr_{97.5}Nb_{1.5}W_{1.0}$ alloys and this oxide has better corrosion protection characteristics than that on Grade 2 CP Ti. $Zr_{97.5}Nb_{1.5}M_{1.0}$ alloys are promising materials for osteo–synthesis prosthetic devices, since corrosion stability is directly associated with biocompatibility and is a necessary condition for applying a material as biomaterial (Rosalbino et al. 2015). The electrochemical

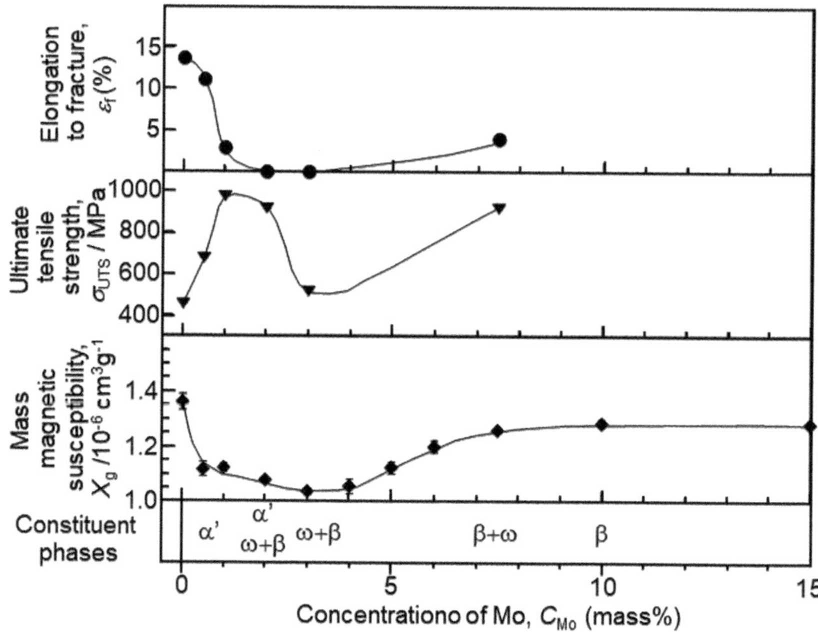

Fig. 9.16. Changes in mass magnetic susceptibility, ultimate tensile strength, and elongation to fracture of Zr-Mo alloy with Mo content and their crystal phases (Reprinted with permission from The Japanese Society for Dental Materials and Devices, Nomura. 2021. J. Jpn. Soc. Dent. Mater. Dev. 40(2): 153–156.). Omega phase decreases magnetic susceptibility, strength, and elongation.

behavior of the ZrTiNbAl alloys is consistent with the formation of passivating oxide films on the surfaces of these materials. The Zr–49Ti–15Nb–4Al alloy, which has the highest Ti (49 wt.%) content, exhibited a larger passive range in the polarization curve and is immune to localized corrosion breakdown in a simulated physiological solution for the range of polarizations (Chelariu et al. 2017).

9.8 High Entropy Alloys

In recent years, a new alloy called "high-entropy alloy (HEA)" (Ranganathan 2003, Cantor et al. 2004, Yeh et al. 2004, Murty et al. 2014, Gao et al. 2016, Miracle and Senkov 2017, George et al. 2019) has been developed. The concept has been proposed and is attracting a lot of attention. HEAs are generally considered to be: (1) a multi-component alloy with five or more constituent elements, (2) a nearly equiatomic composition ratio, and (3) an alloy that forms a single-phase solid medium. Figure 9.17 is a schematic diagram of a high-entropy alloy. HEAs are not formed from conventional alloys in which a specific element contains a small amount of other elements, that is, a "main constituent element" and an "additional element" (or a "solvent" and a "solute"). It is an alloy that forms a single-phase solid solution containing multiple constituent elements at concentrations close to equiatomic composition, and its mechanical and functional properties are also significantly different from conventional alloys. The definition of a HEA varies. However, at the first international conference (International Conference on High-Entropy Materials,

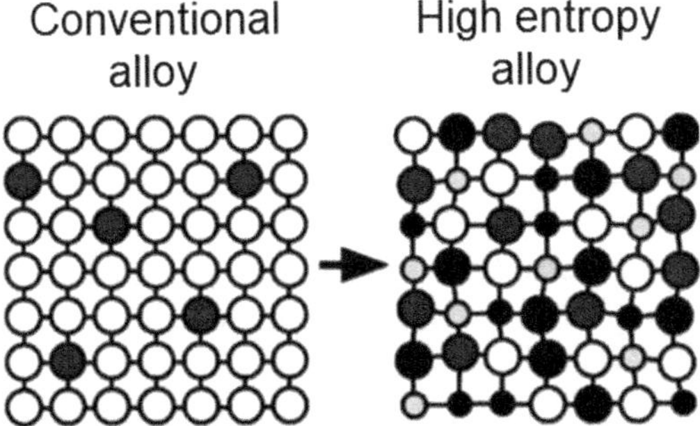

Fig. 9.17. Schematic models of structure of a conventional alloy and a high entropy alloy (Provided by Dr. Takayoshi Nakano, Osaka University). High entropy alloy consists of a single-phase solid solution containing multiple constituent elements at concentrations close to equiatomic composition.

ICHEM 2016) held in 2016, its basic definition was as follows (1) and (2). It was decided to use the formula.

$$\Delta S_{mix} = -R\sum_{i=1}^{n} x_i \ln x_i \tag{9.3}$$

$$\Delta S_{mix} \geq 1.5R(\text{HEA}) \tag{9.4}$$

where ΔS_{mix} is the entropy of the mixture, R is the gas constant (8.314 J/Kmol), x_i is the mole fraction of component i, and n is the number of constituent elements. Furthermore, the concepts of medium entropy alloy (MEA) and low entropy alloy (LEA) using ΔS_{mix} have been proposed, and alloys have been classified based on the size of their entropy. MEA and LEA are defined below.

$$1.0R \leq \Delta S_{mix} \leq 1.5R\ (\text{MEA}) \tag{9.5}$$

$$\Delta S_{mix} \leq 1.0R\ (\text{LEA}) \tag{9.6}$$

In n-element alloys consisting of n elements, ΔS_{mix} is maximum in equiatomic composition alloys. In quaternary equiatomic composition alloys, ΔS_{mix} = 1.39R, and in quinary equiatomic composition ratios. ΔS_{mix} =1.61R. Therefore, even if the criteria shown in equations (1) and (2) are followed, multi-component alloys with five or more components fall into the category of high-entropy alloys, and the atomic composition ratio of the composition ratio is close to equiatomic.

HEAs for biological use is reviewed (George et al. 2019, Geanta et al. 2019). HEAs have been developed as a new class of structural materials that consist of multicomponent elements with an approximately equiatomic ratio for increasing the mixing entropy to stabilize the solid solution phase. Elemental homogenization and functionalization of HEAs for biological use (bioHEAs) are performed by ultra-rapid cooling via laser-powder bed fusion. The characteristics of these BioHEAs, especially focusing on their excellent properties for biomedical applications, are introduced (Ozasa et al. 2023). The newly developed $Ti_{20}Nb_{20}Ta_{20}Zr_{20}Mo_{20}$ alloy with equal atomic composition ratio (numbers are atomic %) exhibits biocompatibility comparable to that of CP Ti. Its mechanical strength is overwhelmingly higher than that of the Ti–6Al–4V alloy, which is highly reliable, and it has high workability (Todai et al. 2017). It is a new material with excellent properties that allows it to be applied to precision casting and three-dimensional additive manufacturing, as it exhibits excellent biocompatibility and mechanical properties even in the cast state. A non-equiatomic Ti, Zr-rich composition stimulated the molecular interaction between biological cells and bioHEA, indicating the possibility of the proposed non-equiatomic Ti–Nb–Ta–Zr–Mo HEM as an advanced biomaterial for bone tissue engineering applications (Hori et al. 2019). TiZrNbTaFe for biomedical applications obtained by powder metallurgy route shows a better mechanical biocompatibility as orthopedic or dental implants (Popescu et al. 2018). A non-equiatomic $Ti_{28.33}Zr_{28.33}Hf_{28.33}Nb_{6.74}Ta_{6.74}Mo_{1.55}$ super-solid solutionized HEA is developed using laser powder bed fusion (LPBF) (Ozkan et al. 2023). Significant suppression of elemental segregation, thus resulting in a single crystalline-like texture by activating layer-to-layer epitaxial growth, is obtained. Relatively low Young's modulus was achieved in the single crystalline-like BioHEA. Moreover, LPBF-fabricated BioHEA exhibits significantly higher yield stress (1355–1426 MPa) due to the effective solid solution hardening compared to as-cast counterpart with marked segregation, and good biocompatibility.

References

ANS/ADA Specification. 1997. No. 5-1997. Dental Casting Alloys. American National Standards Institute, Washington. D.C., USA.

Anusavice, K.J. 2003. Phillips' Science of Dental Materials, 11th ed.: Sanders, St. Louis, MO, USA.

Ashida, M., T. Sugimoto, N. Nomura, Y. Tsutsumi, P. Chen, H. Doi et al. 2015. Microstructure and mechanical properties of large–scale ingots of the Zr–1Mo alloy. Mater. Trans. 56: 1544–1548.

Ashida, M., Y. Tsutsumi, K. Homma, P. Chen, M. Shimojo and T. Hanawa. 2020. Design of zirconium quaternary system alloys and their properties. Mater. Trans. 61: 776–781.

ASTM F560. 2023. Standard Specification for Unalloyed Tantalum for Surgical Implant Applications (UNS R05200, UNS R05400), ASTM International, West Conshohocken, PA, USA.

Bader, R., P. Bergschmidt, A. Fritsche, S. Ansorge, P. Thomas and W. Mittelmeier. 2008. Alternative materials and solutions in total knee arthroplasty for patients with metal allergy. Orthopade 37: 136–142.

Bobyn, J.D., G.L. Stackpool, S.A. Hacking, M. Tanzer and J.J. Krygier. 1999. Characteristics of bone ingrowth and interface mechanics of a new porous tantalum biomaterial. J. Bone Joint Surg. B. 81: 907–914.

Bobyn, J.D., R.A. Poggie, J.J. Krygier, D.G. Lewallen, A.D. Hanssen, R.J. Lewis et al. 2004. Clinical validation of a structural porous tantalum biomaterial for adult reconstruction. J. Bone Joint Surg. Am. 86A: 123–129.

Branzoi, F., M. Iordoc and V. Branzoi. 2017. Evaluation of corrosion behaviour and surface characterization for some biomedical materials. Rev. Roum. Chim. 62: 923–931.

Chelariu, R., L.C. Trinca, C. Munteanu, G. Bolat, D. Sutiman, D. Mareci et al. 2017. Corrosion behavior of new quaternary ZrNbTiAl alloys in simulated physiological solution using electrochemical techniques and surface analysis methods. Electrochim. Acta 248: 368–375.

Cowley, A. and B. Woodward. 2011. A Healthy future: platinum in medical applications. Platinum Met. Rev. 55: 98.

Eisenbarth, E., D. Velten, M. Muller, R. Thull and J. Breme. 2004. Biocompatibility of beta–stabilizing elements of titanium alloys. Biomaterials 25: 5705–5713.

Erbel, R., C. Di Mario, J. Bartunek, J. Bonnier, B. de Bruyne, F.R. Eberli et al. 2007. Temporary scaffolding of coronary arteries with bioabsorbable magnesium stents: a prospective, non-randomised multicentre trial. Lancet 369: 1869–1875.

Frazin-Nia, F. and T. Yoneyama. 2009. Shape memory alloys are suitable for a wide range of biomedical applications, such as dentistry, bone repair and cardiovascular stents. pp. 257–296. *In*: Yoneyama, T. and S. Miyazaki [eds.]. Shape Memory Alloys for Biomedical Applications. Woodhead, Cambridge, UK.

French, R.H., S.J. Glass, F.S. Ohuchi, Y.N. Xu and W.Y. Ching. 1994. Experimental and theoretical determination of the electronic structure and optical properties of three phases of ZrO_2. Phys. Rev. B 49: 5133–5142.

Fukui, Y., T. Inamura, H. Hosoda, K. Wakashima and S. Miyazaki. 2004. Mechanical properties of a Ti–Nb–Al shape memory alloy. Mater. Trans. 45: 1077–1082.

Geanta, V., I. Voiculescu, P. Vizureanu and A.V. Sandu. 2019. High entropy alloys for medical applications. p. 89318. *In:* Sharma, A., Z. Duriagina and S. Kumar [eds.]. Engineering Steels and High Entropy-Alloys. IntechOpen Limited, London, UK.

Gebau, R.C. and R.S. Brown. 2001. Biomedical implant alloy. Adv. Mater. Process. 159: 46–48.

George, E.P., D. Raabe and R.O. Ritchie. 2019. High-entropy alloys. Nature Rev. Mater. 4: 515–534.

Goo, K.W., W.T. Chiu, A. Umise, M. Tahara, M. Sone, K. Kenji Goto et al. 2023. Mechanical properties enhancement of biomedical au-cu-al shape memory alloys by phase manipulation. Mater. Trans. 64: 962–966.

Hanawa, T., O. Okuno and H. Hamanaka. 1992. Compositional change in surface of Ti–Zr alloys in artificial bioliquid. J. Jpn. Inst. Met. 56: 1168–1173.

Hanawa, T. 2019. Overview of metals and applications. pp. 3–30. *In*: Niinomi, M. [ed.]. Metals for Medical Devices, 2nd ed. Wodhead, Duxford, UK.

Hanawa, T. and N. Nomura. 2022. Chapter 4 Zirconium and Zirconium Alloys for Biomedical Use. pp. 107–144. *In*: Wythers, M.C. [ed.]. Advances in Materials Science Research, Vol. 52. Nova Science Publishers, New York, NY, USA.

Heintz, C., G. Riepe, L. Birken, E. Kaiser, N. Chakfe, M. Morlock et al. 2001. Corroded nitinol wires in explanted aortic endografts: an important mechanism of failure? J. Endovasc. Ther. 8: 248–253.

Herber, V., B. Okutan, G. Antonoglou, N.G. Sommer and M. Payer. 2021. Bioresorbable magnesium-based alloys as novel biomaterials in oral bone regeneration: general review and clinical perspectives. J. Clin. Med. 10: 1842.

Hermawan, H., H. Alamdari, D. Mantovani and D. Dube. 2008. Iron-manganese: new class of metallic degradable biomaterials prepared by powder metallurgy. Powder Metall. 51: 38–45.

Hernigou, P., G. Mathieu, A. Poignard, O. Manicom, P. Filippini and A. Demoura. 2007. Oxinium, a new alternative femoral bearing surface option for hip replacement. Eur. J. Orthop. Surg. Trauma. 17: 243–246.

Heublein, B., R. Rohde, V. Kaese, M. Niemeyer, W. Hartung and A. Haverich. 2003. Biocorrosion of magnesium alloys: a new principle in cardiovascular implant technology? Heart 89: 651–656.

Heyse, T.J., D.X. Chen, N. Kelly, F. Boettner, T.M. Wright and S.B. Haas. 2011. Matched–pair total knee arthroplasty retrieval analysis: Oxidized zirconium vs. CoCrMo. Knee 18: 448–452.

Hiromoto, S. and M. Tomozawa. 2010. Corrosion behavior of magnesium with hydroxyapatite coatings formed by hydrothermal treatment. Mater. Trans. 51: 2080–2087.

Hoerth, R.M., M.R. Katunar, A.G. Sanchez, J.C. Orellano, M. Silvia, S.M. Ceré et al. 2014. A comparative study of zirconium and titanium implants in rat: osseointegration and bone material quality. J. Mater. Sci. Mater. Med. 25: 411–422.

Hori, T., T. Nagase, M. Todai, A. Matsugaki and T. Nakano. 2019. Development of non-equiatomic Ti-Nb-Ta-Zr-Mo high-entropy alloys for metallic biomaterials. Scripta Mater. 172: 83–87.

Horiuchi, Y., K. Nakayama, T. Inamura, H.Y. Kim, K. Wakashima, S. Miyazaki et al. 2007. Non-monotonic aging temperature dependence of superelasticity of $Ti_{72}Nb_{15}Zr_{10}Al_3$ quaternary alloys. Mater. Trans. 48: 414–421.

Iijima, Y., T. Nagase, A. Matsugaki, P. Wang, K. Ametama and T. Nakano. 2021. Design and development of Ti–Zr–Hf–Nb–Ta–Mo high-entropy alloys for metallic biomaterials. Mater. Design 202: 109548.

Ikeda, M., S. Komatsu and Y. Nakamura. 2004. Effects of Sn and Zr additions on phase constitution and aging behavior of Ti–50 mass%Ta alloys quenched from β single phase region. Mater. Trans. 45: 1106–1112.

Ikeda, M., D. Sugano, S. Masuda and M. Ogawa. 2005. The influence of aluminum content on shape memory effect of Ti–7Cr–Al alloys fabricated using low grade sponge titanium. Mater. Trans. 46:1604–1609.

Ikeo, N., T. Uemura, A. Taguma and T. Mukai. 2021. Different effects of calcium and zinc as a solute element on the fatigue properties in simulated body fluids of magnesium alloys. Mater. Trans. 62: 1806–1809.

Imai, H., Y. Tanaka, N. Nomura, H. Doi, Y. Tsutsumi, T. Ono et al. 2017. Magnetic susceptibility, artifact volume in MRI, and tensile properties of swaged Zr–Ag composites for biomedical applications. J. Mech. Behav. Biomed. Mater. 66: 152–158.

Imai, H., Y. Tanaka, N. Nomura, Y. Tsutsumi, H. Doi, Z. Kanno et al. 2013. Three–dimensional quantification of susceptibility artifacts from various metals in magnetic resonance image. Acta Biomater. 9: 8433–8439.

Inamura, T., H. Hosoda, K. Wakashima and S. Miyazaki. 2005. Anisotropy and temperature dependence of Young's modulus in textured TiNbAl biomedical shape memory alloy. Mater. Trans. 46: 1597–1603.

ISO 20749:2023. 2023. Dentistry–Pre-capsulated dental amalgam, International Organization for Standardization, Geneva, Switzerland.

ISO 22674:2006. 2006. Dentistry–Metallic materials for fixed and removable restorations and appliances, International Organization for Standardization, Geneva, Switzerland.

ISO 24234:2021. 2021. Dentistry–Dental amalgam, International Organization for Standardization, Geneva, Switzerland.

ISO 9333:2022. 2022. Dentistry—Brazing materials, International Organization for Standardization, Geneva, Switzerland.

Kajima, Y., A. Takaichi, Y. Tsutsumi, T. Hanawa, N. Wakabayashi and A. Kawasaki. 2020. Influence of magnetic susceptibility and volume on MRI artifacts produced by low magnetic susceptibility Zr-14Nb alloy and dental alloys. Dent. Mater. J. 39: 256–261.

Kanetaka, H., Y. Shimizu, H. Hosoda, R. Tomizuka, A. Suzuki, S. Urayama et al. 2007. Orthodontic tooth movement in rats using Ni-free Ti-based shape memory alloy wire. Mater. Trans. 48: 367–372.

Kang, G. and D. Song. 2015. Review on structural fatigue of NiTi shape memory alloys: Pure mechanical and thermo-mechanical ones. Theoret. Appl. Mech. Lett. 5: 245–254.

Kannan, M.B. and O. Wallipa. 2013. Potentiostatic pulse-deposition of calcium phosphate on magnesium alloy for temporary implant applications—an *in vitro* corrosion study. Mater. Sci. Eng. C 33: 675–679.

Kawamura, Y., F. Shimada, K. Hamada, S. Ueno and S. Inoue. 2023. Development of biomedical Mg–1.0Ca–0.5Zn–0.1Y–0.03Mn (at%) alloy by rapidly solidified powder metallurgy processing. Mater. Trans. 64: 2333–2336.

Kielhorn, J., C. Melber, D. Keller and I. Mangelsdorf. 2002. Palladium—A review of exposure and effects to human health. Int. J. Hyg. Environ. Health 205: 417–432.

Kim, B.Y., C.J. Park and H.S. Kwon. 2005. Effect of niobium on the electronic properties of passive films on zirconium alloys. J. Electroanal. Chem. 576: 269–276.

Kim, H.Y., T. Sasaki, K. Okutsu, J.I. Kim, T. Inamura, H. Hosoda et al. 2006. Martensitic transformation and superelastic properties of Ti–Nb base alloys. Acta Mater. 54: 423–433.

Knops, H., R.J. Holliday and C.W. Corti. 2003. Gold in dentistry: alloys, uses and performance. Gold Bull. 36: 93–102.

Kobayashi, E., M. Ando, Y. Tsutsumi, H. Doi, T. Yoneyama, M. Kobayashi et al. 2007. Inhibition effect of zirconium coating on calcium phosphate precipitation of titanium to avoid assimilation with bone. Mater. Trans. 48: 301–306.

Kondo, R., Suyalatu, Y. Tsutsumi, H. Doi, N. Nomura and T. Hanawa. 2011. Microstructure and mechanical properties of Pt–added and Pd–added Zr–20Nb alloys and their metal release in 1 mass% lactic acid solution. Mater. Sci. Eng. C31: 900–905.

Kondo, R., R. Shimizu, N. Nomura, H. Doi, Suyalatu, Y. Tsutsumi et al. 2013. Effect of cold rolling on the magnetic susceptibility of the Zr–14Nb alloy. Acta Biomate. 9: 5795–5801.

Kondo, R., N. Nomura, H. Doi, H. Matsumoto, Y. Tsutsumi and T. Hanawa. 2016. Effect of heat treatment and the fabrication process on mechanical properties of Zr–14Nb alloy. Mater. Trans. 57: 2060–2064.

Kuroda, D., M. Niinomi, M. Morinaga, Y. Kato and T. Yashiro. 1988. Design and mechanical properties of new β type titanium alloys for implant materials. Mater. Sci. Eng. A 243: 244–249.

Levy, G.K., J. Goldman and E. Aghion. 2017. The prospects of zinc as a structural material for biodegradable implants–A review paper: Metals 7: 402.

Li, H., Y. Zheng and L. Qin. 2014. Progress of biodegradable metals. Prog. Nat. Sci. 24: 414–422.

Li, L.Y., R. Zeng, S. Ii, F. Zhang, Y.H. Zou, H.G. Jiang et al. 2018. *In vitro* corrosion of magnesium alloy AZ31—a synergetic influence of glucose and Tris. Front. Mater. Sci. 12: 148–197.

Li, Y., J. Wang, K. Sheng, F. Miao, Y. Wang, Y. Zhang et al. 2022. Optimizing structural design on biodegradable magnesium alloy vascular stent for reducing strut thickness and raising radial strength. Mater. Design 220: 110843.

Liu, C., C. Yang, J. Liu, Y. Tang, Z. Lin, L. Li et al. 2022. Medical high-entropy alloy: Outstanding mechanical properties and superb biological compatibility. Front. Bioeng. Biotechnol. 10: 952536.

Maeshima, T. and M. Nishida. 2004. Shape memory properties of biomedical Ti–Mo–Ag and Ti–Mo–Sn alloys. Mater. Trans. 45: 1096–1100.

Mahtabi, M.J., N. Shamsaei and M.R. Mitchell. 2015. Fatigue of Nitinol: The atate-of-the art and ongoing challenges. J. Mech, Behav. Biomed. Mater. 50: 228–254.

Manaka, T., Y. Tsutsumi, M. Ashida, P. Chen, H. Katayama and T. Hanawa. 2021. Development of electrochemical surface treatment for improvement of localized corrosion resistance of zirconium in chloride environment. Mater. Trans. 62: 788–796.

Mehjabeen, A., T. Song, W. Xu, H.P. Tang and M. Qian. 2018. Zirconium alloys for orthopaedic and dental applications. Adv. Eng. Mater. 20: 1800207.

Mishchenko, O., O. Ovchynnykov, O. Kapustian and M. Pogorielov. 2020. New Zr–Ti–Nb alloy for medical application: development, chemical and mechanical properties, and biocompatibility. Materials 13: 1306.

Mohandas, G., N. Oskolkov, M.T. McMahon, P. Walczak and M. Janowski. 2014. Porous tantalum and tantalum oxide nanoparticles for regenerative medicine. Acta Neurobiol. Exp. 74: 188–196.

Mueller, P.P., T. May, A. Perz, H. Hauser and M. Peuster. 2006. Control of smooth muscle cell proliferation by ferrouos iron. Biomaterials 27: 2193–2200.

Niinomi, M. 2003. Recent research and development in titanium alloys for biomedical applications and healthcare goods. Sci. Technol. Adv. Mater. 4: 445–454.

Niinomi, M., T. Hanawa and T. Narushima. 2005. Japanese research and development on metallic biomedical, dental, and healthcare materials. JOM 57: 18–24.

Niinomi, M. 2019. Design and development of metallic biomaterials with biological and mechanical biocompatibility. J. Biomed. Mater. Res. 107A: 944–954.

Nomura, N., Y. Tanaka, Suyalato, R. Kondo, H. Doi, Y. Tsutsumi et al. 2009. Effects of phase constitution of Zr–Nb alloys on their magnetic susceptibilities. Mater. Trans. 50: 2466–2472.

Nomura, N. 2021. Recent advances in additive manufacturing of metallic dental materials. J. Jpn. Soc. Dent. Mater. Dev. 40: 153–156.

O'Brien, W.J. 2002. Dental materials and their selection. Quintessence Publishing, Batavia, IL, USA 200–209.

Ozasa, R., A. Matsugaki, T. Ishimoto and T. Nakano. 2023. Review—Research and development of titanium-containing biomedical high entropy alloys (BioHEAs) utilizing rapid solidification via laser-powder bed fusion. Mater. Trans. 64: 31–36.

Pfeiffer, P. and H. Schwickerath. 1994. Palladiumionenabgabe von Palladiumlegierungen in Milchsäure/ Kochsalzlösung. Dtsch. Zahnarztl. Z. 49: 616–618.

Pfeiffer, P. and H. Schwickerath. 1995. Vergleigh der Löskichkeiten von MEM- und Palladiumlegierungen. Dtsch. Zahnarztl. Z. 50: 136–140.

Powers, J.M. and R.L. Sakaguchi [eds.]. 2006. Craig's Restorative Dental Materials, 20th ed., Mosly, St. Louis, MO, USA.

Okazaki, Y. 2001. A New Ti–15Zr–4Nb–4Ta alloy for medical applications. Curr. Opin. Solid State Mater. Sci. 5: 45–53.

Patel, A.M. and M. Spector. 1997. Tribological evaluation of oxidized zirconium using an articular cartilage counterface: A novel material for potential use in hemiarthroplasty. Biomaterials 18: 441–447.

Peeters, P., M. Bosiers, J. Verbist, K. Deloose and B. Heublein. 2005. Preliminary results after application of absorbable metal stents in patients with critical limbischemica. J. Endovasc. Ther. 12: 1–5.

Peuster, M., C. Hesse, T. Schloo, C. Fink and C. von Schnakenburg. 2006. Long-term biocompatibility of a corrodible peripheral iron stent in the porcine descending aorta. Biomaterials 27: 4955–4962.

Piconi, C., V. De Santis and G. Maccauro. 2017. Clinical outcomes of ceramicized ball heads in total hip replacement bearings: a literature review. J. Appl. Biomater. Funct. Mater. 15: e1–e9.

Pobertson, R.C.L. and W.G. Peacher. 1943. Symposium on war surgery: use of tantalum wire and foil in repair. Surg. Clin. North Am. 23: 1491–1504.

Popescu, G., B. Ghiban, C.A. Popescu, L. Rosu, R. Truscă, I. Carcea et al. 2018. New TiZrNbTaFe high entropy alloy used for medical applications. IOP Conf. Ser. Mater. Sci. Eng. 400: 022049.

Pudenz, R.H. 1943. The repair of cranial defects with tantalum: an experimental study. J. Am. Med. Assoc. 121: 478–481.

Rao, V.B. and C.R. Houska. 1979. Kinetics of the phase–transformation in a Ti–15Mo–5Zr–3Al alloy as studied by X-ray-diffraction. Metall. Mater. Trans. A 10: 355–358.

Rosalbino, F., D. Maccio, G. Scavino and A. Saccone. 2015. Corrosion behavior of new ternary zirconium alloys as alternative materials for biomedical applications. Mater. Corros. 66: 1125–1132.

Scheinert, D., S. Scheinert, J. Sax, C. Piorkowski, S. Braunlich, M. Ulrich et al. 2005. Prevalence and clinical impact of stent fractures after femoropopliteal stenting. J. Am. Coll. Cardiol. 45: 312–315.

Schinhammer, M., A.C. Hänzi, J.F. Löffler and P.J. Uggowitzer. 2010. Design strategy for Biodegradable Fe-Based alloys for medical applications. Acta Biomater. 6: 1705–1713.

Schnell, I. and R.C. Albers. 2006. Zirconium under pressure: phase transitions and thermodynamics. J. Phys. Condens. Matter. 18: 16.

Shida, T., H. Koseki, I. Yoda, H. Horiuchi, H. Sakoda and M. Osaki. 2013. Adherence ability of Staphylococcus epidermidis on prosthetic biomaterials: an *in vitro* study. Int. J. Nanomed. 8: 3955–3961.

Shimizu, H. and Y. Takeuchi. 2021. Bonding behavior and chemical and mechanical properties of silver-based dental alloys. Jpn. Dent. Sci. Rev. 57: 97–100.

Shinohara, Y., M. Tahara, T. Inamura, S. Miyazaki and H. Hosoda. 2015. Deformation behavior of Ti-4Au–5Cr–8Zr superelastic alloy with or without containing Ti3Au precipitates. Materials Today. pp. S821–S824. Proceedings of International Conference on Martensitic Transformations, ICOMAT-2014.

Sonntag, R., J. Reinders and J.P. Kretzer. 2012. What's next? Alternative materials for articulation in total joint replacement. Acta Biomater. 8: 2434–2441.

Spector, B.M., M.D. Ries, R.B. Bourne, W.S. Sauer, M. Long and G. Hunter. 2001. Wear performance of ultra-high molecular weight polyethylene on oxidized zirconium total knee femoral components. J. Bone Joint Surg. Am. 83-A (Suppl. 2, Pt. 2): 80–86.

Su, Y.H. [ed.]. 2012. Noble Metals. IntecjOpen, London, UK.

Sun, X., W. Zhou, K. Kikuchi, N. Nomura, A. Kawasaki, H. Doi et al. 2017. Fabrication and characterization of a low magnetic Zr–1Mo alloy by powder bed fusion using a fiber laser. Metals 7: 501.

Sun, X., D. Liu, W. Zhou, N. Nomura, Y. Tsutusmi and T. Hanawa. 2020a. Effects of process parameters on the mechanical properties of additively manufactured Zr–1Mo alloy builds. J. Mech. Behavior Biomed. Mater. 104: 103655.

Sun, X., D. Liu, W. Zhou, N. Nomura, H. Doi, Y. Tsutusmi and T. Hanawa. 2020b. Effects of quenching process on microstructure, mechanical properties and magnetic susceptibility in Zr–1Mo alloy fabricated by powder bed fusion process. Mater. Design 187: 108356.

Sun, X.H., D.B. Liu, W.W. Zhou, N. Nomura, Y. Tsutsumi and T. Hanawa. 2020c. Effects of process parameters on the mechanical properties of additively manufactured Zr–1Mo alloy builds. J. Mech. Behav. Biomed. Mater. 104: 103655.

Sun, X.H., D.B. Liu, M.F. Chen, W.W. Zhou, N. Nomura and T. Hanawa. 2020d. Hot isostatic pressing of MRI compatible Zr–1Mo components manufactured by laser powder bed fusion. Mater. Charact. 169: 110657.

Sun, X.H., D.B. Liu, M.F. Chen, W.W. Zhou, N. Nomura and T. Hanawa. 2021a. Combination of hot isostatic pressing and subsequent heat treatment for additively manufactured Zr–1Mo components. Mater. Lett. 285: 129123.

Sun, X.H., Liu, D.B., Chen, M.F., Zhou, W.W., Nomura, N. and T. Hanawa. 2021b. Influence of annealing treatment on the microstructure, Mechanical performance and magnetic susceptibility of low magnetic Zr–1Mo parts manufactured via laser additive manufacturing. Mater. Sci. Eng. A 804: 140740.

Suyalatu, N. Nomura, K. Oya, Y. Tanaka, R. Kondo, H. Doi et al. 2010. Microstructure and magnetic susceptibility of as–cast Zr–Mo alloys. Acta Biomater. 6: 1033–1038.

Suyalatu, R. Kondo, Y. Tsutsumi, H. Doi, N. Nomura and T. Hanawa. 2011. Effects of phase constitution on magnetic susceptibility and mechanical properties of Zr–rich Zr–Mo alloys. Acta Biomater. 7: 4259–4266.

Takada, R., T. Jinno, Y. Tsutsumi, H. Doi, T. Hanawa and A. Okawa. 2017. Inhibitory effect of zirconium coating to bone bonding of titanium implants in rat femur. Mater. Trans. 58: 113–117.

Thompson, S.A. 2000. An overview of nickel-titanium alloys used in dentistry. Int. Endod. J. 33: 297–310.

Todai, M., T. Nagase, T. Hori, A. Matsugaki, A. Sekita and T. Nakano. 2017. Novel TiNbTaZrMo high-entropy alloys for metallic biomaterials. Scripta Mater. 129: 65–68.

Trivedi, P., A.K. Patel, R. Maurya, R. Jayaganthan and K. Balani. 2015. Nanomechanical characterization and protein adsorption of cold–rolled zirconium alloy. JOM 67: 726–732.

Tsutsumi, Y., D. Nishimura, H. Doi, N. Nomura and T. Hanawa. 2009. Difference in surface reactions between titanium and zirconium in Hanks' solution to elucidate mechanism of calcium phosphate formation on titanium using XPS and cathodic polarization. Mater. Sci. Eng. C 29: 1702–1708.

Tsutsumi, Y., T. Nishisaka, H. Doi, M. Ashida, P. Chen and T. Hanawa. 2015. Reaction of calcium and phosphate ions with titanium, zirconium, niobium, and tantalum. Surf. Interface Anal. 47: 1148–1154.

Tsutsumi, Y., I. Muto, S. Nakano, J. Tsukada, T. Manaka, P. Chen et al. 2020. Effect of impurity elements on localized corrosion of zirconium in chloride containing environment. J. Electrochem. Soc. 167: 141507.

Venugopal, B. and T.D. Luckley. 1978. Metal toxicity in mammals. pp. 230–231. *In*: Luckey, T.D. [ed.]. Chemical Toxicity of Metals and Metalloides. Plenum, New York, NY, USA.

Virtanen, S. 2011. Biodegradable Mg and Mg alloys: Corrosion and biocompatibility. Mater. Sci. Eng. B 176: 1600–1608.

Wang, H., S. Zhu, L. Wang, Y. Feng, X. Ma and S. Guan. 2014. Corrosion protection of mesoporous bioactive glass coating on biodegradable magnesium. Appl. Surf. Sci. 307: 92–100.

Weast, R.C. and M.J. Astle. 1981. CRC Handbook of Chemistry and Physics, 62nd ed.: CRC Press, Boca Raton, FL, USA. p. D-135.

Wen, C., S. Guan, L. Peng, C. Ren, X. Wang and Z. Hu. 2009. Characterization and degradation behavior of AZ31 alloy surface modified by bone-like hydroxyapatite for implant applications. Appl. Surf. Sci. 255: 6433–6438.

White, J.B., C.G.M. Kent, H.J. Cloft and D.F. Kallmens. 2006. Behavior of metal implants used in ent surgery in 7 tesla magnetic resonance imaging. Eur. Arch. Otorhinolaryngol 263: 900–905.

Witte, F., V. Kaese, H. Haferkamp, E. Switzer, A. Meyer-Lindenberg, C.J. Wirth et al. 2005. *In vivo* corrosion of four magnesium alloys and the associated bone response. Biomaterials 26: 3557–3563.

Witte, F., H. Ulrich, M. Rudert and E. Willbold. 2007. Biodegradable magnesium scaffolds: Part 1: appropriate inflammatory response. J. Biomed. Mater. Res. 81A: 748–756.

Witte, F. 2010. The history of biodegradable magnesium implants: A review. Acta Biomater. 6: 1680–1692.

Wątroba, M., W. Bednarczyk, J. Kawałko and P. Bała. 2018. Effect of zirconium microaddition on the microstructure and mechanical properties of Zn–Zr alloys. Mater. Charact. 142: 187–194.

Yamamoto, A., R. Honma and M. Sumita. 1998. Cytotoxicity evaluation of 43 metal salts using murine fibroblasts and osteoblastic cells. J. Biomed. Mater. Res. 39: 331–340.

Yoda, I., H. Koseki, M. Tomita, T. Shida, H. Horiuchi, H. Sakoda and M. Osaki. 2014. Effect of surface roughness of biomaterials on Staphylococcus epidermidis adhesion. BMC Microbiol. 14: 234.

Zhang, D.M., C.S. Wong, C. Wen and Y.C. Li. 2017. Cellular responses of osteoblast–like cells to 17 elemental metals. J. Biomed. Mater. Res. 105A: 148–158.

Zhang, L., Y.H. Li, Y.Q. Gu and L.C. Cai. 2019. Understanding controversies in the α-ω and ω-β phase transformations of zirconium form nonhydrostatic thermodynamics. Sci. Rep. 9: 16889.

Zhang, X., Q. Li, L. Li, P. Zhang, Z. Wang and F. Chen. 2012. Fabrication of hydroxyapatite/stearic acid composite coating and corrosion behavior of coated magnesium alloy. Mater. Lett. 88: 76–78.

Zheng, Y.F., X.N. Gu and F. Witte. 2014. Biodegradable metals. Mater. Sci. Eng. R 77: 1–34.

Zhou, F.Y., K.J. Qiu, H.F. Li, T. Huang, B.L. Wang, L. Li and Y.F. Zheng. 2013. Screening on binary Zr–1X (X = Ti, Nb, Mo, Cu, Au, Pd, Ag, Ru, Hf and Bi) alloys with good *in vitro* cytocompatibility and magnetic resonance imaging compatibility. Acta Biomater. 9: 9578–9587.

Zhou, W.W., X.H. Sun, Y. Tsutsumi, N. Nomura and T. Hanawa. 2021. Bioinspired low-magnetic Zr alloy with high strength and ductility. Scripta Mater. 199: 113856.

CHAPTER 10

Surface Treatment and Surface Morphology

10.1 Introduction

The manufacturing process of metals, namely melting, casting, working, and heat treatment, cannot impart biocompatibility or biofunction (Fig. 10.1). Furthermore, there are limits to the ability to improve corrosion resistance by improving the composition. This is the greatest weakness of metals as biomaterials, so surface treatment and surface modification[1] must be performed to impart biocompatibility and biofunction. Surface treatment is a method of changing the composition and structure of the surface and improving only the properties of the surface, while maintaining the mechanical property. As shown in Fig. 10.2, metallic biomaterials are often subjected to surface treatments to improve their corrosion resistance, wear resistance, hard tissue compatibility, and antibacterial properties while maintaining the excellent mechanical properties that metals have. Surface treatment is an effective means to make metal surfaces biocompatible and functional. Surface treatment methods that have been researched for medical applications so far are categorized into dry processes and wet processes, and are summarized in Fig. 10.3. Most of them are applications of methods that have been put into practical use industrially. On the other hand, categorization according to changes in surface morphology and composition by surface coating, modification, and immobilization of molecules, is feasible. Figure 10.4 shows the surface treatment method applied to metallic biomaterials according to controls of surface morphology and surface composition. Since CP Ti and Ti alloys (hereinafter called "Ti materials") have the best biocompatibility among metallic biomaterials, almost all of these are surface treatments for Ti materials (Liu et al. 2004, Hanawa 2019, Xue et al. 2020).

---

[1] In engineering terms, surface treatment and surface modification are sometimes used separately, but since the area is not an eye angle, in this book they are used uniformly as surface treatment.

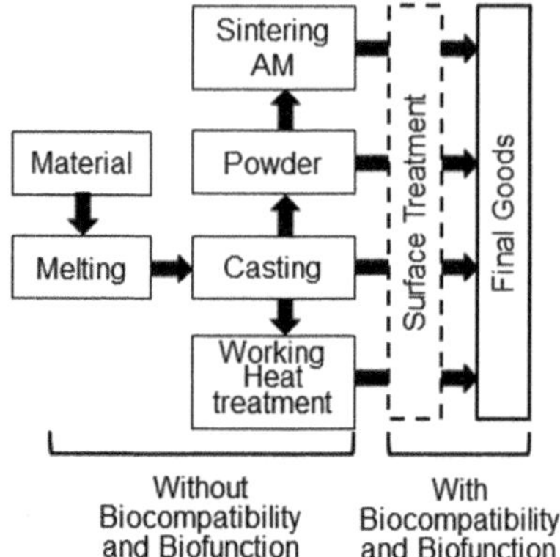

Fig. 10.1. No additional process of biocompatibility and biofunction to metals in the conventional manufacturing process and addition of biocompatibility and biofunction to metals by surface treatment.

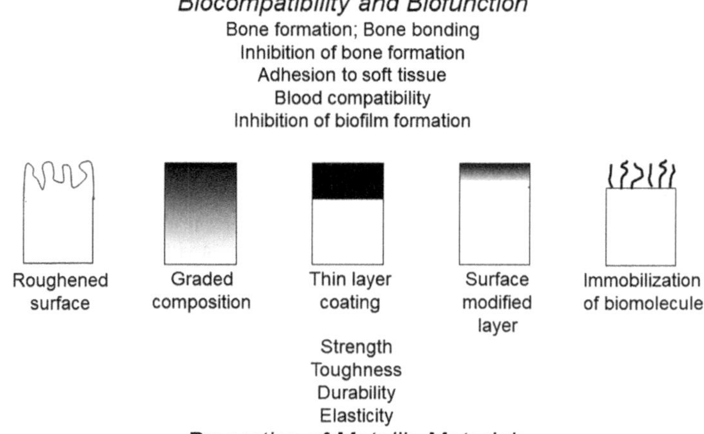

Fig. 10.2. Category of surface treatment of metals to add biocompatibility and biofunction maintaining good mechanical property.

10.2 Dry Process

10.2.1 Outline

A dry process is a process that modifies the surface of a metal using a gas phase or ions, and here it is treated as a process that does not use an aqueous solution. The dry process will be categorized from the viewpoints of surface composition, phase control, and surface morphology control. Surface composition and phase control are expected for the improvement of hard tissue compatibility, improvement of wear resistance, improvement of corrosion resistance, and acquisition of other biocompatibility and biofunction.

The treatment methods currently in practical use include coating Ti materials with thin films of TiO_2, TiN, and HA. HA coating is the mainstream method for promoting bone formation on the surfaces of Ti materials. Plasma spraying has been

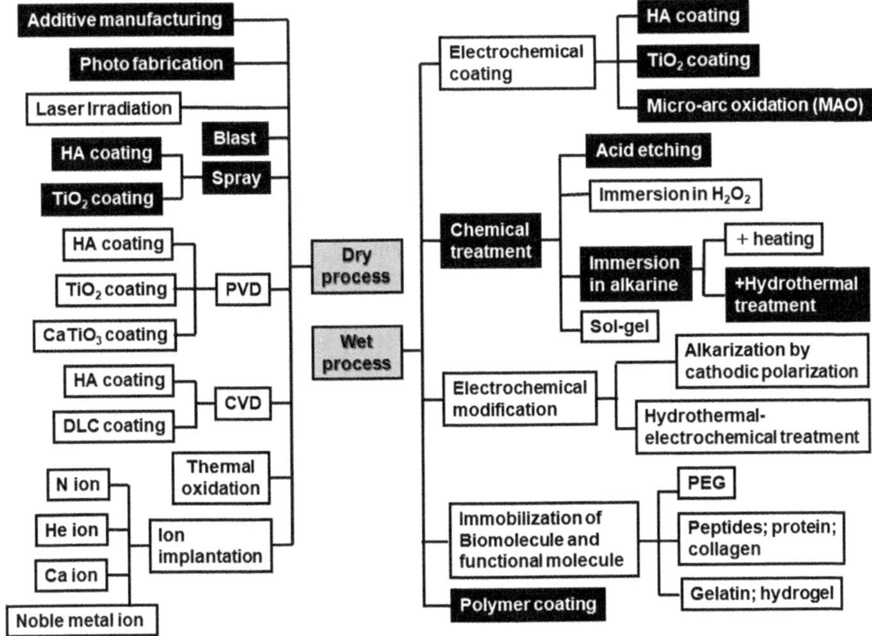

Fig. 10.3. Classification of surface treatment methods into dry process and wet process.

put into practical use (Fig. 4.3B). There are two types of fixation of the stem of an artificial hip joint to the bone: a cemented type that uses poly(methyl methacrylate) (PMMA) bone cement, and a cement-less type that does not use bone cement. In the case of cement fixation, patients may be affected due to polymerization heat and toxicity of residual monomers. In the case of cementless fixation, fine grooves are made on the top of the stem or a porous CP Ti is plasma sprayed to ensure bonding strength with the bone through mechanical anchoring. In addition, with dental implants as shown in Fig. 4.22, Ti materials are implanted into the alveolar bone, and part of it contacts with the soft tissue and is also exposed in the oral cavity, which is semi *in vivo*. Moreover, the periodontal ligament connects the natural tooth and alveolar bone and acts as a buffer, but does not exist between the implant and the alveolar bone. For this reason, hard tissue compatibility, soft tissue compatibility, and antibacterial properties are required depending on the area of contact, and surface treatments are actively being studied.

It uses physical or chemical methods to change the composition and phase of the metal implant surface to improve its compatibility with hard tissue, soft tissue, and blood compatibility, as well as its wear resistance and corrosion resistance. These treatments are usually studied for Ti materials, so Ti materials are mainly discussed. Ti materials have the property of direct bonding with bone tissue at the optical microscopic level (osseointegration), but (1) it takes a relatively long period of about 3 mon for Ti to become fixed in bone tissue. It is known that (2) sufficient fixation may not always be obtained depending on the condition of the bone; therefore, it is necessary to further improve hard tissue compatibility. Surface treatment will be considered from this perspective. As shown in Fig. 10.4, surface treatments aimed at

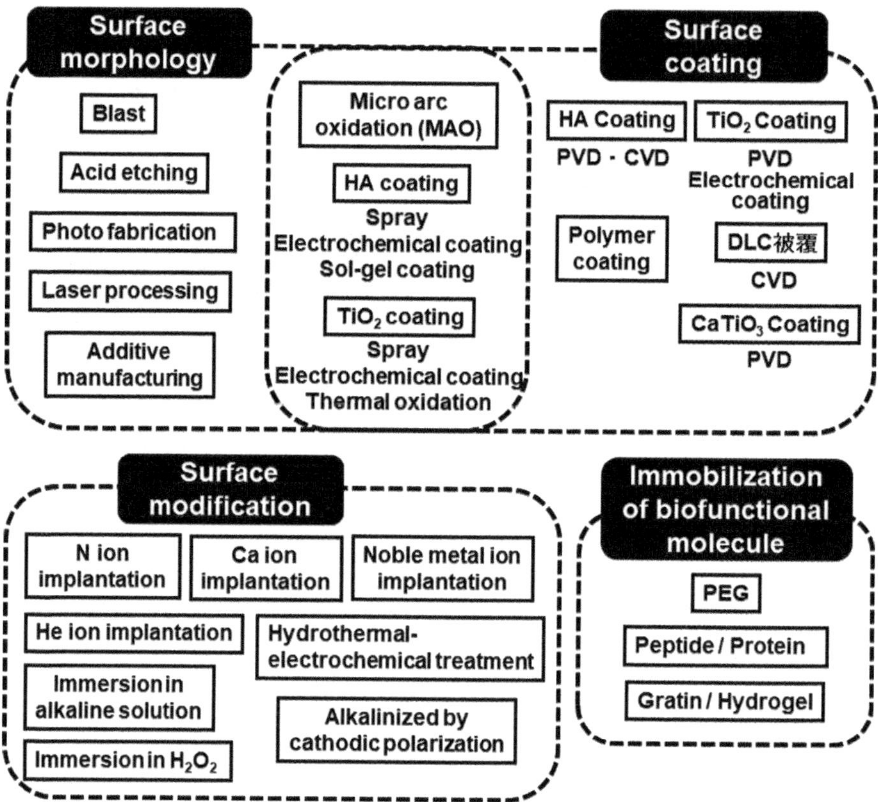

Fig. 10.4. Category of surface treatment techniques of metals for medical application according to controls of surface morphology and surface composition.

improving bone formation ability without HA coating include methods for directly producing apatite on the surface that can bond with bone (apatite formation) and methods for promoting apatite formation by a surface composition and a phase formed on the surface.

10.2.2 Spraying

It would be good if HA bulk bodies could be used as implants because they can be directly bonded to bone and can be synthesized artificially, but they do not have sufficient mechanical properties such as strength and ductility, so it is difficult to use in areas where large loads are applied. Therefore, research has been conducted since the 1970s to apply HA coating, which has the property of adhesion to bone, on the surface of metallic biomaterials with excellent mechanical properties. Ti–6Al–4V alloy coated with HA by spraying is used clinically for orthopedics (deGroot et al. 1987, LeGeros 1988, Yankee et al. 1991).

The thermal spraying forms a coating layer by continuously spraying metal or ceramic particles heated to a molten or semi-molten state onto a substrate at high speed (Fig. 10.5). A heat source is required to melt the raw materials and kinetic

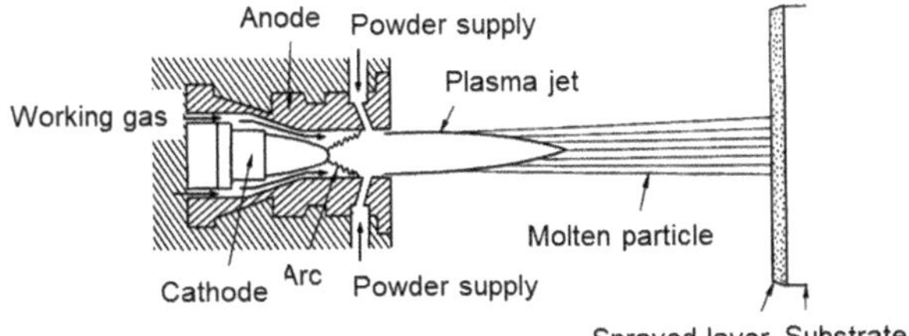

Fig. 10.5. Schematic diagram of plasma spray.

Table 10.1. Comparison of spray methods.

Condition	**Method**		
	Flame spray	**Arc spray**	**Plasma spray**
Heat source	Gas combustion energy	Electric energy	Electric energy
Temperature (K)	3000 – 3300	5000	15000
Particle speed (m s^{-1})	80 – 600	50	200
Material shape	Powder; Wire; Rod	Wire	Powder; Wire

energy is required to increase the speed. Depending on the energy supply, these methods are classified into flame spraying, arc spraying, plasma spraying, etc. (Table 10.1) (Brunette et al. 2001). Since the raw material for HA coating is powder, flame spraying and plasma spraying are mainly used. In direct current (DC) plasma spraying, HA particles are melted by a plasma flame of approximately 10,000 K or higher and impact to metal implants at a velocity of 100–200 m s^{-1}, forming an HA coating layer. HA coating by thermal spraying has been put into practical use for artificial hip joints and dental implants. Calcium phosphate coatings other than HA using thermal spraying are also being considered.

This method has a long history of HA coating on the surface of Ti material implants, has been used extensively, has a high deposition rate, and is relatively low cost, while it also involves a high-temperature process, making it easy to control the coating phase and layer thickness. However, problems have also been pointed out, such as the substrate temperature rising, and the difficulty of improving adhesion when the HA coating layer that is formed is more than a few tens of μm thick.

10.2.3 Vapor Deposition

In light of the problems with thermal spraying, vapor deposition is investigated. Vapor deposition includes physical vapor deposition (PVD) and chemical vapor deposition (CVD).

The PVD is a method of converting a solid raw material (target) into a thin coating layer on a substrate. A solid raw material is vaporized using energy such as heat, plasma, or laser to create a coating layer on a substrate. The composition of the coating layer has a composition that is chemically the same as or similar to that of the solid raw material. Examples of a schematic diagram of each method of PVD include vacuum evaporation, sputtering, ion plating, and laser ablation are shown in Fig. 10.6

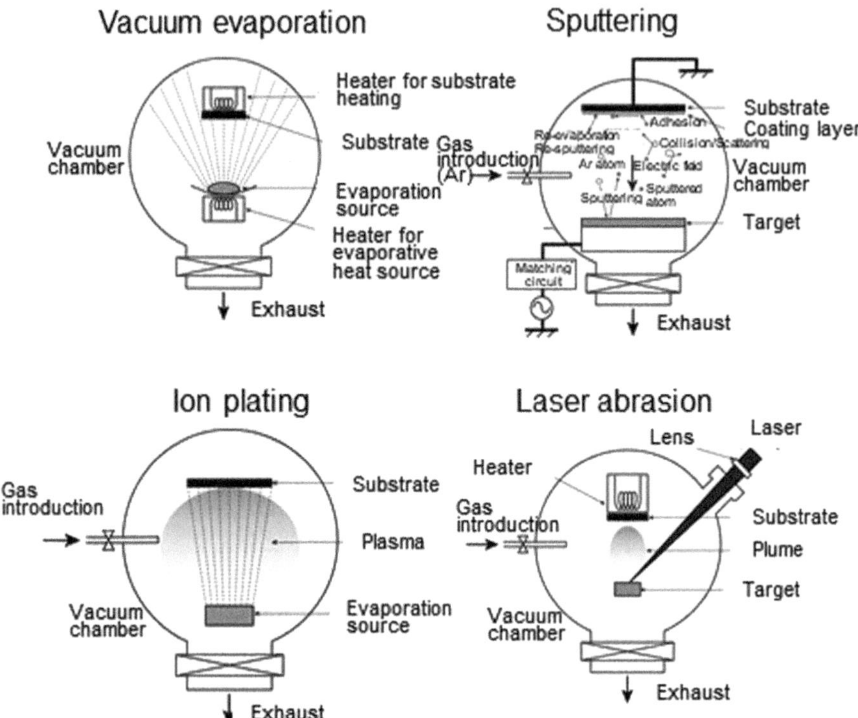

Fig. 10.6. Category of PVD methods and their principles (Reprinted with permission from CRC Press, *Biological and Biomedical Coatings Handbook: Processing and Characterization, Advances in Materials Science and Engineering* (Goto et al.: Chapter 7 Bio-ceramic coating on titanium by physical and chemical vapor deposition, 2011) 299–332.).

(Goto et al. 2011). HA coating using the PVD has been performed on Ti materials from the perspective of application to metal implants (Yoshinari et al. 1991, Wolke et al. 1994, Wang et al. 1997, Yamashita et al. 1998, Narushima et al. 2005).

"Sputtering" is a thin layer forming method that is widely used industrially, and it uses atoms and clusters that fly out when high kinetic energy particles such as argon ions impact with a solid target to deposit them on a substrate. "Ion plating" is a method of forming a film on a substrate by ionizing or exciting evaporated particles generated from a solid surface using thermal energy by plasma. "Laser ablation," also known as pulsed laser deposition (PLD), is a method that uses laser with a pulse width to decompose and vaporize a solid target. Targets for the PVD include HA sintered bodies (Yoshinari et al. 1991, Wolke et al. 1994, Wang et al. 1997), tricalcium phosphate (TCP) sintered bodies (Narushima et al. 2005), calcium phosphate glass (Yamashita et al. 1998), etc. The HA and calcium phosphate layer formed by these PVD have a thickness of several μm or less and have high adhesion force. In particular, the sputtering method, which is expected to remove adsorbed gases from the substrate surface, has yielded HA coatings with adhesion strengths exceeding 60 MPa. Figure 10.7 shows a calcium phosphate layer fabricated by RF magnetron sputtering on the surface of a blasted Ti–6Al–4V alloy and its cross section after implantation in a rabbit femur for 4 weeks. The surface roughness of

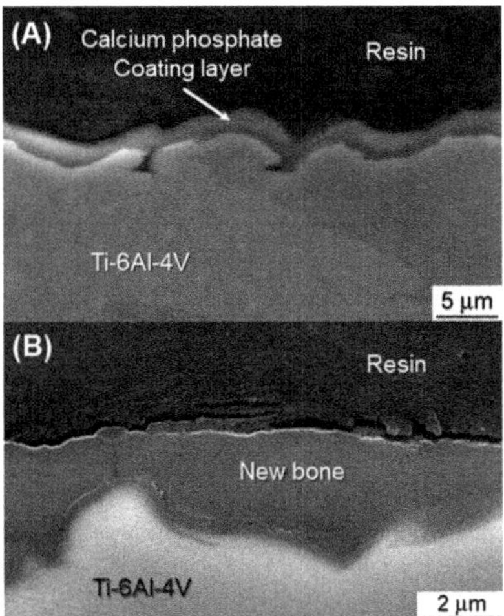

Fig. 10.7. (A) Cross section of a calcium phosphate layer coated on a blasted Ti-6Al-4V surface by RF magnetron sputtering and (B) cross section after 4 wk of implantation into a rabbit femur (Provided by Dr. Takayuki Narushima, Tohoku University).

the blasted Ti–6Al–4V plate is maintained even after coating, and the dense and uniform coating layer covers the complex surface irregularities well (Fig. 10.7A). The maintenance of the surface roughness of the Ti material substrate demonstrates the superiority of thin layer coating using the PVD over methods such as thermal spraying, which form relatively thick calcium phosphate coatings. In addition, new bone has invaded the irregularities formed by the blasting process (Fig. 10.7B). From the perspective of improving corrosion resistance, TiO_2 coating has also been applied to Ti materials and stainless steel using the PVD. Corrosion resistance is improved by forming a defect-free TiO_2 layer that is thicker than the passive film (Pan et al. 1997). To further improve adhesion strength, there is also the ion beam dynamic mixing (IBDM), which combines the PVD layer formation process with ion implantation. A method has been reported that combines the formation of an HA film by the PVD using electron beams and Ca ion implantation (Yoshinari et al. 1994). Figure 10.8 shows a comparison of previously reported methods for forming HA on Ti material surfaces from the viewpoints of substrate temperature, coating layer thickness, coating area, and adhesion. The PVD is considered to be a promising method as an HA coating process for metallic biomaterials from the viewpoint of decreasing the process temperature and thinning the layer (Goto et al. 2011). The presence of rutile structures in the TiO_2 films formed through PVD is associated with a higher dielectric constant, which induced the activation of factor XII of blood coagulation, the formation of fibrin network, and platelet adhesion (Huang et al. 2022).

The CVD is a process in which raw materials supplied as a gas become thin layers or powders through chemical reactions such as thermal decomposition and hydrogen reduction (Goto et al. 2011) as shown in Fig. 10.9. The PVD uses a solid raw material with a chemical composition similar to that of the target material, whereas the CVD involves a chemical reaction, so the raw material gas has a different chemical composition from the target material. In addition, CVD usually

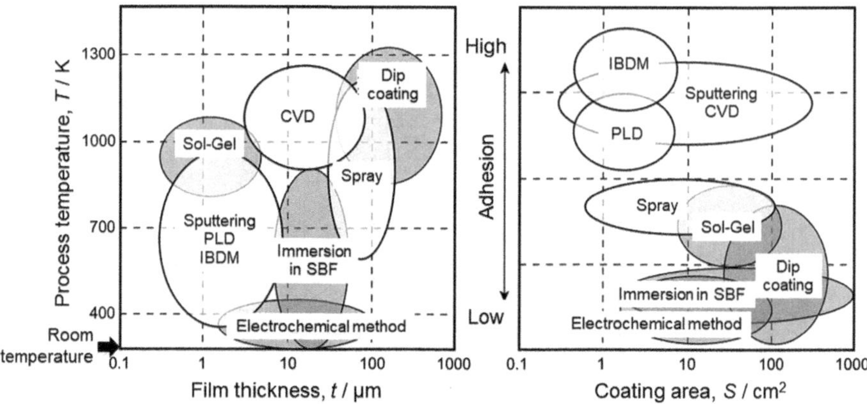

Fig. 10.8. (A) Relationship process temperature and layer thickness and (B) relationship between adhesion strength and coating area of apatite layer formation methods on Ti (Reprinted with permission from CRC Press, *Biological and Biomedical Coatings Handbook: Processing and Characterization, Advances in Materials Science and Engineering* (Goto et al.: Chapter 7 Bio-ceramic coating on titanium by physical and chemical vapor deposition, 2011) 299–332.).

require higher process temperatures than PVD. However, it is easier to control the orientation and morphology of the coating layer than with the PVD. The CVD also requires excitation energy such as heat, plasma, or laser to cause a chemical reaction. At present, CVD coatings have rarely been applied to metallic biomaterials, but the formation of HA coatings using metalorganic (MO) as raw materials has been reported. Heat (Sato et al. 2006a) and laser (Sato et al. 2006b) are used to activate the raw material gas. CVD that uses organometallic compounds is called metalorganic chemical vapor deposition (MOCVD). Bis-dipivaloylmethanato-calcium ($Ca(DPM)_2$) and triphenylphosphate ($(C_6H_5O)_3PO$) are used as raw materials for HA formation on Ti materials using the MOCVD. The cause of toxicity in metals is released metal ions. To prevent this ion release, metals implanted in the body are required to have high corrosion resistance, therefore passive metals or noble metals and their alloys have been used. It is known that the TiO_2 and HA coatings mentioned above improve the corrosion resistance of Ti materials. Electron cyclotron resonance plasma oxidation is used for octacalcium phosphate (OCP) coating (Orii et al. 2010).

$CaTiO_3$ coating is also being considered for surface treatment of Ti materials using PVD and CVD. $CaTiO_3$ is thought to promote hyaluronan formation under biologically simulated environments (Asami et al. 2003, Sato et al. 2007). On the other hand, research is being conducted to improve lubricity by depositing DLC using CVD (Liza et al. 2017).

10.2.4 Ion Implantation

When ions are impacted onto a solid surface, if their kinetic energy exceeds a threshold, the ions will be implanted into the solid. This phenomenon is "ion implantation." As shown in Fig. 10.10, when atoms or ions are impacted to a solid surface, deposition, sputtering, or implantation occurs according to the increase of the kinetic energy of the atoms or ions (Goto et al. 2011). While the PVD uses a phenomenon where the kinetic energy is less than 10^3 eV, the ion implantation uses a larger kinetic energy

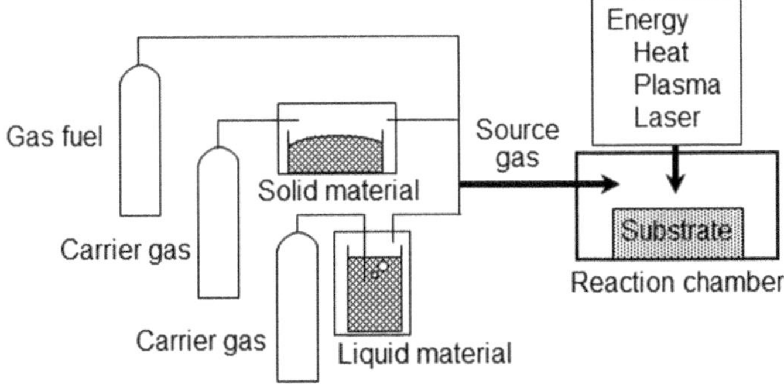

Fig. 10.9. Schematic diagram of CVD methods (Reprinted with permission from CRC Press, *Biological and Biomedical Coatings Handbook: Processing and Characterization, Advances in Materials Science and Engineering* (Goto et al.: Chapter 7 Bio-ceramic coating on titanium by physical and chemical vapor deposition, 2011) 299–332.).

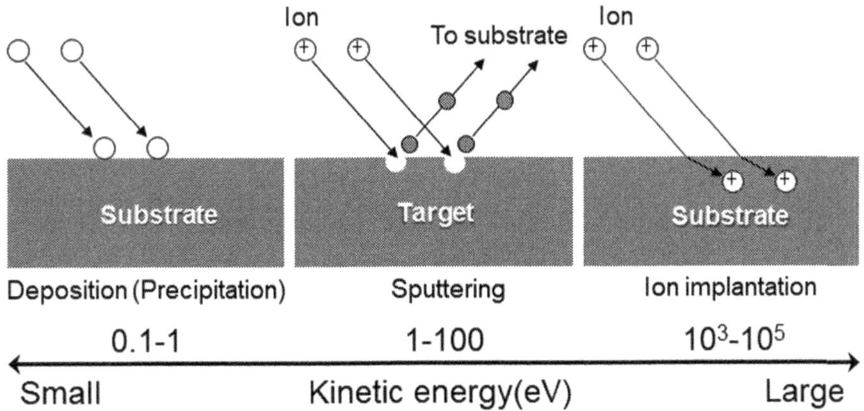

Fig. 10.10. Surface reactions by impacted particles depending on the kinetic energy (Reprinted with permission from CRC Press, *Biological and Biomedical Coatings Handbook: Processing and Characterization, Advances in Materials Science and Engineering* (Goto et al.: Chapter 7 Bio-ceramic coating on titanium by physical and chemical vapor deposition, 2011) 299–332.).

of ions. It is possible to control the concentration distribution of implanted ions near the solid surface by adjusting the ion kinetic energy and dose. Furthermore, it has advantages such as excellent process controllability, room temperature process, and no peeling of the reaction layer. By implanting Ca ions into CP Ti, $CaTiO_3$ and TiO_2 layer are formed on the CP Ti surface, resulting in rapid apatite formation on the Ti surface in simulated body fluids, active formation of osteogenic tissue in the presence of osteoblasts, and promotion of bone formation in rat tibia (Hanawa et al. 1994, 1997a).

10.2.5 Gas Treatment

The gas treatment method is known as an easy process and mass-produced process because it can treat a large number of parts without using special equipment and restriction of the shape of the material. An oxide layer formed by atmospheric oxidation on Ti–6Al–4V alloy and type 316L stainless steel has been shown to improve the adhesion between the metals and the bone in a rat femur (Hazan et al. 1993). These oxidation treatments are performed at a relatively low temperature of 553 K.

10.2.6 Blasting

Blasting is performed by impacting hard particles (abrasives) such as alumina (Al_2O_3) or titania (TiO_2) against the surface of the metal using centrifugal force or compressed air. For implant bodies such as artificial hip joint stems and dental implants, surface roughening is intended to improve the adhesion force with bone and bone contact rate associated with mechanical anchoring (Wong et al. 1995, Ivanoff et al. 2001). Surface roughness can be controlled by the diameter of the abrasive material, and an average surface roughness of about 0.5 to 6 μm can be obtained on CP Ti surfaces by blasting using alumina particles of tens to hundreds of μm. As an example, Fig. 10.11 shows the surface of a Ti-6Al-4V alloy substrate with an average surface roughness of 4.6 μm that was blasted using ceramic particles. In blasting, there is some concern about the residual abrasive on the metal surface. Since HA abrasives are maintained on CP Ti by blasting, these residual HA particles work to improve bone formation (Ishikawa et al. 1997).

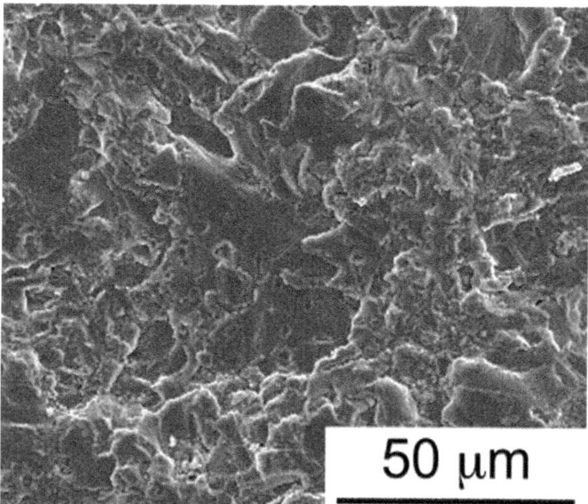

Fig. 10.11. Blast treated surface of Ti-6Al-4V alloy.

10.2.7 Hard Film Coating by PVD

TiN (Streicher et al. 1991, Kola et al. 1996, Paschoal et al. 2003) and diamond-like carbon (DLC) (Streicher et al. 1991, Kola et al. 1996, Li and Gu 2002, Paschoal et al. 2003) coatings by sputtering and ion plating are performed. In particular, TiN coating improves wear properties of type 316L stainless steel, Co–Cr–Mo alloy, Ti–6Al–4V alloy, and Ti–6Al–7Nb alloy against ultra-high molecular weight polyethylene (UHMWPE) (Streicher et al. 1991) and corrosion resistance of them (Kola et al. 1996,

Paschoal et al. 2003). TiN coatings have been put to practical use in bone fixators and artificial hip joints.

Improving wear resistance reduces metal ion release rate, because generation of wear debris decreases, preventing phagocytosis by macrophages. In addition, the corrosion resistance of metallic biomaterials is governed by the passive film formed on the surface, so if the passive film is damaged by wear, ion release will be accelerated, causing allergies and cytotoxicity. From this point of view, it is important to improve wear resistance and corrosion resistance. Surface treatments for metallic biomaterials aimed at improving wear resistance and corrosion resistance include forming a coating film and forming a reaction layer by adding interstitial solid solution elements. Surface treatments aimed at improving hard tissue compatibility of the anterior segment have mainly targeted CP Ti, while stainless steel and Co–Cr–Mo alloys have also been applied to improve wear and corrosion resistance. Ti materials have low wear resistance due to its physical and chemical essential properties (Buckley and Miyoshi 1984), while stainless steel and Co–Cr–Mo alloys have inferior corrosion resistance compared to Ti materials.

10.2.8 Ion Implantation of Nitrogen and Noble Metals

Nitrogen ion implantation is used to improve the wear resistance against UHMWPE and wear-related corrosion resistance of Ti materials and type 316L stainless steel (Buchanan et al. 1987, Röstlund et al. 1989, Rieu et al. 1991). Ion implantation conditions are important. Fretting wear is closely related to the thickness of the modified layer formed by ion implantation (Vadirai et al. 2007).

As can be seen from the existence of a corrosion-resistant alloy such as Ti–0.15Pd, the coating of noble metals or noble metal oxides to Ti materials is effective for improving corrosion resistance. An example of noble metal ion implantation into Ti materials is Ir ion implantation into Ti–6Al–4V alloy, and Ir ion implantation should be performed so that the maximum concentration is 2.5–5.0 at%. As a result, corrosion resistance close to that of Ir has been obtained (Buchanan et al. 1990).

10.2.9 Heat Diffusion Treatment

Since interstitial elements such as O, N, and C cause solid solution hardening of CP Ti, these elements are thermally diffused into the CP Ti surface to harden the surface and improve wear resistance. In particular, the solubility of O in the α phase of CP Ti is extremely high at 14 mass% at around 1000 K, so significant solid solution hardening can be expected by allowing oxygen to diffuse into the CP Ti surface. Thermal diffusion treatment is mainly performed by gas treatment. The typical method is to use the atmosphere (Borgioli et al. 2004), while a method using CO gas has also been used to suppress the formation of an oxide film on the surface (Kim et al. 2006). Figure 10.12 shows changes in maximum surface hardness and hardened layer depth of CP Ti (α type), Ti–4.5Al–3V–2Fe–2Mo (α+β type), and Ti-15Mo-5Zr-3Al (β type) alloys with diffusion treatment time in Ar-5%CO atmosphere at 1073 K (Kim et al. 2009). The higher the proportional of the α phase, which has a higher oxygen solubility, the greater the surface hardness. On the other hand, the

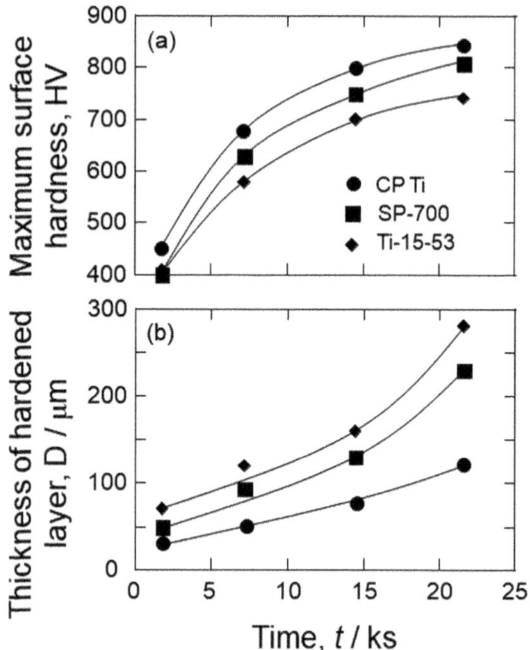

Fig. 10.12. Changes in (a) maximum surface hardness and (b) hardened layer depth with diffusion treatment time at 1073 K in Ar-5%CO atmosphere (Reprinted with permission from The Japan Institute of Metals and Materials, Kim et al. 2009. Mater. Trans. 50: 2763–2771.).

more the β phase increases, which has a higher oxygen diffusion, the deeper the hardened layer becomes.

10.2.10 Laser Irradiation

Laser irradiation has been used to modify the surface of dental implants using lasers (Saran et al. 2023). Patterning of Ti surfaces on the micrometer order and submicrometer order has been performed using femtosecond lasers (Shinonaga et al. 2014, Chen et al. 2017, 2018) to accelerate differentiation of stem cells. TiN can be formed on Ti alloys by laser pattern irradiation, improving wear resistance (Liu et al. 2023).

10.2.11 Thermal Oxidation

The visible-light-responsive antibacterial activity of a single-phase rutile TiO_2 film doped C and N on CP Ti by thermal oxidation is feasible (Koizumi et al. 2023). The TiO_2 film exhibited excellent bonding strength with the CP Ti substrate, indicating its high potential as an antibacterial active coating in combination with visible-light irradiation for CP Ti implants. The band gap of TiO_2 co-doped with C and N is 2.28 eV, working as a visible-light-response photocatalyst (Ishikawa et al. 2023). TiO_2 layers with antibacterial activity under visible-light irradiation by combining Au-sputtering and thermal oxidation of CP Ti is formed (Ueda et al. 2021, 2023).

10.3 Wet Process

10.3.1 Outline

Wet process is a treatment carried out in an aqueous solution, and is an inexpensive treatment method that does not require large-scale capital investment. The basic method is immersion in an aqueous solution and electrochemical treatment in an aqueous solution, while many methods have been attempted by changing the composition and pH of the aqueous solutions, as well as the electric potential and current density. Recently, micro-arc oxidation (MAO) or micro plasma oxidation (MPO) has been actively researched. Regarding chemical treatments, immersion in alkaline solution, combination of immersion and heating, hydrothermal treatment, and acid etching are being studied. Most wet processes aim to promote bone formation and improve bonding with bone tissue.

10.3.2 Electrochemical HA Coating

Electrochemical methods are commonly used to coat HA. Electrochemical methods have been developed to form carbonate apatite into plates, needles, and granules (Ban et al. 1997, Ban and Maruno 1998). It has the advantage that HA can be coated on any shape of substrate as long as it is electroconductive. In addition, heating the substrate during electrochemical treatment allows for efficient coating of HA (Yuda et al. 2005, Kuroda et al. 2008). A method using cathodic current involves precipitation of β-TCP to immobilize collagen (Hosaka et al. 2006). There is also a method that uses low-potential alternating current (Tanaka et al. 2007a), and this method is effective for processing thin materials such as meshes and fibers. A method using pulses has also been attempted. On the other hand, methods have also been devised in which nanometer-sized HA particles are precipitated in an acidic solution (Narayanan et al. 2007, Hayakawa et al. 2008, Narayanan et al. 2008a) and a method in which HA layers are precipitated using potentiodynamics (Meng et al. 2008).

It has been found that bare Mg alloy implants suffer from rapid corrosion. Therefore, surface coating is applied to improve the corrosion resistance and biocompatibility of Mg alloys. Electrodeposition of HA on Mg alloys have been studied (Guan and Brown 2001, Wen et al. 2009, Hiromoto and Tomozawa 2010, Kannan et al. 2013).

10.3.3 Electrochemical TiO_2 Coating

Titanium oxide layer formation has been performed by anodic polarization in solutions of calcium glycerophosphate and calcium acetate (Zhu et al. 2001). Recently, it has been used for the spontaneous formation of TiO_2 tubes in Na_2SO_4 electrolytes containing NaF (Narayanan et al. 2008b) and NH_4-containing electrolytes (Jang et al. 2008). In this method, the diameter, length, and wall thickness are influenced by voltage, current, and treatment time. Recently, research has been underway to form a porous uniform layer on the Ti surface using high-voltage MAO or MPO, and to immobilize biofunctional molecules on the surface (Vadirai et al. al. 2007). MAO is effective for forming a porous uniform layer on metal surfaces. A uniform layer of

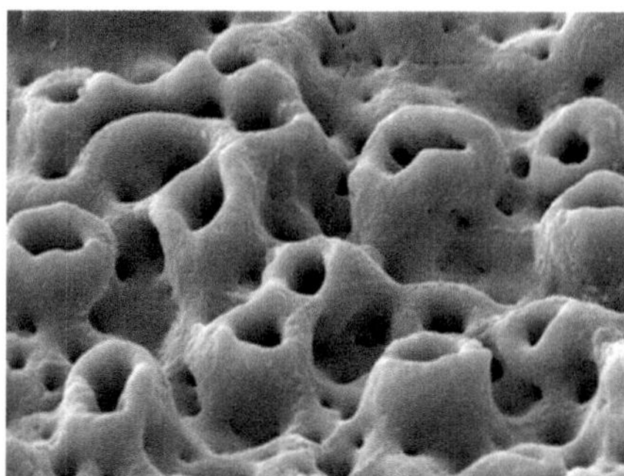

Fig. 10.13. Formation of porous TiO_2 layer on Ti surface by micro-arc oxidation (Reprinted with permission from Nobel Biocare, provided by Dr. Peter Schüpbach.).

connected pores can be formed even on surfaces with complex shapes (Fig. 10.13). The distinction from anodic oxidation is not strict, and the case where connecting pores are formed due to oxygen generation due to high-voltage anodic oxidation is called MAO. Ultraviolet (UV) irradiation improves the bioactivity of TiO_2 formed with MAO (Han et al. 2008). MAO has also been applied to form thick porous HA layers (Ishizawa and Ogino 1995, Han et al. 2003, Liu et al. 2005, Ma et al. 2008, Meng et al. 2008). It has also been applied to the production of ZrO_2 on Zr (Yan and Han 2007, Han et al. 2009). HA formation on Ti–Nb–Sn alloy is also accelerated by MAO (Tanaka et al. 2016). Using MAO techniques, a surface with two functions appearing hard tissue compatibility and antibacterial property on CP Ti are created by the addition of antibacterial elements, such as Ag, Cu, and Zn, in the electrolyte (Shimabukuro et al. 2019a, b, c, 2020a). The conditions to appear two functions become clear (Shimabukuro et al. 2020b, Tsutsumi et al. 2021, 2023).

On the other hand, in order to improve the corrosion resistance and safety of Ni–Ti shape memory and superelastic alloys, a titanium oxide film without Ni can be formed by applying a potential in a mixture of glycerol, lactic acid, sulfuric acid, and ethanol (Fukushima et al. 2006, Yoneyama and Hanawa 2021). The electrochemical process of the formation of Ni-free surface oxide film is illustrated in Fig. 10.14. During application of the potential, Ni is released from the surface oxide and simultaneously oxide is grown without Ni. This process eliminates Ni from the surface oxide completely. Pulsed anodization also allows to form a Ni-free TiO_2 layer on Ni–Ti alloy (Tate et al. 2023).

10.3.4 Immersion and Precipitation

By immersion of CP Ti in NaOH or KOH alkaline solution, a hydrated titania gel containing alkali ions (gelled titanium oxide containing hydroxyl groups) with a thickness of about 1 μm is formed on the surface (Kim et al. 1996). When this is heat-treated, the gel layer becomes denser, and an amorphous layer of alkali titanate is firmly bonded to the substrate. When this is immersed in a simulated body fluid (SBF), alkali ions are released and hydronium ions enter instead, forming a titania hydrogel on the surface. As a result, the released alkali ions increase the degree of supersaturation of the surrounding SBF with respect to H^+, and the gel on the surface

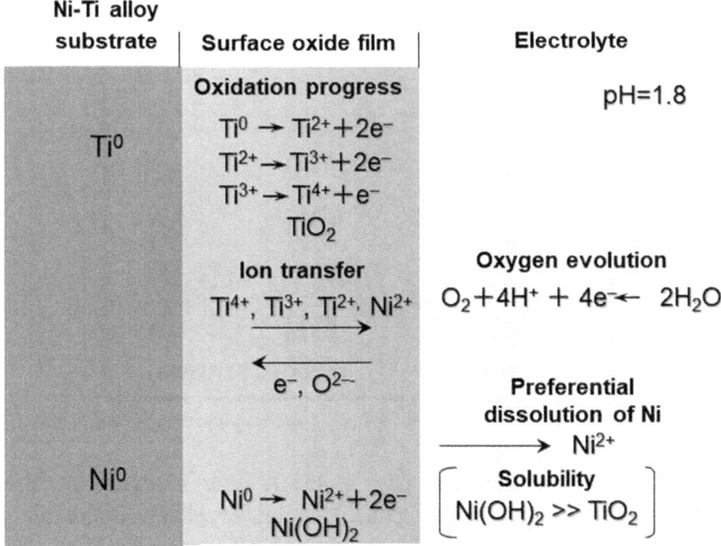

Fig. 10.14. The electrochemical process of the formation of Ni-free surface oxide film.

induces nucleation of HA, resulting in the rapid formation of HA layer on the surface. This method has already been put into practical use with artificial hip joint stems.

When CP Ti is immersed in a Ca-containing aqueous solution, a titanium oxide layer containing calcium hydroxide is formed. When immersed in SBF, this oxidized layer promotes calcium phosphate precipitation (Kono et al. 2007). As mentioned above, the most effective treatment is immersion in an alkaline solution. Hydrothermal treatment in a similar solution (Hanawa et al. 1997b) or under high pressure (Hamada et al. 2002) further accelerates HA formation. Hydrothermally Ca-coated surfaces have synergic effects in enhancing osseointegration of Ti and Ti–6Al–4V alloy due to their micron-scaled surface properties and biologically active surface chemistry (Park et al. 2007, Suh et al. 2007). On the other hand, this method is not effective for metals that are difficult to generate calcium phosphate, such as Zr. Therefore, a method has been devised to cathodically polarize Zr to create an alkaline environment on the surface (Fig. 10.15), alkalizing the Zr surface (increasing the surface OH concentration) and accelerating HA formation (Tsutsumi et al. 2010).

Immersion of CP Ti in H_2O_2 containing $TaCl_2$ accelerates HA formation in SBF (Ohtsuki et al. 1997). Implantation into the rabbit tibia revealed good bonding with the bone.

A dissolution-precipitation reaction is used for achieving robust carbonate apatite (CA) coating to CP Ti (Shi et al. 2020) that is utilized as a dental implant.

10.3.5 Acid Etching

Acid treatment is effective in increasing the cellular activity of CP Ti (Ban et al. 2006, Iwaya et al. 2008), and the combination of acid etching and alkaline treatment also accelerates HA precipitation (Kono et al. 2007). Furthermore, treatment at

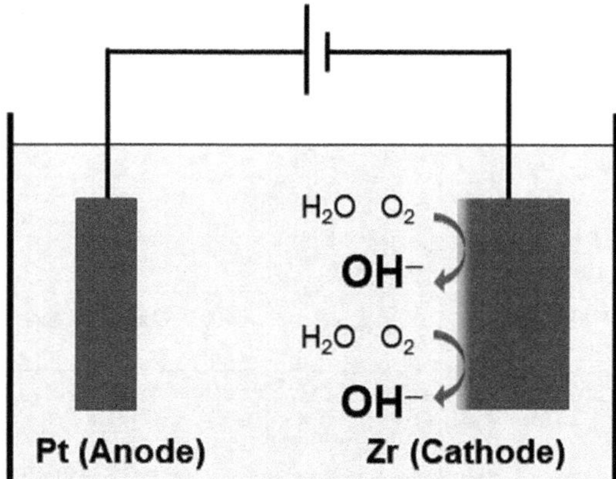

Fig. 10.15. Local alkalinization of Ti surface by cathodic polarization in a supporting electrolyte solution.

353 K in H_2O_2/HNO_3 solution and 12 h at 453 K in an autoclave accelerates the precipitation of HA (Sultana et al. 2006). Heating in calcium hydroxide slurry is also effective to form titanium oxide containing $CaTiO_3$ layer (Ohtsu et al. 2007, Ueda et al. 2009). Phosphate ion-incorporated Ti surfaces hydrothermally treated with various concentrations of phosphoric acid improve the biocompatibility of Ti implants by enhancing osteoblast attachment, differentiation, and biomechanical anchorage (Park et al. 2010).

10.3.6 Immobilization of Biofunctional Molecules

It is a natural idea that by immobilizing biomolecules involved in bone formation on the surface of a material, it is possible to promote bone formation on the material surface and strengthen the bonding with bone, and much research has been carried out at present. Attempts have also been made to promote soft tissue adhesion.

Type I collagen (Streicher et al. 1991, Nagai et al. 2002, Viornery et al. 2002, Chang et al. 2008), bone morphogenetic protein-4 (BMP-4) (Puleo et al. 2002), fibronectin (Kola et al. 1996, Pugdee et al. 2007), etc., are immobilized. Arg-Gly-Asp (RDG) peptide is motif of cell adhesion (Pierschbacher and Ruoslahti 1984), and immobilization of RDG peptide (Pierschbacher and Ruoslahti 1984) promotes cell expansion and accelerates bone formation (Rezania et al. 1997, Schliephake et al. 2002, Paschoal et al. 2003). There is a method of immobilization via zwitterion poly(ethylene glycol), PEG (NH_2-PEG-COOH), electrodeposited on the CP Ti surface (Oya et al. 2009, Tanaka et al. 2009, Park et al. 2011). In addition, GRGDS is known as a cell adhesion peptide (Yamanouchi et al. 2008) and peptides with cysteine as residues are also effective (Xiao et al. 1997, 1998, Rezania et al. 1999). On the other hand, peptide sequences that specifically adhere to CP Ti surfaces have been synthesized (Pan et al. 1997, Yoshinari et al. 2010). Immobilization of BMPs is also effective (Li and Gu 2002). The subgroup of BMPs was the most favorable to coating. Surface modification of CP Ti implants by the subgroup of BMPs seems to favor osseointegration in the early stages of healing (López-Valverde et al. 2022).

In order to use metals for stents, guide wires, artificial valves, etc., biofunction such as the inhibition of platelet adhesion, bacterial adhesion, and blood lubricity is required. In addition, in order to prevent infections caused by implantation, it is necessary to inhibit bacterial adhesion and biofilm formation on the material surface. One way to inhibit platelet adhesion, and bacterial adhesion is to inhibit protein adsorption. This is also effective to inhibit nonspecific adsorption of peptides, DNA, and antibodies. Since PEG is a functional molecule that inhibits protein adsorption, the immobilization of PEG on the surface of a material may improve the above-mentioned biofunctions. As a method for immobilizing polymers on metal surfaces, thiol (−SH) groups on the Au surface have been known for a long time, and currently the immobilization of PEG on Au nanoparticles is performed. However, this method can only be used on noble metal surfaces.

Copolymers of poly(L-lysine)-g-poly(ethylene glycol) (PLL-g-PEG) have been synthesized for blood contact materials and biosensors. PLL-g-PEG instantly adsorbs to TiO_2, $Si_{0.4}Ti_{0.6}O_2$, and Nb_2O_5 from aqueous solution (Kenausis et al. 2000, Huang et al. 2001). In another example, protein adsorption to TiO_2 and Au surfaces can be reduced by more than 70% by the immobilization of poly(ethylene glycol)-poly(DL-lactic acid) (PEG-PLA) copolymer micelles (Huang et al. 2002). The surface of stainless steel is silanized with a silane coupling agent, activated with argon plasma, and graft-polymerized poly(ethylene glycol) methacrylate (PEGMA) by ultraviolet irradiation, resulting in the PEGMA being grafted at a high concentration. This surface is effective in preventing the adsorption of bovine serum albumin and γ-globulin (Zhang et al. 2001). Photo-immobilization of photoactive PEG onto CP Ti has been carried out (To et al. 2007). On the other hand, as shown in Fig. 10.16, PEG whose

(A)

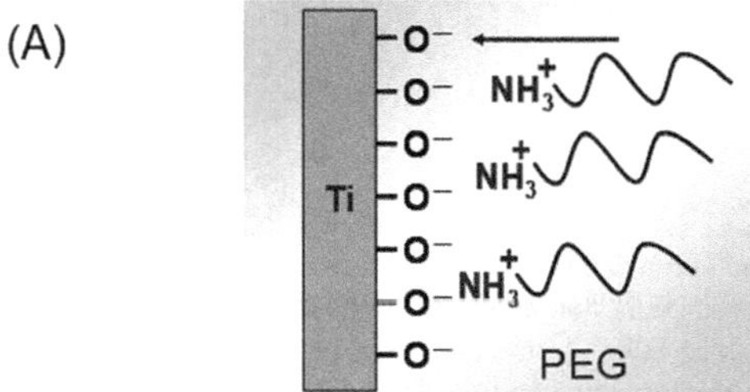

(B)

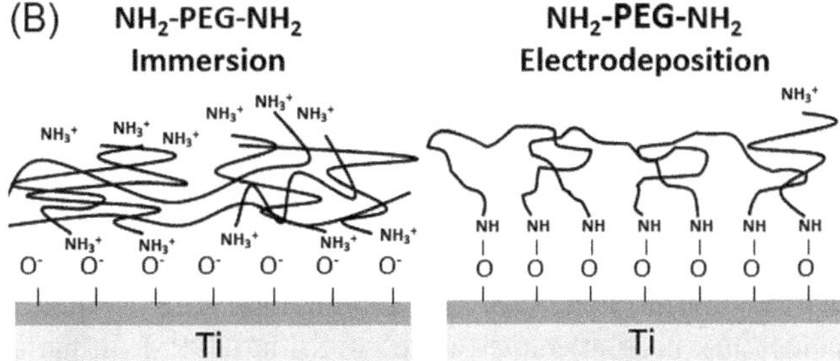

Fig. 10.16. The immobilization of NH_2-PEG-NH_2 by electrodeposition. The terminated PEGs electrically migrate to and are immobilized on the Ti cathode (A). More terminated amines combine with Ti oxide as an NH-O bond by electrodeposition, while more amines randomly exist as NH_3^+ in the PEG molecule by immersion (B).

terminal is modified with amine so that it has a charge in an aqueous solution can be immobilized on CP Ti surface by electrodeposition (Tanaka et al. 2007b, c, 2008). This surface can inhibit protein adsorption, platelet adhesion, and biofilm formation (Fig. 10.17). Bonding of PEG-diamine with the CP Ti surface by electrodeposition was strong with no detachment from Ti. PEG-diamine was immediately adsorbed onto the CP Ti surface by the weak electrostatic force and bonded randomly via this force. Subsequent rearrangement and condensation occurred alongside an electrochemical reaction between the molecules and the Ti surface due to cathodic charge. Consequently, PEG-diamine molecules are strongly immobilized on the CP Ti surface under electrodeposition (Fukushima et al. 2020). This process is roughly illustrated in Fig. 10.18. A unique surface treatment to provide a protective surface film over 3D-printed interconnected porous biomedical Ti–24Nb–4Zr–8Sn alloy scaffolds under simulated inflammatory environment is attempted (Wen and Huang 2022).

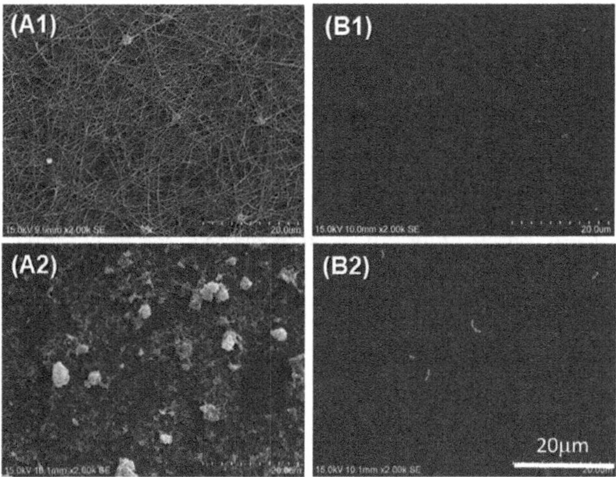

Fig. 10.17. Inhibition of platelet adhesion and biofilm formation on Ti by immobilization of NH_2-PEG-NH_2 by electrodeposition. (a1) Platelet adhesion and fibrin network on untreated Ti, (b1) inhibition of platelet adhesion on PEG-immobilized Ti by electrodeposition, (a2) biofilm formation on untreated Ti, and (b2) inhibition of biofilm formation on PEG-immobilized Ti by electrodeposition.

10.3.7 Adhesion Improvement with Polymers

Not only in the field of dentistry but also other field of medicine, the bonding strength of metals with polymers is important. Therefore, factors influencing adhesion and surface treatments is investigated.

In dentistry, the interfacial chemical structure governing the bonding strength, especially at the nanometer level, is one of the most challenging aspects to the development of composite materials. The combination of a Ti alloy with a resin for crown facings has been attempted (Taira and Imai 1995). In particular, silane coupling agents containing S-H groups and Si-O-CH_3 groups are comprehensively used to combine dental alloys with resins (Smith et al. 2004). The S-H groups work as a bonding agent with polymers; the Si-O-CH_3 works as a bonding agent with metals.

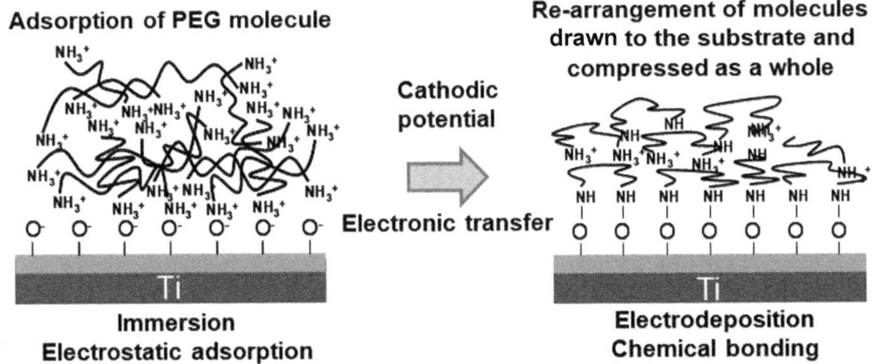

Fig. 10.18. Schematic illustration of electrodeposition process of PEG molecules to CP Ti surface by cathodic potential.

The mechanical properties and durability of composite resin increases with silanized filler (Abbound et al. 2000, Ferracane et al. 1998, Kanie et al. 2004, Yoshida et al. 2001). However, in most studies about materials using silane coupling agents in the field of dentistry, only the bonding strength is evaluated and discussed, and there are few reports that examine and discuss the chemical structures at the bonding interface and how they influence the bonding strength.

Several studies on silane coupling agents to combine polymers with metals have been performed in other fields. An aluminum-vegetable oil composite using a silane coupling agent has been developed (Bexell et al. 2003, 2004). Rubber-to-metal bonding by a silane coupling agent was investigated (Jayaseelan and Ooji 2001). In addition, the surface modification of stainless steel by grafting of poly(ethylene glycol) using a silane coupling agent has been reported (Zhang et al. 2001). However, only the chemical structure is investigated in these studies. In other words, the relationship between the bonding strength and the interfacial chemical structure containing a silane coupling agent layer has not been studied.

The unequivocal relationship between the shear bonding strength and the chemical structure at the bonding interface of a CP Ti-segmented polyurethane (SPU) composite through a silane coupling agent (γ-mercaptopropyl trimethoxysilane) is investigated (Sakamoto et al. 2007). On the other hand, the shear bond strength of the Ti/SPU interface increased with ultraviolet (UV) irradiation according to the increase of the cross-linkage in SPU. UV irradiation to a CP Ti-SPU composite is clearly a factor governing the shear bond strength of the Ti/SPU interface (Sakamoto et al. 2008a). In addition, active hydroxyl groups on the surface oxide film are clearly factors governing the shear bond strength (Sakamoto et al. 2008b). After good bonding between metal and polymer is produced, biofunctionalization techniques developed in the field of polymers could be applied to the composite materials.

A silane coupling agent is considered a reliable, good adhesion promoter to silica-based (or silica-coated) indirect restorations. Surface pre-treatment steps, e.g., acid etching for porcelain and tribo-chemical silica-coating for metal alloys, is used before silanization to attain strong, durable bonding of the substrate to resin composite. In clinical practice, however, the main problem of resin bonding using silanes and other coupling agents is the weakening of the bond (degradation) in the wet oral environment over time. A silane coupling agent is a justified and popular adhesion promoter (adhesive primer) used in dentistry. The commercial available silane coupling agents can fulfil the requirements in clinical practice for durable bonding. Development of new silane coupling agents, their optimization, and surface treatment methods are in progress to address the long term resin bond durability and are highly important (Matinlinna et al. 2018). For adhesion of metals to adhesives in dentistry, refer to Subsection 4.5.8.

10.4 Surface Morphology Control

The purpose of controlling the surface morphology is to roughen the surface of metallic biomaterials. The roughening of the surface is intended to improve the adhesion between the metal implant and the bone tissue through mechanical anchoring. Currently, methods of surface morphology control that are widely used in practical use include spraying CP Ti onto the surface of alloy artificial joint stems consisting of Ti–6Al–4V alloy (Fig. 10.19). Sand-blasted large-grit acid-etched surface (SLA), which combines blasting and acid etching, is applied to dental implants (Fig. 10.20). A hydrothermally produced $SrTiO_3$ coating improves the osteoconductivity of the SLA-treated Ti surface by enhancing both the early and late cell response of bone marrow stromal cells (Park et al. 2012). MAO is also effective for forming connective porous TiO_2 layer and has been practically used for dental implants (Fig. 10.13). The bond strength between bone and material is also affected by the morphology of the material surface. Various morphologies of material surfaces such as beads, grooves, fibrous meshes, and pores have been designed. Large-pore bodies are made by casting to replace plastic beads. At this time, the pore size is 0.4–1.5 mm and the porosity is 70%. Porous bodies with pore sizes of 0.1–0.4 mm and porosity of 35–50% are manufactured by sintering metal beads or diffusion welding of metal fibers. Furthermore, a porous body with micro-pores with a pore size of 0.02–0.2 mm is made by plasma spraying of CP Ti powder. Bonding of bone to the material surface is the fastest and most effective when the thickness is 50–400 μm. The surface roughness of a material affects the expression of cell functions during the wound healing process and remodeling. It has been confirmed

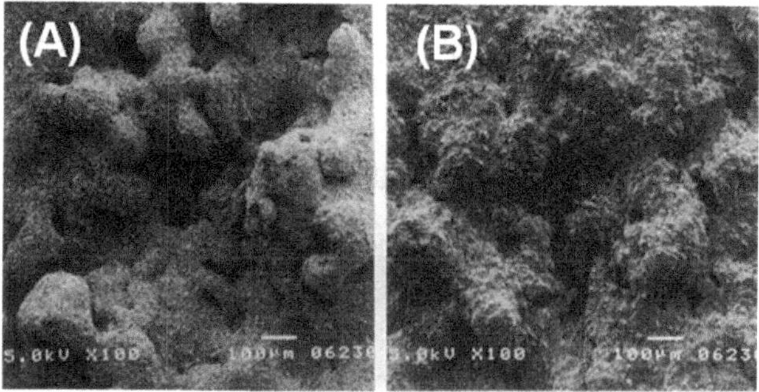

Fig. 10.19. Surface of Ti (A) and HA (B) plasma sprayed on Ti-6Al-4V alloy substrate (Reprinted with permission from Japanese Society for Biomaterials, Hayashi, K. 1995. J. Jpn. Soc. Biomater. 13: 81–87.).

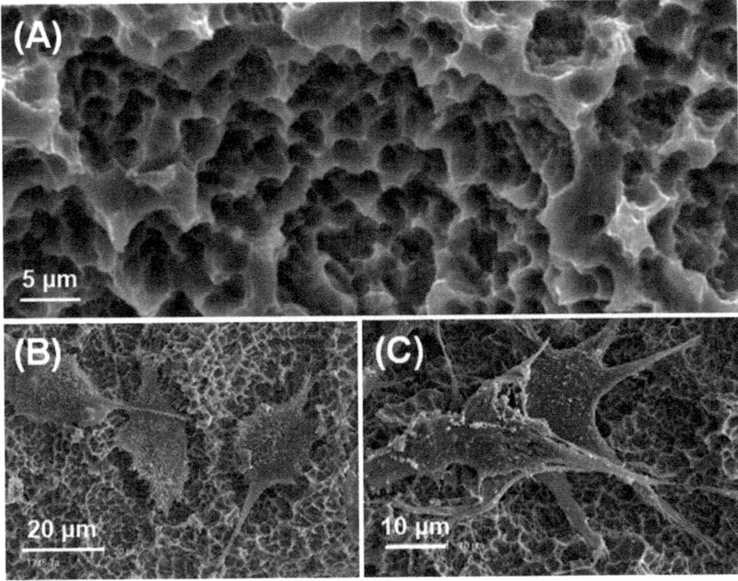

Fig. 10.20. (A) Blasted and acid etched surface (SLA), (B, C) Osteoblasts are engrafted on the SLA surface (Provided by Straumann Co., Ltd.).

that osteogenic cells strongly adhere to rough metal surfaces *in vitro* (Hazan et al. 1993). Furthermore, surface roughness plays an important role in the cell differentiation. Osteoblasts produce more collagen and promote mineralization on rough surfaces than on smooth surfaces (Buckley and Miyoshi 1984). Even *in vivo*, a rough surface has better bone integration than a smooth surface, and the rougher the surface, the greater the shear strength between the material and the bone tissue. As described above, the roughness of the material surface is an important factor that influences the bonding with living tissue.

A variety of methods have been used to make pores in the implant surface. Typical examples include metal bead treatment (Röstlund et al. 1989), CP Ti plasma spray (Buchanan et al. 1987), and fiber mesh coating (Rieu et al. 1991). Figure 10.21 shows photographs of the surfaces of artificial hip joint stems with various porous treatments (Ratner et al. 2004). Roughened surface is formed by bonding spherical metal powders (beads) with an organic binder and sintering them (Davis 2003) (Fig. 10.21A). A special electrode-type powder production device is used to produce metal beads, and CP Ti and Co–Cr–Mo alloy powders with particle sizes of approximately 100–700 μm can be obtained. In this case, long-term sintering in a high-temperature inert or reducing atmosphere increases the bonding strength between the beads and the substrate material (Pillar et al. 1975). Fiber mesh coating roughens the surface by diffusion bonding metal wires to the substrate material (Fig. 10.21B). CP Ti powder is attached to the implant surface using plasma spraying (Fig. 10.21C). The degree of increase in the surface area of the implant body due to Ti plasma spray is significant to improve the bonding strength to the bone (Schroeder et al. 1981). Another method has been used to improve biocompatibility by thermally spraying hyaluronan onto roughened surfaces (Fig. 10.21D). It has also been reported

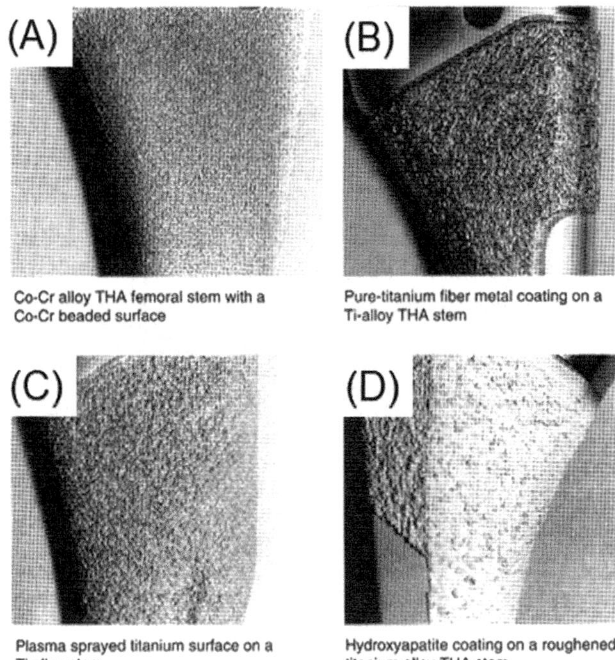

Fig. 10.21. Various porous treatments applied to the surface of the artificial hip joint stem (A) Metal bead treatment, (B) fiber mesh coating, (C) titanium plasma spray, (D) hydroxyapatite coating (Reprinted with permission Elsevier Academic Press, *Biomaterials Science* (Ratner et al., 2004) 539.).

that forming a thin HA film on a mesh coating promotes bone growth into the coating (Ducheyne et al. 1980). The possibility of biofilm formation is decreased by 80–90% for flat substrates versus untreated and non-optimized plasma-sprayed porous Ti, but also by 65–95% for other porous Ti coatings. Moreover, these porous surfaces are shown to lead to a 10–50% enhanced cell proliferation and gene expression versus state-of-the-art vacuum plasma sprayed porous Ti coatings (Gasik et al. 2012). It has been shown that grain size influences cell compatibility. The superior osteoblast cell compatibility of microroughened Ti surface made of equal channel angular pressing process is induced with ultrafine-grain substrates over coarse-grain CP Ti and Ti-6Al-4V alloy substrates (Park et al. 2009).

10.5 Biofunctional Surface Morphology

The evolution of surface morphogenesis technology is considered to be the formation of surface structures at the micrometer or nanometer level, and in recent years there have been a number of reports that this structure is effective for bone formation. One is to form nanotubes such as TiO_2 on the surface, which promote cell adhesion, bone formation, etc., due to the nanometer-size effect (Allam et al. 2008, Narayanan et al. 2009, Brammer et al. 2012). Regarding the effect of nanostructures, although circumstantial evidence of promoting bone formation has been obtained, the scientific mechanism has not yet been elucidated. On the other hand, periodic nanostructures on the surface have been shown to promote bone formation (Shinonaga et al. 2014, Matsugaki et al. 2015). Furthermore, it has been confirmed that periodic nanostructures influence not only stem cell adhesion but also its differentiation, promoting differentiation into osteoblasts and chondrocytes (Chen et al. 2017, 2018), as shown in Fig. 10.22. Differentiation of hMSC is accelerated on submicron grid pattern. Multilayer TiO_2 nano-network has excellent biocompatibility and surface bioactivity, promoting human bone marrow mesenchymal stem cells (hBMSCs) toward the osteogenic differentiation pathway (Yang and Huang 2019). The bioactive TiO_2 nano-network structure introduced in this study has considerable potential for applications in implant dentistry. On the other hand, based on the result that not only bone density but also orientation is important for bone quality (Ishimoto et al. 2013), it is possible to control the orientation of bone structure by forming grooves with consideration to the direction of the principal stress vector applied during bone formation. The technology to do this has been established: orientation induction by promoting principal stress transfer through shape control (Noyama 2013). Optimization of metal implant surface shape that enables bone orientation control based on principal stress vector distribution, as shown in Fig. 10.23. This method has been put into practical use as a surface treatment for dental implants. Additive manufacturing is an effective means for forming surfaces with such minute and complex structures, and it is expected that it will continue to be used for surface morphology control in the future. In addition, there is an increasing number of studies on preventing bacterial adhesion using periodic microstructures at the micrometer level (Anselme et al. 2010, Orapirlyakul et al. 2018, Mas-Moruno et al. 2019), as shown in Fig. 10.24.

10.6 Cleaning and Hydrophilic Treatment

Surface contamination of dental implants is known to interfere with bone formation and osseointegration (Ueno et al. 2012). Therefore, devices that perform photoactivation treatments such as ultraviolet ray irradiation or plasma irradiation before implantation are in the market. These photoactivation treatments remove surface contamination, exposing more surface hydroxyl groups on the surface and making it hydrophilic, promoting cell adhesion and promoting bone formation. In this regard, it has been shown that osteogenic ability can be determined by surface wettability (Yamamoto et al. 2012). Chair-side treatment of implants with UV or non-thermal plasma appear to be effective for improving osseointegration (Pesce 2020).

10.7 Time Transient of Surface Treatment

Surface treatments to improve biocompatibility and biofunction have undergone the following changes at the research level, as shown in Fig. 10.25.

First generation (untreated surface): Grinding and polished surface

Second generation (morphological surface): Grooving, blasting, acid etching, anodizing, laser ablation

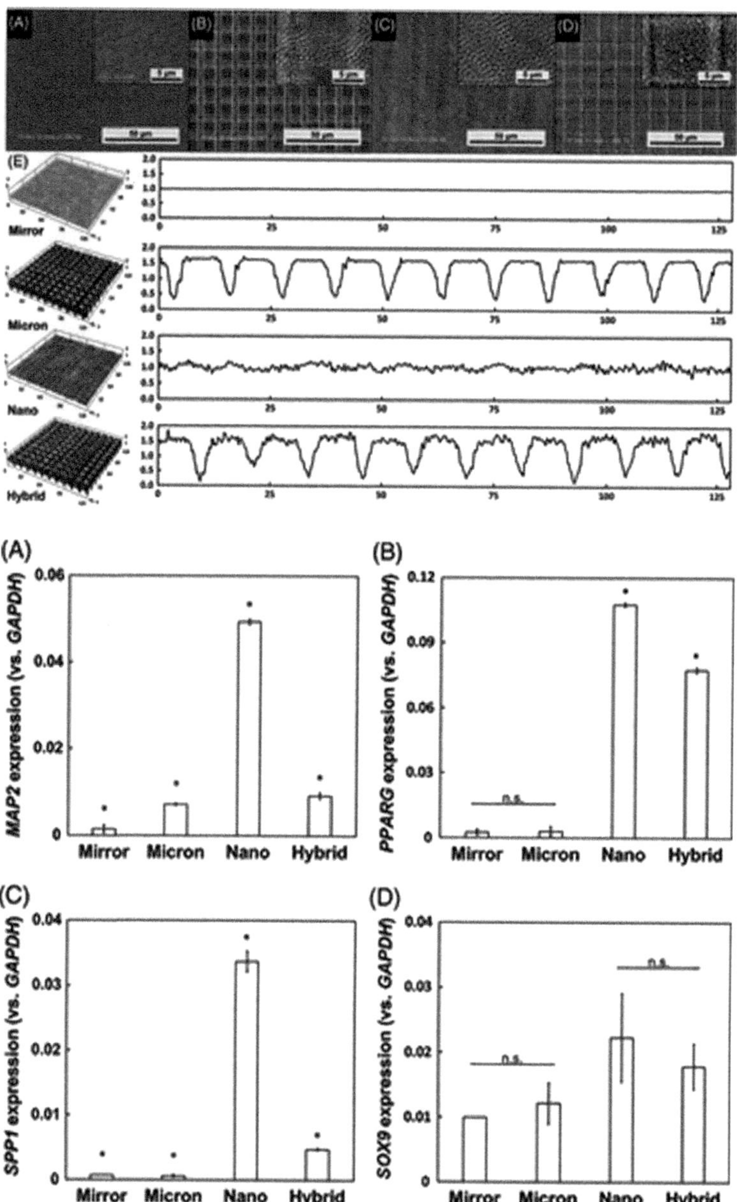

Fig. 10.22. Top: Surface morphology of Ti with or without femtosecond laser processing. SEM images of all specimens. Scale bar denotes 50 μm. (a) Mirror, (b) micron Ti, (c) nano Ti, and (d) hybrid Ti. (e) Images and cross-sectional profiles of all specimens acquired by 3D-LM. Detected surface area is 128 × 128 μm. Bottom: Evaluation of the effects of the grid topographies on cell multifunctional differentiation concerning intracellular gene expression after 3 days of induction of differentiation. Histograms of expression levels of selected target genes in hMSCs cultured on Ti surfaces 3 days after the induction of differentiation. (a) *MAP2* (Neurogenic differentiation), (b) *PPARG* (Adipogenic differentiation), (c) *SPP1* (Osteogenic differentiation), and (d) *SOX9* (Chondrogenic differentiation). Results were statistically analyzed. $*p < 0.05$. (Reproduced with permission from Wiley, Chen et al. 2018. J. Biomed. Mater. Res. Part A 106: 2735–2743.).

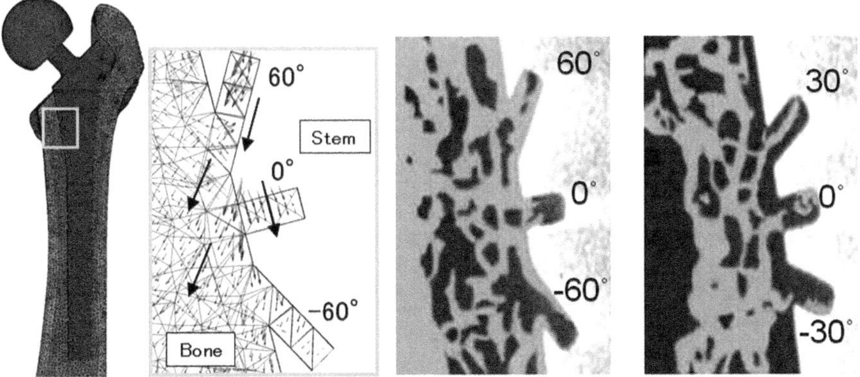

Fig. 10.23. Orientation induction by promoting principal stress transfer through shape control. Optimization of metal implant surface shape that enables bone orientation control based on principal stress vector distribution. The principal stress vector of the bone within the groove angle of 60° is distributed parallel to the groove and almost parallel to the principal stress vector of the surrounding bone. Bone is most abundant in the 60° groove (white color area is new bone). (Reproduced with permission from Elsevier, Noyma et al. 2013. Bone 52: 659–667).

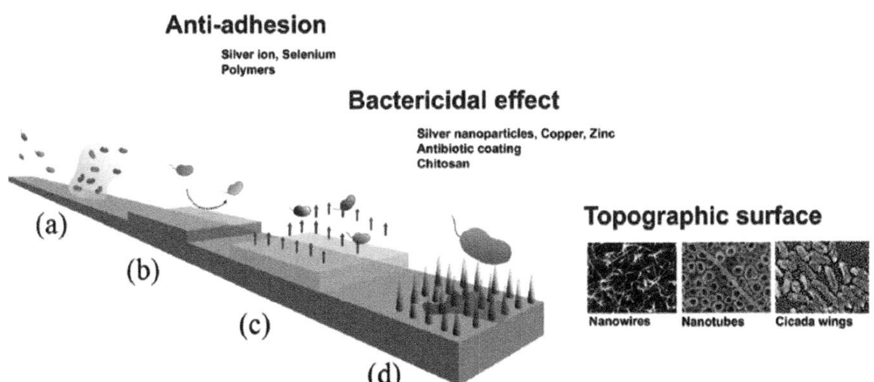

Fig. 10.24. Planktonic bacteria attach on material surface and form biofilms. (a) Various techniques were used as antibacterial strategies. Anti-adhesive surface coats using concepts of surface chemistry and functionality including ions and polymer coats. (b) Material surface can be coated with bactericidal substances such as antibiotics and silver. (c) Nanotopographic surface modifications were also effective strategies used as either anti-adhesives or bactericidal. (d) Examples of nanotopography, such as nanowires promoting osteoblastogenesis and have bactericidal. (Reprinted with permission from SAGE open access, Orapiriyakul et al. 2018. J. Tissue Eng. 9: 2041731418789838.).

Third generation (physicochemically active surface): HA and calcium phosphate coating

Fourth generation (biochemically active surface): Immobilization of biofunctional molecules.

Fifth generation (biological surface): Stem cells or tissue coating.

Advanced second generation (morphological biofunctional surface): Micrometer/ nanometer size cyclic patterns.

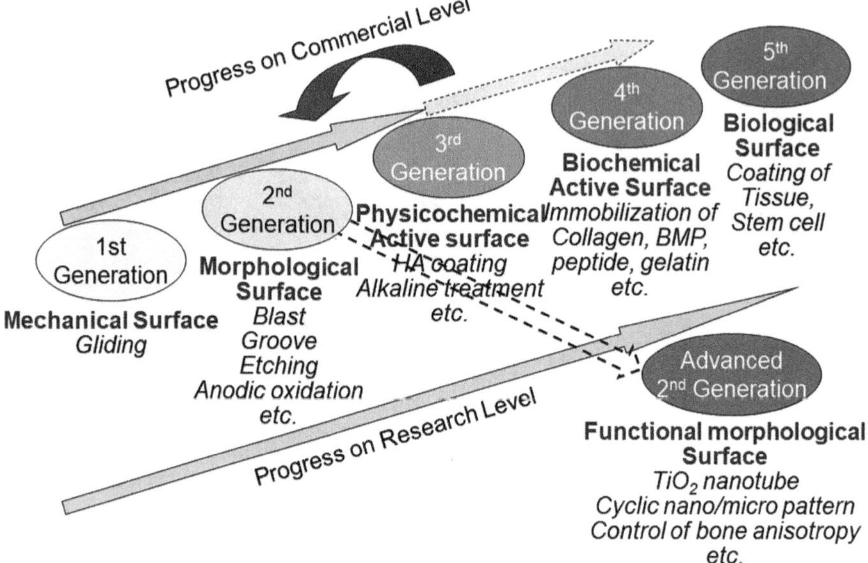

Fig. 10.25. Time transition of progress of surface treatment techniques and estrangement between research and commercialization.

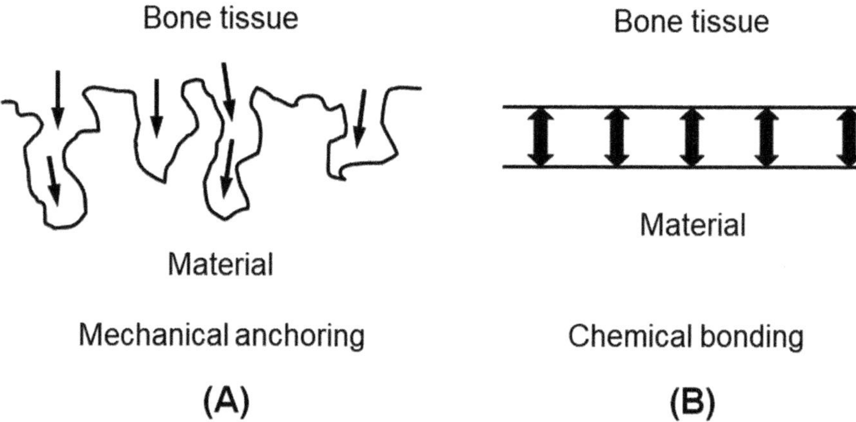

Fig. 10.26. Mechanical anchoring (a) and chemical bonding (b) between bone and material.

In the second generation, as shown in Fig. 10.26, it is difficult to chemically bond bone tissue and materials in the human body. Therefore, roughened surface is fabricated and bone tissue can invade into the irregularities and pores during the healing process and mechanically anchored after healing. This is the second generation.

In the third generation, HA is the basic inorganic component of teeth and bone, and it has been thought that bone formation is promoted on the HA surface. Therefore, surface treatments coating HA is popular technique in order to promote bone tissue formation on the material surface. On the other hand, coatings such as bioactive glass, TCP, CA, and OCP, which have higher osteogenic ability than HA, are also being used. Furthermore, it is possible to perform surface treatment that promotes bone formation by spontaneously forming through surface activity alone, without coating of HA or calcium phosphate. The earliest method devised was Ca ion implantation. On the other hand, when Ti is immersed in an alkaline solution such as NaOH or KOH and heated, bone formation is promoted on the surface. This method has been put into practical use for artificial hip joints. A method is applied to cathodic polarization to create an alkaline environment on the surface of the electrode, thereby performing alkali treatment more efficiently than immersion in an alkaline solution.

In the fourth generation, many researches have been conducted up to now. Immobilization of type I collagen, fibronectin, and peptides with the RGD sequence, which is involved in cell adhesion, promotes cell expansion and, as a result, accelerates bone formation. Immobilization of BMP is also effective. On Ti electrodeposited with PEG, protein adsorption platelet adhesion, bacterial adhesion, and biofilm formation can also be suppressed. It is natural to think that by immobilizing biomolecules involved in bone formation on the material surface, as in the fourth generation, it would be possible to promote bone formation on the material surface and strengthen the bond with bone tissue. Much research has been done on it, and it is generally received favorably. However, in order to widely disseminate the immobilization of biological functions, it is necessary to guarantee its safety, maintain quality, and verify the durability of the immobilization layer during storage term. Without it, it will not be put into practical use.

Fifth generation is not attempted yet at present. Much more time is required to complete this treatment technique.

After all, most of the second-generation products are currently in practical use, and there are only a few examples of third-generation products being put into practical use. When it comes to the fourth generation, there is almost no prospect of practical use. Looking at the products that have actually been put into practical use and are widely used, those that aim at bonding by roughening the surface and allowing living tissue to penetrate there have achieved considerably better results than those that aim for surface chemical compatibility. This is also one of the reasons why the practical application of the third generation and beyond has not progressed.

In the advanced second generation, many excellent results are obtained by researchers. However, the mechanism of the nanometer-sized effects is not clear at present as described in section 10.5. Periodic nanostructures on the surface have been shown to promote bone formation, and in addition, it has been confirmed that they promote not only stem cell adhesion but also differentiation. In addition, a technology has been established to control the orientation of bone structures by forming grooves with consideration to the direction of the principal stress vector applied during bone formation. Additive manufacturing process may be an effective means for creating such surfaces.

10.8 Optimal Surface Treatment

If good biocompatibility and biofunction can be imparted to metals, the range of their use will greatly expand. As mentioned above, due to recent advances in surface functionalization technology and its evaluation technology, biocompatibility and biofunction of material surfaces have made progress that could not have been predicted 20 years ago at the research level. The biocompatibility and biofunction also enable the application of metals as scaffold materials for regenerative medicine. Biodegradable polymers, bio-derived polymers, calcium phosphate ceramics, and composite materials of these have been studied as scaffolds used in regenerative medicine. These disappear or become integrated with the living tissue after the regeneration of the living tissue is completed or during the regeneration process. In this regard, metals have nothing to do with regenerative medicine. However, when reconstructing living tissue, it may be easier to regenerate using stronger materials, and tissue regeneration may be easier. Research has begun on surface-treating Ti fibers and porous Ti materials to modify them with biomolecules and applying them as scaffolding materials for regenerative medicine (Vehof et al. 2001). Since metallic biomaterials remain in the body semi-permanently, Ti materials, which have relatively high biocompatibility, are used. In order to use metal as a scaffold material, cell adhesion and tissue compatibility are required. Recently, in regenerative medicine, it has become widely recognized that the ideal surface is one that induces cell function and tissue through the functions of the material surface, rather than implanting cells and tissues. Extending this idea, inorganic chemical processing and morphology control by surface treatment that do not use biomolecules, cells, or tissues are preferable for approval, authentication, and practical application.

References

Abboud, M., L. Casaubieilh, F. Morval, M. Fontanille and E. Duguet. 2000. PMMA-based composite materials with reactive ceramic fillers: IV. Radiopacifying particles embedded in PMMA beads for acrylic bone cements. J. Biomed. Mater. Res. 53: 728–736.

Allam, N.K., K. Shankar and C.A. Grimes. 2008. A general method for the anodic formation of crystalline metal oxide nanotube arrays without the use of thermal annealing. Adv. Mater. 20: 3942–3946.

Anselme, K., P. Davidson, A.M. Popa, M. Giazzon, M. Liley and I. Ploux. 2010. The interaction of cells and bacteria with surfaces structured at the nanometre scale. Acta Biomater. 6: 3824–3846.

Asami, K., K. Saito, N. Ohtsu, S. Nagata and T. Hanawa. 2003. Titanium-implanted $CaTiO_3$ films and their changes in Hanks' solution. Surf. Interface Anal. 35: 483–488.

Ban, S., S. Maruno, N. Arimoto, A. Harada and J. Hasegawa. 1997. Effect of electrochemically deposited apatite coating on bonding of bone to the HA-G-Ti composite and titanium. J. Biomed. Mater. Res. 36: 9–15.

Ban, S. and S. Maruno. 1998. Morphology and microstructure of electrochemically deposited calcium phosphates in a modified simulated body fluid. Biomaterials 19: 1245–1253.

Ban, S., Y. Iwaya, H. Kono and H. Sato. 2006. Biofunctionalization of titanium for dental implant. Dent. Mater. 22: 115–1120.

Bexell, U., M. Olsson, M. Jhansson, J. Samuelsson and P.E. Sundell. 2003. A tribological study of a novel pre-treatment with linseed oil bonded to mercaptosilane-treated aluminum. Surf. Coat. Technol. 166: 141–152.

Bexell, U., M. Olsson, P.E. Sundell, M. Jhansson, P. Carlsson and M.A. Hellsing. 2004. ToF-SIMS study of linseed oil bonded to mercaptosilane-treated aluminum. Appl. Surf. Sci. 231–232: 362–365.

Borgioli, F., E. Galvanetto, A. Fossati and G. Pradelli. 2004. Glow-discharge and furnace treatments of Ti-6Al-4V. Surf. Coat. Tech. 184: 255–262.

Brammer, K.S., C.J. Frandsen and S. Jin. 2012. TiO_2 nanotubes for bone regeneration. Trend. Biotechnol. 30: 315–322.

Brunette, D.M., P. Tergvall, M. Textor and P. Thomsen. 2001. Titanium in Medicine: Springer, Berlin, Germany. pp. 231–455.

Buchanan, R.A., E.D. Rigney Jr. and J.M. Williams. 1987. Wear-accelerated corrosion of Ti-6Al-4V and nitrogen-ion-implanted Ti-6Al-4V: Mechanisms and influence of fixed-stress magnitude. J. Biomed. Mater. Res. 21: 367–377.

Buchanan, R.A., I.S. Lee and J.M. Williams. 1990. Surface modification of biomaterials through noble metal ion implantation. J. Biomed. Mater. Res. 24: 309–318.

Buckley, D.H. and K. Miyoshi. 1984. Friction and wear of ceramics. Wear 100: 333–353.

Chang, W.J., K.L. Qu, S.Y. Lee, J.Y. Chen, Y. Abiko, C.T. Lin et al. 2008. Type I collagen grafting on titanium surfaces using low-temperature glow discharge. Dent. Mater. J. 27: 340–346.

Chen, P., T. Aso, R. Sasaki, Y. Tsutsumi, M. Ashida, H. Doi et al. 2017. Micron/submicron hybrid topography of titanium surfaces influences adhesion and differentiation behaviors of the mesenchymal stem cells. J. Biomed. Nanotechnol. 13: 324–336.

Chen, P., T. Aso, R. Sasaki, M. Ashida, Y. Tsutsumi, H. Doi et al. 2018. Adhesion and differentiation behaviors of mesenchymal stem cells on titanium with micrometer and nanometer-scale grid patterns produced by femtosecond laser irradiation, J. Biomed. Mater. Res. 106A: 2736–2743.

Li, D.J. and H.Q. Gu. 2002. Cell attachment on diamond-like carbon coating. Bull. Mater. Sci. 25: 7–13.

Davis, J.R. 2003. Coatings. pp. 179–194. *In*: Handbook of Materials for Medical Devices: ASM International, Materials Park, OH, USA.

deGroot, K., R. Geesink, C.P.A.T. Klein and P. Serekian. 1987. Plasma sprayed coatings of hydroxylapatite. J. Biomed. Mater. Res. 21: 1375–1381.

Ducheyne, P., L.L. Hench, A. Kagan II, M. Martens, A. Bursens and J.C. Mulier. 1980. Effect of hydroxyapatite impregnation on skeletal bonding of porous coated implants. J. Biomed. Mater. Res. 14: 225–237.

Ferracane, J.L., H.X. Berge and J.R. Condon. 1998. In vitro aging of dental composites in water-Effect of degree of conversion, filler volume, and filler matrix coupling. J. Biomed. Mater. Res. 42: 465–472.

Fukushima, O., Y. Tsutsmi and T. Hanawa. 2020. Mechanism of electrodeposition process of poly(ethylene glycol) diamine to titanium surface. Mater. Trans. 61: 1346–1354.

Gasik, M., L. Van Mellaert, D. Pierron, A. Braem and D. Hofmans. 2012. Reduction of biofilm infection risks and promotion of osteointegration for optimized surfaces of titanium implants. Adv. Healthc. Mater. 1: 117–127.

Gebau, R.C. and R.S. Brown. 2001. Biomedical implant alloy. Adv. Mater. Process. 159: 46–48.

Goto, T., T. Narushima and K. Ueda. 2011. Chapter 7 Bio-ceramic coating on titanium by physical and chemical vapor deposition. pp. 299–332. *In:* Zang, S. [ed.]. Biological and Biomedical Coatings Handbook: Processing and Characterization, Advances in Materials Science and Engineering, CRC Press, Boca Raton, FL, USA.

Hamada, K., M. Kon, T. Hanawa, K. Yokoyama, Y. Miyamoto and K. Asaoka. 2002. Hydrothermal modification of titanium surface in calcium solutions. Biomaterials 23: 2265–2272.

Han, Y., D. Chen, J. Sun, Y. Zhang and K. Xu. 2008. UV-enhanced bioactivity and cell response of micro-arc oxidized titania coatings. Acta Biomater. 4: 1518–1529.

Han, Y., S.H. Hong and K.W. Xu. 2003. Formation mechanism of biomedical apatite coatings on porous titania layer. Surf. Coat. Technol. 168: 249–258.

Han, Y., Y. Yan and C. Lu. 2009. Ultraviolet-enhanced bioactivity of ZrO_2 films prepared by micro-arc oxidation. Thin Solid Film 517: 1577–1581.

Hanawa, T., K. Murakami and S. Kihara. 1994. Calcium phosphate precipitation on calcium-ion-implanted titanium in electrolyte. pp. 170–184. *In*: Horowitz, E. and J.E. Parr [eds.]. Characterization and Performance of Calcium Phosphate Coatings for Implants, ASTM STP 1196. American Society for Testing and Materials, Philadelphia, PA, USA.

Hanawa, T., Y. Kamiura, S. Yamamoto, T. Kohgo, A. Amemiya, H. Ukai et al. 1997a. Early bone formation around calcium-ion-implanted titanium inserted into rat tibia. J. Biomed. Mater. Res. 36: 131–136.

Hanawa, T., M. Kon, H. Ukai, K. Murakami, Y. Miyamoto and K. Asaoka. 1997b. Surface modification of titanium in calcium-ion-containing solutions. J. Biomed. Mater Res. 34: 273–278.

Hanawa, T. 2019. Titanium-tissue interface reaction and its control with surface treatment. Front. Bioeng. Biotechnol. 7: 170.

Hayakawa, T., M. Kawashita and G.H. Takaoka. 2008. Coating of hydroxyapatite films on titanium substrates by electrodeposition under pulse current. J. Ceram. Soc. Jpn. 116: 68–73.

Hayashi, K. 1995. Effect of grooves at the titanium surface on the formation of calcified materials by osteoblast-like cells. J. Jpn. Soc. Biomater. 13: 81–87.

Hazan, R., R. Brener and U. Oron. 1993. Bone growth to metal implants is regulated by their surface chemical properties. Biomaterials 14: 570–574.

Hiromoto, S. and M. Tomozawa. 2010. Corrosion behavior of magnesium with hydroxyapatite coatings formed by hydrothermal treatment. Mater. Trans. 51: 2080–2087.

Hosaka, M., Y. Shibata and T. Miyazaki. 2006. Preliminary β-tricalcium phosphate coating prepared by discharging in a modified body fluid enhances collagen immobilization onto titanium. J. Biomed. Mater. Res. 78B: 237–242.

Huang, H.H., Z.H. Zhi-Hwa Chen, D.T. Nguyen, C.M. Tseng, C.S. Chen and J.H. Chang. 2022. Blood coagulation on titanium dioxide films with various crystal structures on titanium implant surfaces. Cells 11: 2623.

Huang, N.P., R. Michel, J. Vörös, M. Textor, R. Hofer and A. Rossi. 2001. Poly (L-lysine)-g-poly(ethylene glycol) layers on metal oxide surfaces: surface-analytical characterization and resistance to serum and fibrinogen adsorption. Langmuir 17: 489–498.

Huang, N.P., G. Csucs, K. Emoto, Y. Nagasaki, K. Kataok and M. Textor. 2002. Biotin-derivatized poly (L-lysine)-g-poly (ethylene glycol): A novel polymeric interface for bioaffinity sensing. Langmuir 18: 252–258.

Ishikawa, K., Y. Miyamoto, M. Nagayama and K. Asaoka. 1997. Blast coating method: New method of coating titanium surface with hydroxyapatite at room temperature. J. Biomed. Mat. Res. 38: 129–134.

Ishikawa, T., R. Sahara, K. Ohno, K. Ueda and T. Narushima. 2023. Electronic structure analysis of light-element-doped anatase TiO_2 using all-electron GW approach. Comp. Mater. Sci. 220: 112059.

Ishimoto, T., T. Nakano, Y. Umakosh, M. Yamamoto and Y. Tabata. 2013. Degree of biological apatite c-axis orientation rather than bone mineral density controls mechanical function in bone regenerated using recombinant bone morphogenetic protein-2. J. Bone Miner. Res. 28: 1170–1179.

Ishizawa, H. and M. Ogino. 1995. Characterization of thin hydroxyapatite layers formed on anodic titanium oxide films containing Ca and P by hydrothermal treatment. J. Biomed. Mater. Res. 29: 1071–1079.

Ito, Y., H. Hasuda, M. Sakuragi and S. Tsuzuki. 2007. Surface modification of plastic, glass and titanium by photoimmobilization of polyethylene glycol for antibiofouling. Acta Biomater. 3: 1024–1032.

Ivanoff, C.J., C. Hallgren, G. Widmark, L. Sennerby and A. Wennerberg. 2001. Histologic evaluation of the bone integration of TiO(2) blasted and turned titanium microimplants in humans. Clin. Oral. Impl. Res. 12: 128–134.

Iwaya, Y., M. Machigashira, K. Kanbara, M. Miyamoto, K. Noguchi and Y. Izumi. 2008. Acid etching of titanium for bonding with veneering composite resins. Dent. Mater. J. 27: 415–421.

Jang, J.M., S.J. Park, G.S. Choi, T.W. Kwon and K.H. Kim. 2008. Chemical state and ultra-fine structure analysis of biocompatible TiO_2 nanotube-type oxide film formed on titanium substrate. Metal. Mater. Int. 14: 457–463.

Jayaseelan, S.K. and W.J.V. Ooji. 2001. Rubber-to-metal bonding by silanes. J. Adhes. Sci. Technol. 15: 967–991.

Kanie, T., H. Arikawa, K. Fujii and K. Inoue. 2004. Physical and mechanical properties of PMMA resins containing γ-methacryloxyproplytrimethoxysilane. J. Oral Rehabil. 31: 161–171.

Kannan, M.B. and O. Wallipa. 2013. Potentiostatic pulse-deposition of calcium phosphate on magnesium alloy for temporary implant applications—an *in vitro* corrosion study. Mater. Sci. Eng. C 33: 675–679.

Kenausis, G.L., J. Vörös, D.L. Elbert, N. Huang, R. Hofer and L. Ruiz-Taylor. 2000. Poly(l-lysine)-g-poly(ethylene glycol) layers on metal oxide surfaces: attachment mechanism and effects of polymer architecture on resistance to protein adsorption. J. Phys. Chem. B104: 3298–3309.

Kim, H.M., F. Miyaji, T. Kokubo and T. Nakamura. 1996. Preparation of bioactive Ti and its alloys via simple chemical surface treatment. J. Biomed. Mater. Res. 32: 409–417.

Kim, Y.Z., T. Konno, T. Murakami, T. Narushima and C. Ouchi. 2009. Surface hardening method for titanium materials using Ar-5%CO gas in combination with post heat treatment under vacuum. Mater. Trans. 50: 2763–2771.

Koizumi, R., K. Ueda, K. Ito, K. Ogasawara, H. Kanetaka, T. Mokudai et al. 2023. Visible-light-induced antibacterial activity of carbon and nitrogen co-doped rutile TiO_2 films. Thin Solid Film 780: 139944.
Kola, P.V., S. Daniels, D.C. Cameron and M.S.J. Hashmi. 1996. Magnetron sputtering of tin protective coatings for medical applications. J. Mater. Proc. Tech. 56: 422–430.
Kono, H., M. Miyamoto and S. Ban. 2007. Bioactive apatite coating on titanium using an alternate soaking process. Dent. Mater. J. 26: 186–193.
Kuroda, K., M. Moriyama, R. Ichino, M. Okido and A. Seki. 2008. Formation and *in vivo* evaluation of carbonate apatite and carbonate apatite/$CaCO_3$ composite films using the thermal substrate method in aqueous solution. Mater. Trans. 49: 1434–1440.
LeGeros, R.Z. 1988. Calcium phosphate materials in restorative dentistry: a review. Adv. Dent. Res. 2: 164–180.
Li, D.J. and H.Q. Gu. 2002. Cell attachment on diamond-like carbon coating. Bull. Mater. Sci. 25: 7–13.
Liu, X., P.K. Chu and C. Ding. 2004. Surface modification of titanium, titanium alloys, and related materials for biomedical applications. Mater. Sci. Eng. R 47: 49–121.
Liu, X., Y. Tanaka, F. Fujiwara, S. Maegawa, S. Ono and F. Itoigawa. 2023. Surface modification technique of titanium alloy to improve the tribological properties using sub-ns laser irradiation in PAO oil. J. Adv. Mech. Design System. Manuf. 17: JAMDSM0014.
Liu, F., F.P. Wang, T. Shimizu, K. Igarashi and L.C. Zhao. 2005. Formation of hydroxyapatite on Ti–6Al–4V alloy by microarc oxidation and hydrothermal treatment. Surf. Coat. Technol. 199: 220–224.
Liza, S., J. Hieda, H. Akasaka, N. Ohtake, Y. Tsutsumi, A. Nagai and T. Hanawa. 2017. Deposition of boron doped DLC films on TiNb and characterization of their mechanical properties and blood compatibility. Sci. Technol. Adv. Mater. 18: 76–87.
López-Valverde, N., J. Aragoneses, A. López-Valverde, N. Quispe-López, C. Rodríguez and J.M. Aragoneses. 2022. Effectiveness of biomolecule-based bioactive surfaces, on os-seointegration of titanium dental implants: A systematic review and meta-analysis of *in vivo* studies. Frot. Bioeng. Biotechnol. 10: 986112.
Ma, W., J.H. Wei, Y.Z. Li, X.M. Wang, H.Y. Shi, S. Tsutsumi and D.H. Li. 2008. Histological evaluation and surface componential analysis of modified micro-arc oxidation-treated titanium implants. J. Biomed. Mater. Res. 86B: 162–169.
Mas-Moruno, C., B. Su and M.J. Dalby. 2019. Multifunctional coatings and nanotopographies: Toward cell instructive and antibacterial implants. Adv. Healthcare Mater. 8: 1801103.
Matinlinna, J.P., C.Y.K. Lung and J.K.H. Tsoi. 2018. Silane adhesion mechanism in dental applications and surface treatments: A review. Dent. Mater. 34: 13–28.
Matsugaki, A., G. Aramoto, T. Ninomiya, H. Sawada, S. Hata and T. Nakano. 2015. Abnormal arrangement of a collagen/apatite extracellular matrix orthogonal to osteoblast alignment is constructed by a nanoscale periodic surface structure. Biomaterials 37: 134–143.
Meng, X.W., T.Y. Kwon and K.H. Kim. 2008. Hydroxyapatite coating by electrophoretic deposition at dynamic voltage. Dent. Mater. J. 27: 666–671.
Nagai, M., T. Hayakawa, A. Fukatsu, M. Yamamoto, M. Fukumoto and F. Nagahama. 2002. *In vitro* study of collagen coating of titanium implants for initial cell attachment. Dent. Mater. J. 21: 250–260.
Narayanan, R., S.K. Seshadri, T.Y. Kwon and K.H. Kim. 2007. Electrochemical nano-grained calcium phosphate coatings on Ti-6Al-4V for biomaterial applications. Scripta Mater. 56: 229–232.
Narayanan, R., T.W. Kwon and K.H. Kim. 2008a. Calcium phosphate–based coatings on titanium and its alloys. J. Biomed. Mater. Res. 85B: 231–239.
Narayanan, R., J.Y. Ha, T.Y. Kwon and K.H. Kim. 2008b. Structure and properties of self-organized TiO_2 nanotubes from stirred baths. Metall. Mater. Trans. B 39: 493–499.
Narayanan, R., T.W. Kwon and K.H. Kim. 2009. TiO_2 nanotubes from stirred glycerol/NH4F electrolyte: Roughness, wetting behavior and adhesion for implant applications. Mater. Chem. Phys. 117: 460–464.
Narushima, T., K. Ueda, T. Goto, H. Masumoto, T. Katsube, H. Kawamura et al. 2005. Preparation of calcium phosphate films by radiofrequency magnetron sputtering. Mater. Trans. 46: 2246–2252.
Noyama, Y., T. Nakano, T. Ishimoto, T. Sakai and H. Yoshikawa. 2013. Design and optimization of the oriented groove on the hip implant surface to promote bone microstructure integrity. Bone 52: 659–667.

Ohtsu, N., T. Ashino, M. Ishihara, F. Skamoto and T. Hanawa. 2007. Calcium-phosphate formation on titanium modified with newly developed calcium-hydroxide-slurry treatment. Mater. Trans. 48: 105–110.

Ohtsuki, C., H. Iida, H. Hayakawa and A. Osaka. 1997. Bioactivity of titanium treated with hydrogen peroxide solutions containing metal chlorides. J. Biomed. Mater. Res. 35: 39–47.

Orapiriyakul, W., P.S. Young and L. Damiati. 2018. Antibacterial surface modification of titanium implants in orthopaedics. J. Tissue Eng. 9: 2041731418789838.

Orii, Y., H. Masumoto, Y. Honda, T. Anada, T. Goto, K. Sasaki et al. 2010. Enhancement of octacalcium phosphate deposition on a titanium surface activated by electron cyclotron resonance plasma oxidation. J. Biomed. Mater. Res. B Appl. Biomater. 93: 476–483.

Oya, K., Y. Tanaka, H. Saito, K. Kurashima, K. Nogi, H. Tsutsumi et al. 2009. Calcification by MC3T3-E1 cells on RGD peptide immobilized on titanium through electrodeposited PEG. Biomaterials 30: 1281–1286.

Pan, J., C. Leygraf, D. Thierry and A.M. Ektessabi. 1997. Corrosion resistance for biomaterial applications of TiO_2 films deposited on titanium and stainless steel by ion-beam-assisted sputtering. J. Biomed. Mater. Res. 35: 309 318.

Park, J.W., K.B. Park and J.Y. Suh. 2007. Effects of calcium ion incorporation on bone healing of Ti6Al4V alloy implants in rabbit tibiae. Biomaterials 28: 3306–3313.

Park, J.W., Y.J. Kim, C.H. Park, D.H. Lee, Y.G. Ko, J.H. Jang et al. 2009. Enhanced osteoblast response to an equal channel angular pressing-processed pure titanium substrate with microrough surface topography. Acta Bimater. 5: 3272–3280.

Park, J.W., Y.J. Kim, J.H. Jamg, T.G. Kwon, Y.C. Bae and J.Y. Suh. 2010. Effects of phosphoric acid treatment of titanium surfaces on surface properties, osteoblast response and removal of torque forces. Acta Biomater. 6: 1661–1670.

Park, J.W., K. Kurashima, Y. Tsutsumi, C.H. An, J.Y. Suh, H. Doi et al. 2011. Bone healing of commercial oral implants with RGD immobilization through electrodeposited poly(ethylene glycol) in rabbit cancellous bone. Acta Biomater. 7: 3222–3229.

Park, J.W., Y.J. Kim, J.H. Jang and J.Y. Suh. 2012. Surface characteristics and primary bone marrow stromal cell response of a nanostructured strontium-containing oxide layer produced on a microrough titanium surface. J. Bimed. Mater. Res. Part A 100: 1477–1487.

Paschoal, A.L., E.C. Vanâncio, L. de Campos Franceschini Canale, O.L. da Silva, D. Huerta-Vilca and A. de Jesus Motheo. 2003. Metallic biomaterials TiN-coated: corrosion analysis and biocompatibility. Artif. Org. 27: 461–464.

Pesce, P., M. Menini, G. Santori, E. De Giovanni, F. Bagnasco and L. Canullo. 2020. Photo and plasma activation of dental implant titanium surfaces. A systematic review with meta-analysis of pre-clinical studies. J. Clin. Med. 31: 2817.

Pierschbacher, M.D. and E. Ruoslahti. 1984. Cell attachment activity of fibronectin can be duplicated by small synthetic fragments of the molecule. Nature 309: 30–33.

Pillar, R.M., H.U. Cameron and I. Macnab. 1975. Porous surface layered prosthetic devices. Biomed. Eng. 10: 126–131.

Pugdee, K., Y. Shibata, N. Yamamichi, H. Tsutsumi, M. Yoshinari and Y. Abiko. 2007. Gene expression of MC3T3-E1 cells on fibronectin immobilized titanium using tresyl chloride-activation technique. Dent. Mater. J. 26: 647–655.

Puleo, D.A., R.A. Kissling and M.S. Sheu. 2002. A technique to immobilize bioactive proteins, including bone morphogenetic protein-4 (BMP-4), on titanium alloy. Biomaterials 23: 2079–2087.

Ratner, B.D., A.S. Hoffman, F.J. Schoen and J.E. Lemons [eds.]. 2004. Biomaterials Science, 2nd ed. Elsevier Academic Press, San Diego, CA, USA. p. 539.

Rezania, A., R. Johnson, A.R. Lefkow and K.E. Healy. 1999. Bioactivation of metal oxide surfaces. 1. Surface characterization and cell response. Langmuir 15: 6931–6939.

Rezania, A., C.H. Thomas, A.B. Branger, C.M. Waters and K.E. Healy. 1997. The detachment strength and morphology of bone cells contacting materials modified with a peptide sequence found within bone sialoprotein. J. Biomed. Mater. Res. 37: 9–19.

Rieu, J., A. Pichat, L.M. Rabbe, A. Rambert, C. Chabrol and M. Robelet. 1991. Ion implantation effects on friction and wear of joint prosthesis materials. Biomaterials 12: 139–143.

Röstlund, T., B. Albrektsson, T. Albrektsson and H. McKellop. 1989. Wear of ion-implanted pure titanium against UHMWPE. Biomaterials 10: 176–181.
Sakamoto, H., H. Doi, E. Kobayashi, T. Yoneyama, Y. Suzuki and T. Hanawa. 2007. Structure and strength at the bonding interface between a titanium-segmentated polyurethane composite through 3-(trimethoxysilyl) propyl methacrylate for artificial organs. J. Biomed. Mater. Res. 82A: 52–61.
Sakamoto, H., Y. Hirohashi, H. Saito, H. Doi, Y. Tsutsumi, Y. Suzuki et al. 2008a. Effect of active hydroxyl groups on the interfacial bond strength of titanium with segmented polyurethane through γ-mercaptopropyl trimethoxysilane. Dent. Mater. J. 27: 81–92.
Sakamoto, H., Y. Hirohashi, H. Doi, Y. Tsutsumi, Y. Suzuki, K. Noda et al. 2008b. Effect of UV irradiation on the shear bond strength of titanium with segmented polyurethane through γ-mercapt propyl trimethoxysilane. Dent. Mater. J. 27: 124–132.
Saran, R., K. Ginjupalli, S.D. George, S. Chidangil and V.K. Unnikrishnan. 2023. LASER as a tool for surface modification of dental biomaterials: A review. Heliyon 9: e17457.
Sato, M., R. Tu and T. Goto. 2006. Preparation conditions of $CaTiO_3$ film by metal-organic chemical vapor deposition. Mater. Trans. 47: 1386–1390.
Sato, M., R. Tu, T. Goto, K. Ueda and T. Narushima. 2007. Hydroxyapatite formation on $CaTiO_3$ film prepared by metal-organic chemical vapor deposition. Mater. Trans. 48: 1505–1510.
Schliephake, H., D. Scharnweber, M. Dard, S. Rössler, A. Sewing and J. Meyer. 2002. Effect of RGD peptide coating of titanium implants on periimplant bone formation in the alveolar crest. An experimental pilot study in dogs. Clin. Oral Implant. Res. 13: 312–319.
Schroeder, A., E. Van der Zypen, H. Stich and F. Shutter. 1981. The reactions of bone, connective tissue, and epithelium to endosteal implants with titanium-sprayed surfaces. J. Maxilofacial. Surg. 9: 15–25.
Shi, R., K. Hayashi and K. Ishikawa. 2020. Rapid osseointegration bestowed by carbonate apatite coating of rough titanium. Adv. Mater. Interface 7: 2000636.
Shimabukuro, M., Y. Tsutsumi, R. Yamada, M. Ashida, P. Chen, H. Doi et al. 2019a. Investigation of realizing both antibacterial property and osteogenic cell compatibility on titanium surface by simple electrochemical treatment. ACS Biomater. Sci. Eng. 5: 5623–5630.
Shimabukuro, M., H. Ito, Y. Tsutsumi, K. Nozaki, P. Chen, R. Yamada et al. 2019b. The effects of various metallic surfaces on cellular and bacterial adhesion. Metals 9: 1145.
Shimabukuro, M., Y. Tsutsumi, K. Nozaki, P. Chen, R. Yamada, M. Ashida et al. 2019c. Chemical and biological toles of zinc in a porous titanium dioxide layer formed by micro-arc oxidation. Coatings 9; 705.
Shimabukuro, M., Y. Tsitsumi, K. Nozaki, P. Chen, R. Yamada, M. Ashida et al. 2020a. Investigation of antibacterial effect of copper introduced titanium surface by electrochemical treatment against facultative anaerobic bacteria. Dent. Mater. J. 39: 639–647.
Shimabukuro, M., A. Hiji, T. Manaka, K. Nozaki, P. Chen, M. Ashida et al. 2020b. Time-transient effects of silver and copper in the porous titanium dioxide layer on antibacterial properties. J. Funct. Biomater. 11: 44.
Shinonaga, T., M. Tsukamoto, A. Nagai, K. Yamashiata, T. Hanawa, N. Matsushita et al. 2014. Cell spreading on titanium dioxide film formed and modified with aerosol beam and femtosecond laser. Appl. Surf. Sci. 288: 649–653.
Smith, N.A., G.G. Antoun, A.B. Ellis and W.C. Crone. 2004. Improved adhesion between nickel-titanium shape memory alloy and polymer matrix via silane coupling agents. Composite Part A S 35: 1307–1312.
Streicher, R.M., H. Weber, R. Schön and M. Semlitsch. 1991. New surface modification for Ti-6Al-7Nb alloy: oxygen diffusion hardening. Biomaterials 12: 125–129.
Suh, J.Y., O.C. Jeung, B.J. Choi and J.W. Park. 2007. Effects of a novel calcium titanate coating on the osseointegration of blasted endosseous implants in rabbit tibiae. Clin. Oral Impl. Res. 18: 362–369.
Sultana, R., M. Kon, L.M. Hirakata, E. Fujihara, K. Aasoka and T. Ichikawa. 2006. Surface modification of titanium with hydrothermal treatment at high pressure. Dent. Mater. J. 25: 470–479.
Taira, Y. and Y. Imai. 1995. Primer for bonding resin to metal. Dent. Mater. 11: 2–6.
Tanaka, H., Y. Mori, A. Noro, A. Kogure, M. Kamimura, N. Yamada et al. 2016. Apatite formation and biocompatibility of a low young's modulus Ti-Nb-Sn alloy treated with anodic oxidation and hot water. Plos One 11: e0150081.

Tanaka, Y., E. Kobayashi, S. Hiromoto, K. Asami, H. Imai and T. Hanawa. 2007a. Calcium phosphate formation on titanium by low-voltage electrolytic treatments. J. Mater. Sci. Mater. Med. 18: 797–806.

Tanaka, Y., Doi, H., Iwasaki, Y., Hiromoto, S., Yoneyama, T., Asami, K., Imai, H. and T. Hanawa. 2007b. Electrodeposition of amine-terminatedpoly(ethylene glycol) to titanium surface. Mater. Sci. Eng. C 27: 206–212.

Tanaka, Y., H. Doi, E. Kobayashi, T. Yoneyama and T. Hanawa. 2007c. Determination of the immobilization manner of amine-terminated poly(ethylene glycol) on a titanium surface with XPS and GD-OES. Mater. Trans. 48: 287–292.

Tanaka, Y., H. Saito, Y. Tsutsumi, H. Doi, H. Imai and T. Hanawa. 2008. Active hydroxyl groups on surface oxide film of titanium, 316l stainless steel, and cobalt-chromium-molybdenum alloy and its effect on the immobilization of poly(ethylene glycol). Mater. Trans. 49: 805–811.

Tanaka, Y., H. Saito, Y. Tsutsumi, H. Doi, N. Nomura, H. Imai et al. 2009. Effect of pH on the interaction between zwitterions and titanium oxide. J. Colloid Interface Sci. 330: 138–143.

Tate, K., Y. Matsui, R. Kawakami, A. Tsuruta and N. Ohtsu. 2023. Endothelium cell responses on pulsed-anodized NiTi alloy with HNO_3, NH_4NO_3, H_2SO_4, and $(NH_4)_2SO_4$ as electrolytes. Mater. Trans. 64: 1265–1270.

Tsutsumi, H., Y. Tsutsumi, M. Shimabukuro, T. Manaka, P. Chen, M. Ashida et al. 2021. Investigation of the long-term antibacterial properties of titanium by two-step micro-arc oxidation treatment. Coatings 11: 798.

Tsutsumi, Y., D. Nishimura, H. Doi, N. Nomura and T. Hanawa. 2010. Cathodic alkaline treatment of zirconium to give the ability to form calcium phosphate. Acta Biomater. 6: 4161–4166.

Tsutsumi, Y., H. Tsutsumi, T. Manaka, P. Chen, M. Ashida, H. Katayama et al. 2023. Development of a surface treatment to achieve long-lasting antimicrobial properties and non-cytotoxicity through simultaneous incorporation of Ag and Zn via two-step micro-arc oxidation. Coatings 13: 627.

Ueda, M., M. Ikeda and M. Ogawa. 2009. Chemical–hydrothermal combined surface modification of titanium for improvement of osteointegration. Mater. Sci. Eng. C 29: 994–1000.

Ueda, T., N. Sato, R. Koizumi, K. Ueda, K. Ito, K. Ogasawara et al. 2021. Formation of carbon-added anatase-rich TiO_2 layers on titanium and their antibacterial properties in visible light. Dent. Mater. 37: e37–e46.

Ueda, T., R. Koizumi, K. Ueda, K. Ito, K. Ogasawara, H. Kanetaka et al. 2023. Antibacterial properties of TiO_2 layers formed by Au-sputtering and thermal oxidation of titanium under visible light. Mater. Trans. 64: 155–164.

Ueno, T., M. Takeuchi, N. Hori, F. Iwasa, H. Minamikawa, Y. Igarashi et al. 2012. Gamma ray treatment enhances bioactivity and osseointegration capability of titanium. J. Biomed. Mater. Res. 100B: 2279–2287.

Vadiraj, A., M. Kamaraj and R. Gnanamoorthy. 2007. Fretting wear studies on PVD TiN coated, ion implanted and thermally oxidised biomedical titanium alloys. Surf. Eng. 23: 209–215.

Vehof, J.W.M., A.E. deRuijter, P.H.M. Spauwen and J.A. Jansen. 2001. Influence of rhBMP-2 on rat bone marrow stromal cells cultures on titanium fiber mesh. Tissue Eng. 7: 373–383.

Viornery, C., H.L. Guenther, B.O. Aronsson, P. Péchy, P. Descouts and M. Grätzel. 2002. Osteoblast culture on polished titanium disks modified with phosphonic acids. J. Biomed. Mater. Res. 62: 149–155.

Wang, C.K., J.H.C. Lin, C.P. Ju, H.C. Ong and R.P.C. Chang. 1997. Structural characterization of pulsed laser-deposited hydroxyapatite film on titanium substrate. Biomaterials 18: 1331–1338.

Wen, C., S. Guan, L. Peng, C. Ren, X. Wang and Z. Hu. 2009. Characterization and degradation behavior of AZ31 alloy surface modified by bone-like hydroxyapatite for implant applications. Appl. Surf. Sci. 255: 6433–6438.

Wen, J.Y. and H.H. Huang. 2022. Surface film characterizations and electrochemical behavior of type I collagen-immobilized interconnected porous Ti–Nb–Zr–Sn alloy scaffolds in simulated inflammatory environment. J. Mater. Res. Technol. 21: 5081–5097.

Wolke, J.C.G., K. van Dijk, H.G. Schaeken, K. de Groot and J.A. Jansen. 1994. Study of the surface characteristics of magnetron-sputter calcium phosphate coatings. J. Biomed. Mater. Res. 28: 1477–1484.

Wong, M., J. Eulenberger, R. Schenk and E. Hunziker. 1995. Effect of surface topology on the osseointegration of implant materials in trabecular bone. J. Biomed. Mat. Res. 29: 1567–1575.

Xiao, S.J., M. Textor, N.D. Spencer and H. Sigrist. 1998. Covalent attachment of cell-adhesive (Arg-Gly-Asp)-containing peptides to titanium surfaces. Langmuir 114: 5507–5516.

Xiao, S.J., M. Textor, N.D. Spencer, M. Wieland, B. Keller and H. Sigrist. 1997. Immobilization of the cell-adhesive peptide Arg-GlyAsp-Cys (RGDC) on titanium surfaces by covalent chemical attachment. J. Mater. Sci. Mater. Med. 8: 867–872.

Xue, T., S. Attarilar, S. Liu, J. Liu, X. Song, L. Li et al. 2020. Surface modification techniques of titanium and its alloys to functionally optimize their biomedical properties: Thematic review. Front. Bioeng. Biotechnol. 8: 603072.

Yamamoto, D., T. Iida, K. Arii, K. Kuroda, R. Ichino, M. Okido et al. 2012. Surface hydrophilicity and osteoconductivity of anodized Ti in aqueous solutions with various solute Ions. Mater. Trans. 53: 1956–1961.

Yamanouchi, N., K. Pugdee, W.J. Chang, S.Y. Lee, M. Yoshinari, T. Hayakawa et al. 2008. Gene expression monitoring in osteoblasts on titanium coated with fibronectin-derived peptide. Dent. Mater. J. 27: 744–750.

Yamashita, K., M. Matsuda, T. Arashi and T. Umegaki. 1998. Crystallization, fluoridationand some properties of apatite thin films prepared through RF-sputtering from CaO-P_2O_5 glasses. Biomaterials 19: 1239–1244.

Yan, Y. and Y. Han. 2007. Structure and bioactivity of micro-arc oxidized zirconia films. Surf. Coat. Technol. 201: 5692–5695.

Yang, W.E. and H.H. Huang. 2019. Multiform TiO_2 nano-network enhances biological response to titanium surface for dental implant applications. Appl. Surf. Sci. 471: 1041–1052.

Yankee, S.J., B.J. Pletka, R.L. Salsbury and W.A. Johnson. 1991. Historical development of plasma sprayed hydroxylapatite biomedical coatings. pp. 261–270. *In*: Sudarshan, T.S., D.G. Bhat and M. Jeandin [eds.]. Surface Modification Technologies IV. TMS, Warrendale, PA, UAS.

Yoneyama, T. and T. Hanawa. 2021. Reduction in nickel content of the surface oxide layer on Ni-Ti alloy by electrolytic treatment. J. Oral Sci. 63: 50–53.

Yoshida, K., M. Tanagawa and M. Atsuta. 2001. Effects of filler composition and surface treatment on the characteristics of opaque resin composites. J. Biomed. Mater. Res. 58: 525–530.

Yoshinari, M., T. Kato, K. Matsuzaka, T. Hayakawa and K. Shiba. 2010. Prevention of biofilm formation on titanium surfaces modified with conjugated molecules comprised of antimicrobial and titanium-binding peptides. Biofouling 26: 103–110.

Yoshinari, M., Y. Ohtsuka and T. Dérand. 1994. Thin hydroxyapatite coating produced by the ion beam dynamic mixing method. Biomaterials 15: 529–535.

Yoshinari, M., K. Ozeki and T. Sumii. 1991. Properties of hydroxyapatite-coated Ti-6Al-4V alloy produced by the ion-plating method. Bull. Tokyo Dent. Coll. 32: 147–156.

Yuda, A., S. Ban and Y. Izumi. 2005. Biocompatibility of apatite-coated titanium mesh prepared by hydrothermal-electrochemical method. Dent. Mater. J. 24: 588–595.

Zhang, F., E.T. Kang, K.G. Neoh, P. Wang and K.L. Tan. 2001. Surface modification of stainless steel by grafting of poly(ethylene glycol) for reduction in protein adsorption. Biomaterials 22: 1541–1548.

Zhu, X.L., K.H. Kim and Y.S. Jeong. 2001. Anodic oxide films containing Ca and P of titanium. Biomaterial. Biomaterials 22: 2199–2206.

Appendix
Specifications of Metallic Biomaterials

Table A1. Chemical composition of CP Ti and Ti alloy in ISO and ASTM standards (mass%) (Data from ISO and ASTM).

	Zr	**Nb**	**Ta**	**Al**	**V**	**Fe**	**O**	**N**	**H**	**C**	**Ti**
Unalloyed Ti (ISO 5832 – 2:2018) Grade1						< 0.15	< 0.18	< 0.03	< 0.0125	< 0.1	Bal.
Unalloyed Ti (ISO 5832 – 2: 2018) Grade2						< 0.2	< 0.25	< 0.03	< 0.0125	< 0.1	Bal.
Unalloyed Ti (ISO 5832 – 2: 2018) Grade3						< 0.25	< 0.35	< 0.05	< 0.0125	< 0.1	Bal.
Unalloyed Ti (ISO 5832 – 2: 2018) Grade4						< 0.3	< 0.45	< 0.05	< 0.0125	< 0.1	Bal.
Wrought Ti – 6Al – 4V (ISO 5832 – 3:2021)				5.5 – 6.75	3.5 – 4.5	< 0.3	< 0.2	< 0.05	< 0.015	< 0.08	Bal.
Wrought Ti – 5Al – 2.5Fe (ISO 5832 – 10:1996)				4.5 – 5.5		2 – 3	< 0.2	< 0.05	< 0.013	< 0.08	Bal.
Wrought Ti – 6Al – 7Nb (ISO 5832 – 11:2014)		6.5 – 7.5	< 0.5	5.5 – 6.5		< 0.25	< 0.2	< 0.05	< 0.009	< 0.08	Bal.
Unalloyed Ti (ASTM F67 – 13) Grade1						< 0.2	< 0.18	< 0.03	< 0.0125	< 0.1	Bal.
Unalloyed Ti (ASTM F67 – 135) Grade2						< 0.3	< 0.25	< 0.03	< 0.0125	< 0.1	Bal.

Table A1 contd. ...

...Table A1 contd.

	Zr	**Nb**	**Ta**	**Al**	**V**	**Fe**	**O**	**N**	**H**	**C**	**Ti**
Unalloyed Ti (ASTM F67 – 13) Grade3						< 0.3	< 0.35	< 0.05	< 0.0125	< 0.1	Bal.
Unalloyed Ti (ASTM F67 – 13) Grade4						< 0.5	< 0.40	< 0.05	< 0.0125	< 0.1	Bal.
Wrought Ti – 6Al – 4V (ASTM F136 – 13(2021)e1)				5.5 – 6.5	3.5 – 4.5	< 0.25	< 0.13	< 0.05	< 0.012	< 0.08	Bal.
Wrought Ti – Al – 7Nb (ASTM F1295 – 16)		6.5 – 7.5	< 0.5	5.5 – 6.5		< 0.25	< 0.2	< 0.05	< 0.009	< 0.08	Bal.
Wrought Ti – 13Nb – 13Zr (ASTM F1713 – 08(2021)e1)	12.5 – 14	12.5 – 14				< 0.25	< 0.15	< 0.05	< 0.012	< 0.08	Bal.

Table A2. Mechanical property of CP Ti and Ti alloy in ISO and ASTM standards (Data from ISO and ASTM).

	Heat treatment	**0.2% offset yield strength (MPa)**	**Ultimate tensile strength (MPa)**	**Elongation to fracture (%)**	**Reduction of area (%)**
Unalloyed Ti (IS0 5832-2:2018) Grade1	Annealing	170	240	24	30
Unalloyed Ti (IS0 5832-2: 2018) Grade2	Annealing	230	345	20	30
Unalloyed Ti (IS0 5832-2: 2018) Grade3	Annealing	300	450	18	30
Unalloyed Ti (IS0 5832-2: 2018) Grade4	Annealing (A) Cold working (B)	440 520	550 680	15 10	25 18
Wrought Ti-6Al-4V (IS0 5832-3:2021)	Annealing	780	860	10	25
Wrought Ti-5Al-2.5Fe (IS0 5832-10:1996)	Annealing	800	900	10	25
Wrought Ti-6Al-7Nb (IS0 5832-11:2014)	Annealing	800	900	10	25
Unalloyed Ti (ASTM F67-13) Grade1	Annealing	310	240	24	
Unalloyed Ti (ASTM F67-135) Grade2		450	345	20	
Unalloyed Ti (ASTM F67-13) Grade3		550	450	18	
Unalloyed Ti (ASTM F67-13) Grade4		655	550	15	
Wrought Ti-6Al-4V (ASTM F136-13(2021)e1)	Annealing	795	860	10	
Wrought Ti-Al-7Nb (ASTM F1295-16)	Annealing	800	900	10	25
Wrought Ti-13Nb-13Zr (ASTM F1713-08(2021)e1)	Aging Solution treated Non-annealing	725 345 345	860 550 550	8 15 8	15 30 15

Table A3. Chemical composition of Co-based alloy in ISO and ASTM standards (mass%).(Data from ISO and ASTM).

	C	Si	W	S	P	Be	Cr	Mo	Mn	Ni	Ti	N	B	Fe	Co
Co – Cr – Mo Casting Alloy (ISO5832 – 4:2014)	< 0.35	< 1.0					26.5 – 30	4.5 – 7.0	< 1.0	< 1.0				< 1.0	Bal.
Wrought Co – Cr – W – Ni Alloy (ISO5832 – 5:2022)	< 0.15	< 1	14 – 16				19 – 21		< 2	9 – 11				< 3	Bal.
Wrought Co – Ni – Cr – Mo Alloy (ISO5832 – 6:2022)	< 0.025	< 0.15		< 0.01	< 0.015		19 – 21	9 – 10.5	< 0.15	33 – 37	< 1.0			< 1.0	Bal.
Co – Cr – Ni – Mo – Fe Alloy (ISO5832 – 7:2016)	< 0.15	< 1		< 0.015	< 0.015	< 0.001	18.5– 21.5	6.5 – 8	1 – 2.5	14 – 18				Bal.	39 – 42
Wrought Co – Ni – Cr – Mo – W – Fe Alloy (ISO5832 – 8:1997)	< 0.05	< 0.5	3 – 4	< 0.01			18 – 22	3 – 4	< 1.0	15 – 25	0.5 – 3.5			4 – 6	Bal.
Wrought Co – Cr – Mo Alloy (ISO5832 – 12:2019)	< 0.35	< 1.0					26 – 30	5 – 7	< 1.0	< 1.0		< 0.25		< 0.75	Bal.
Cast Co – Cr – Mo A11oy (ASTM F75 – 23)	< 0.35	< 1.0					27 – 30	5 – 7	< 1.0	< 1.0				< 0.75	Bal.
Wrought Co – Cr – W – Ni Alloy (ASTM F90 – 23)	0.05 – 0.15	< 0.4	14 – 16	< 0.03	< 0.04		19 – 21		1.0 – 2.0	9 – 11				< 3	Bal.
Wrought Co – 35Ni – 20Cr – 10Mo Alloy (ASTM F562 – 22)	< 0,025	< 0.15		< 0.01	< 0.015		19 – 21	9 – 10.5	< 0.15	33 – 37	< 1.0		< 0.015	< 1.0	Bal.
Wrought Co – Ni – Cr – Mo – W – Fe Alloy (ASTM F563 – 00)	<0.05	< 0.5	3 – 4	< 0.01			18 – 22	3 – 4	< 1.0	15 – 25	0.5 – 3.5			4 – 6	Bal.
Co – 28Cr – 6Mo Alloy (ASTM F799 – 19)	< 0.35	< 1.0					26 – 30	5 – 7	<1.0	< 1.0		< 0.25		< 0.75	Bal.

Table A4. Mechanical property of Co-based alloy in ISO and ASTM standards (Data from ISO and ASTM).

		0.2% Offset yield strength (MPa)	Ultimate tensile strength (MPa)	Elongation to fracture (%)	Reduction of area (%)
Co-Cr-Mo Casting Alloy (ISO5832-4:2014)		450	665	8	
Wrought Co-Cr-W-Ni Alloy (ISO5832-5:2022)	Annealing	310	860	10	
Wrought Co-Ni-Cr-Mo Alloy (ISO5832-6.2022)	Annealing Cold working	300 650 – 1000	800 1000 – 1200	40 10 – 20	
Forgeable and Cold-Formed Co-Cr-Ni-Mo-Fe Alloy (ISO5832-7:2016)	Annealing 30% cold working	450 1300	950 1450	65 8	
Wrought Co-Ni-Cr-Mo-W-Fe Alloy (ISO5832-8:1997)	Annealing Cold working	275 830 – 1310	600 1000 – 1580	50 5 – 18	
Wrought Co-Cr-Mo Alloy (ISO5832-12:2019)	Annealing Hot working Cold working	550 700 827	750 1000 1172	16 12 12	
Cast Co-Cr-Mo A1loy (ASTM F75-23)		450	655	8	8
Wrought Co-Cr-W-Ni Alloy (ASTM F90-23)	Annealing	310	860	30-45	
Wrought Co-35Ni-20Cr-10Mo Alloy (ASTM F562-22)	Annealing Cold working	241 – 448 1586	793 – 1000 1793	50.0 8.0	65.0 35.0
Wrought Co-Ni-Cr-Mo-W-Fe Alloy (ASTM F563-00)	Annealing Cold working	276 827 – 1310	600 1000 – 1586	50 12 – 18	65 45
Co-28Cr-6Mo Alloy (ASTM F799-19)		827	1172	12	35

Table A5. Chemical composition of stainless steel in ISO and ASTM standards (mass%) (Data from ISO and ASTM).

	C	N	Si	Mn	P	S	Cu	Cr	Ni	Mo	Nb	V	Fe
Wrought – Stainless Steel (ISO5832–1:2016)D	< 0.03	< 0.1	< 1.0	< 2.0	< 0.025	< 0.01	< 0.5	17 – 19	13 – 15	2.25 – 3.5			Bal.
Wrought – Stainless Steel (ISO5832–1:2016)E	< 0.03	0.1 – 0.2	< 1.0	< 2.0	< 0.025	< 0.01	< 0.5	17 – 19	14 – 16	2.35 – 4.2			Bal.
Wrought – High Nitrogen Stainless Steel (ISO5832–9:2016)	< 0.08	0.25 – 0.5	< 0.75	2 – 4.25	< 0.025	< 0.01	< 0.25	19.5 – 22	9 – 11	2 – 3	0.25 – 0.8		Bal.
Stainless Steel (ASTM F138 – 19) Grade 1	< 0.08	< 0.1	< 0.75	< 2.0	< 0.025	< 0.01	< 0.5	17 – 19	13.0 – 15.5	2 – 3			Bal.
Stainless Steel (ASTM F138 – 19) Grade 2	< 0.03	< 0.1	< 0.75	< 2.0	< 0.025	< 0.01	< 0.5	17 – 19	13.0 – 15.5	2 – 3			Bal.
Stainless Steel (ASTM F745 – 95)	< 0.06		< 1.0	< 2.0	< 0.045	< 0.03		17 – 19	11 – 14	2 – 3			Bal.
Stainless Steel (ASTM F1314 – 18)	< 0.03	0.2 – 0.4	< 0.75	4 – 6	< 0.025	< 0.01	< 0.5	20.5 – 23.5	11.5 – 13.5	2 – 3	0.1 – 0.3	0.1 – 0.3	Bal.
Stainless Steel (ASTM F – 1586 – 21)	< 0.08	0.25 – 0.5	< 0.75	2 – 4.25	< 0.025	< 0.01	< 0.25	19.5 – 22.0	9 – 11	2 – 3	0.25 – 0.8		Bal.

Table A6. Mechanical property of stainless steel in ISO and ASTM standards (Data from ISO and ASTM).

	Heat treatment	**02% offset yield strength (MPa)**	**Ultimate tensile strength (MPa)**	**Elongation to fracture (%)**
Wrought Stainless Steel (ISO5832-1:2016)D	Annealing Cold working	190 690	490 – 690 860 – 1100	40 12
Wrought Stainless Steel (ISO5832-1:2016)E	Annealing Cold working	285 690	590 – 800 860 – 1100	40 12
Wrought High Nitrogen Stainless Steel (ISO5832-9:2016)	Annealing	430	740	35
Stainless Steel (ASTM F138-19) Grade1	Annealing Cold working	205 690	515 860	40 12
Stainless Steel (ASTM F138-19) Grade2	Annealing Cold working	170 690	480 860	40 12
Stainless Steel (ASTM F745-95)	Solution treated Annealing	205	485	30
Stainless Steel (ASTM F1314-18)	Annealing Cold working	380 862	690 1035	35 12
Stainless Steel (ASTM F1586-21)	Annealing	430	740	35

Index

A

α” phase 153
α+β type Ti alloy 148, 150, 154, 155, 173, 174
acid etching 261, 263, 267, 268, 271
active oxygen 162
additive manufacturing 162, 186, 205, 208
Ag alloy 213, 217, 218
AISI numbering 193, 194
alkaline solution 261–263, 275
allotropic transformation 183
alloy 26–28, 33, 44, 48, 54, 56
AM 162, 186, 190, 205, 206
animal experiment 59, 60, 80, 89, 91
anode 39, 44–46
anodic polarization test 67
anodic reaction 38, 39, 42
antibacterial property 262
antithrombotic evaluation 89
artificial hip joint 98–101
artificial joint 211, 234, 235, 237
artificial knee joint 100, 101
artificial valve 96, 97, 112, 113
Au alloy 211–215, 217–219
austenitic stainless steel 200, 201
austenitic transformation 220
austenitic-ferritic stainless steel 194

B

β transus 152, 153, 155
β type Ti alloy 148, 150, 154–157, 173, 174
bacteria 128, 130, 131, 134
bacterial adhesion 90
band gap energy 170–172
biocompatibility 4, 10, 15, 16, 18, 19, 22, 54, 128, 148–150, 159, 167, 171–173
biodegradable metal 211, 229, 230
biofilm 129, 130
biofilm formation 90, 91
biofunction 4, 5, 10, 12, 15, 16, 18, 19
biofunctional molecule 261, 264, 273
biological environment 126, 127
biological evaluation 59, 79, 80
biomaterials 1–6, 8–19
biomolecule 264, 275, 276
blasting 255, 258, 268, 271
blood compatibility 54–56
BM 229, 230, 233
body fluid 126–129, 143
bone bonding 17, 54, 119, 165, 167
bone fixator 95, 97, 98, 101
bone formation 250, 252, 257, 258, 261, 264, 270, 271, 274, 275
brazing alloy 213, 218
bridge 96, 116, 117, 119, 121

C

calcium phosphate formation 170, 171
carbon 196, 203
carcinogenicity 126
cardiology 96, 105
catheter 96–97, 105–108, 110, 111
cathode 39, 42, 44–47
cathodic reaction 38–40, 42, 47, 50
cell culture 59, 68, 79–83, 87
ceramics 2, 4–10, 13, 17
cerebral aneurysm clip 97, 110, 111
chemical bond 7–9
chromium 202
clasp 96, 117, 120
cleaning 271
Co–27Cr–6Mo alloy 184
cobalt-based alloy 180, 182, 183, 186, 188
Co–Cr–Mo alloy 134, 140, 143, 144, 180–183, 186
Co–Cr–Ni–Mo alloy 182
Co–Cr–W–Ni alloy 180, 181, 184
commercially pure titanium 150, 151
Co–Ni–Cr–Mo alloy 180, 182, 185
coronary artery intervention 107
corrosion 22, 27, 35–51, 59, 62, 67–77, 126–128, 133–136
corrosion potential 69–71, 73, 74
corrosion rate 231

corrosion resistance 148, 149, 160–162, 167, 170–172, 180, 182, 186–188, 190, 193–195, 197, 199, 200, 202–209, 212–215, 218–219, 228, 229, 231, 234, 235, 237, 249–251, 255, 256, 258, 259, 261, 262
CP Ti 148–151, 153–155, 159–162, 164–171, 173, 174
crack initiation 141, 142
crack propagation 141, 142
crevice corrosion 42–44, 50, 135–137, 202, 206, 208
crown 96, 114–119, 121
crystal structure 25–29, 31, 35, 152, 153
CVD 253, 255–257

D

demand 1, 4, 13, 14
dental amalgam 213, 219
dental archwire 120
dental casting alloy 117, 213, 215, 216
dental implant 96, 97, 114, 118, 119, 121
dentistry 96, 97, 114, 121, 122
denture 96, 116–120
DES 98–100, 104, 106, 107, 109, 110, 114, 115, 117, 119, 121
dislocation 28, 31–35
dissolution of cobalt 188
dissolution test 72
drug eluting stent 110

E

ε phase 182–184, 186, 186
EBM 186, 189
electrochemical coating 261, 262
electron beam melting 186
electron orbital band 23
electrostatic force 168, 169, 172
Elgiloy 181, 186
embolization coil 110–112
endodontic file 97, 120, 121
endoscope 96, 97, 123
equilibrium phase 152, 153, 159
equilibrium phase diagram 29, 30

F

fatigue 126, 127, 136, 139–144, 155–158
fatigue test 60, 62–64
Fe–Cr system 194
Fe–Cr–Ni system 194
Fe–Cr–Ni–Mn system 194
Fermi level energy 24, 25
ferritic stainless steel 207, 208
fracture 127, 133, 136, 140–145
free electron 25, 26
fretting fatigue 126, 140, 142–144
fretting fatigue test 62, 63
friction wear 139

G

γ phase 182–186, 189
Galvanic corrosion 42, 44, 45, 135
gas treatment 257, 259
guidewire 105, 106

H

HA 250, 252, 253–256, 258, 261–263, 268, 270, 273–275
hard film coating 258
hard material 9, 10, 14, 15
hard tissue compatibility 54, 55, 87, 88, 249–251, 259, 262
heat diffusion treatment 259
heat treatment 22, 27, 29, 34
high entropy alloy 211, 240, 241
hip joint simulator 66, 67
history 1, 4, 9–11
HS25 181, 182
human error 144, 145
hydrogen peroxide 263, 264

I

imaging equipment 123
immobilization 249, 264–266, 273, 275
implantable cardioverter defibrillator 113
infectious disease 130
inflammation 129, 138, 139
inlay 96, 115, 121
intergranular corrosion 45
intermetallic compound 27, 28
ion implantation 255, 256, 259, 275
iron 193

K

knee joint simulator 65, 66

L

L-605 182, 185, 190
laser irradiation 260
life element 52
localized corrosion 42, 43, 45, 46, 48
low-nickel containing Co–Cr alloy 189

M

macrophage 162
magnesium alloy 230
magnetic alloy 233
magnetic resonance imaging 132
magnetic susceptibility 133
magnetism 200, 208
manganese 202
MAO 261, 262, 268
market 1, 13, 14
martensitic 29, 30
martensitic stainless steel 200, 201
martensitic transformation 29, 220, 221
mechanical property 59, 150, 151, 155, 158, 195–197
medical devices 1, 2, 4, 5, 9, 10, 12–15, 17, 19
metal allergy 137–139
metal-ceramic restoration 211, 216, 217
metallic biomaterials 1, 2, 8–11, 13–17
metallic bond 22, 23, 25–27
metallosis 182, 189
metals 1, 2, 4–10, 12–15, 18, 19
micro arc oxidation 261, 262
molybdenum 196
MP35N 181, 182, 185, 188, 190
MRI artifact 132–134, 211, 237, 238

N

Nb 211, 213, 221, 222, 229, 234–236, 238, 239, 242
Nernst equation 40
nickel 185, 189, 203
nickel-free stainless steel 207
Ni–Ti alloy 227
nitrogen 202, 207, 208
noble metal 212–214, 216–218
noble metal alloy 212–214, 216–218,
n-type semiconductor 167, 168, 171, 172

O

orthodontics 114, 119, 120
orthopedics 96, 97
osseointegration 165–167
osteolysis 130, 131

P

pace maker 96, 112
palladium alloy 218
parent phase transformation 220
passive film 36, 37, 42–48, 50, 56, 69, 70, 73–76, 151, 161–165, 167–172, 188, 189, 193, 194, 196, 202, 203, 205, 206, 208, 235, 236
passivity 37, 41
patch test 139
percutaneous coronary intervention PCI 107
percutaneous transluminal coronary angioplasty 107
pitting corrosion 42, 43, 45, 46, 48, 136, 199, 202, 205–208
plastic deformation 31–33, 35
PLIF 103
plif lumbar interbody fusion 103
point of zero charge 169
polarization resistance 70, 71
polymers 2, 4–10, 13, 17
potential-pH diagram 40–42
Pourbaix diagram 40, 41
precipitation hardening stainless steel 194, 196
property 7, 9, 17, 19
Pt 211–220, 238
Pt alloy 213
PTCA 106, 107
pure iron 233
PVD 253–256, 258

R

regenerative medicine 1–3, 9, 10, 12–14
restoration 96, 97, 114–118, 121
reverse transformation 221, 223, 225, 226

S

safety 50, 54
Schaeffler diagram 194, 207
selective laser melting 186
shape memory effect 221, 223, 225, 226, 229
simulated body fluid 59, 65, 67, 68, 72, 74, 78, 79
slip deformation 31–33, 35
SLM 186, 188
S-N curve 141, 142
soft material 8–10
soft tissue adhesion 264
soft tissue compatibility 54, 55
solid solution 27–29, 33, 34
spinal fixator 97, 98, 102
stacking fault energy 185, 189
stainless steel 193, 194–209
steel 26, 29, 35, 43–46, 48–50, 54, 56
stent 95–97, 105–110
stent graft 97, 107, 109
stress corrosion cracking 42, 45
stress shielding 127, 145, 146
stress-strain curve 6, 8, 60–62
striation 141, 142
superelasticity 221, 223, 226, 229
surface charge 168
surface hydroxyl group 168, 169, 172

surface modification 249, 264, 273
surface morphology 249, 250, 252, 268, 270–272
surface structure 22, 36
surface treatment 249–252, 256, 259, 266, 268, 271, 274–276
surgical robot 96, 97, 123

T

Ta 211, 229, 234–236, 242
Tafel extrapolation 70, 71
tarnish 135
tensile test 60, 61, 67
THA 98, 99
thermal oxidation 260
Ti–13Nb–13Zr alloy 149, 150
Ti–6A–4V alloy 154
Ti–6Al–7Nb alloy 150, 154, 156
TiO_2 250, 255–258, 260–262, 265, 268, 270, 271
titanium material 154
titanium-zirconium alloy 159
TLIF 103
Total hip arthroplasty 98
toxicity 50–54
toxicity test 80, 81
transforaminal lumbar interbody fusion 103
transformation 22, 27–29
tribocorrosion 74, 75
twin deformation 32, 35
type 304 stainless steel 199, 200, 202–204
type 316L stainless steel 193, 196–198, 200, 202, 205–207

U

UHMWPE 140, 181
ultra high molecular weight polyethylene 140, 181
unequilibrium phase 30, 34

V

vapor deposition 253, 254, 256, 257
Vitallium 180–183, 186

W

wear debris 126, 127, 139, 181
wear resistance 180, 182, 211, 249–251, 259, 260
wear test 60, 64–66
working 22, 29, 30, 35

X

XPS 76–78
X-ray photoelectron spectroscopy 76

Y

Young's modulus 145

Z

zinc alloy 233
zirconium alloy 235, 239
zirconium oxide 236, 262